Ophthalmic Anaesthesia

Ophthalmic Anaesthesia

A practical handbook

Second Edition

G BARRY SMITH MB BS FFA(RCS Eng) ——————————
Honorary Consultant Anaesthetist,
Moorfields Eye Hospital,
London, UK

ROBERT C HAMILTON MB BCh FRCPC ——————————
Clinical Professor of Anaesthesia,
The University of Calgary and
Consultant Anaesthetist, Gimbel Eye Centre,
Calgary, Alberta, Canada

CAROLINE A CARR MA MB BS FRCA ——————————
Consultant Anaesthetist,
Moorfields Eye Hospital and Eastman Dental Hospital,
London, UK

A member of the Hodder Headline Group
LONDON • SYDNEY • AUCKLAND
Co-published in the USA by
Oxford University Press, Inc., New York

Arnold is a member of the Hodder Headline Group
338 Euston Road, London NW1 3BH

First published in Great Britain 1983
Second Edition 1996

Co-published in the United States of America by
Oxford University Press, Inc.,
198 Madison Avenue, New York, NY10016
Oxford is a registered trademark of Oxford University Press

Whilst the advice and information in this book is believed to be true and
accurate at the date of going to press, neither the authors nor the publisher
can accept any legal responsibility or liability for any errors or omissions
that may be made. In particular (but without limiting the generality of the
preceding disclaimer) every effort has been made to check drug dosages;
however it is still possible that errors have been missed. Furthermore,
dosage schedules are constantly being revised and new side-effects
recognized. For these reasons the reader is strongly urged to consult the
drug companies' printed instructions before administering any of the drugs
recommended in this book.

British Library Cataloguing in Publication Data
A catalogue record for this book is available from the British Library

Library of Congress Cataloging-in-Publication Data
A catalog record for this book is available from the Library of Congress

ISBN 0 340 56757 0 (hb)

1 2 3 4 5   96 97 98 99

Editorial and Production Services Fisher Duncan, 10 Barley Mow Passage, London W4 4PH
Typeset in 10/11 Times, with Optima by Phoenix Photosetting, Chatham, Kent
Printed and Bound in Great Britain by St Edmundsbury Press, Bury St Edmunds, Suffolk and
J W Arrowsmith Ltd, Bristol

Contents

Preface

During the last 10 years, the practice of eye surgery has changed radically and ophthalmic anaesthesia has been obliged to adapt and change to suit new circumstances. Economic pressures and medico-legal hazards have brought pressure on anaesthetists to demonstrate the arguments for and against any particular technique and to bolster those arguments by estimates of relative risk and quality assurance. Many patients come for 'walk-in surgery' leaving little opportunity for preoperative assessment and they expect to leave shortly after surgery having had a not-unpleasant experience and without any sequel more than some minor discomfort. Patient expectations fostered by the media are raised to ever less attainable heights; indeed, some patients believe that cataract extraction is a simple, uncomplicated, minor procedure – woe betide surgeons or anaesthetists who think the same, a humbling experience awaits them.

At the time when the first edition of this book was published, it was unusual to monitor vital functions routinely during local anaesthesia. Even under general anaesthesia, only pulse rate, blood pressure and cardiogram were measured. A choice of physiological variables to measure poses problems of choosing the best equipment, financing expensive items with a short service life and arranging for them to be updated and replaced as new products appear on the market. Every new monitor requires additional time in preparation while the electrodes, probes or sensors are attached to the patient and the instrument is turned on, checked and adjusted. This increases time between patients and reduces the number of operations.

In the same way that eye surgery has become subdivided into many minor subspecialties dealing with different parts of the eye, so anaesthesia has tended to divide along lines in which some anaesthetists put in local blocks, and others specialize in children, motility, adnexal surgery or diabetes. It is rapidly becoming the case in the larger centres that the all-round general ophthalmic anaesthetist is becoming a rarity. For this reason, it is no longer appropriate for a single author to write a book on ophthalmic anaesthesia, but for subspecialists in their own field to be asked to contribute their specialist knowledge. Dr Roy Hamilton brings his wealth of experience of local anaesthesia provided for patients at the Gimbel Eye Centre, Calgary, Canada. In spite of his prodigious workload, he maintains a personal interest in each patient and observes the effects of his drugs on the different orbital structures and relates this to his very detailed knowledge of anatomy. He believes that the ophthalmic anaesthetist should be more skilled in the use of local anaesthesia than his surgical colleague and just as familiar with the anatomy.

In asking Dr Caroline Carr to approach the problems of strabismus surgery, paediatrics and day-case anaesthesia, I knew I was asking a rising star of ocular anaesthesia and, with the highly specialized and immense clinical diversity available at

Moorfields, I thought her contribution could not fail to be interesting and of unique value for other hospitals where ophthalmic work is more limited in its scope.

Finally, I hope that surgeons and anaesthetists will accept the challenge of this book, the aim of which is to make surgery safer and more successful for patients.

Barry Smith
1995

CHAPTER 1

Anatomy of the eye and orbit

ROBERT C HAMILTON ───────────────────────────────

INTRODUCTION

A detailed knowledge of appropriate anatomy is essential for practitioners of the art and science of ophthalmic anaesthesia. To embark on orbital regional anaesthesia blocks without this, is to subject patients to unacceptable risk of serious sequelae. For those who wish to pursue this thoroughly, cadaver dissection is an excellent means of gaining necessary insights into the three dimensional aspects of the anatomy of this small but vital part of the human body.[16, 21] In reading this chapter, an atlas of orbital anatomy (e.g. Doxanas and Anderson[5]) and a human skull are worthwhile resources.

PLANES OF THE HEAD AND ORBIT

The planes of the head and orbit are depicted in Fig. 1.1.

Planes of the head

Coronal planes of the head are those planes parallel to the frontal plane of the face (e.g. if one's nose were sliced off, the slice would be in the coronal plane). Sagittal planes of the head are at right angles to the coronal planes and in the long axis of the body (e.g. if one's ear were sliced off, the slice would be in the sagittal plane). Transverse planes are at right angles to both coronal and sagittal planes (e.g. if one's head were chopped off at eyebrow level, the chop would be in the transverse plane).

One important sagittal plane of the head is the mid-sagittal plane of the eye while held in primary gaze. It corresponds with the visual axis of the globe in primary gaze (Fig. 1.2) Visualization of this plane is important in the safe placement of needles in the intracone space (see Chapters 7 and 8).

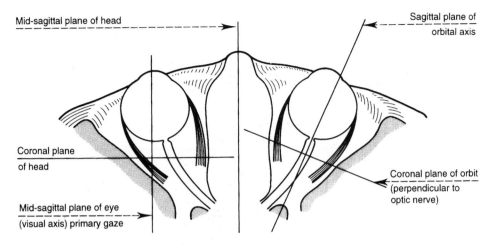

Fig. 1.1.   Sagittal and coronal planes of the head (left) and orbit (right).

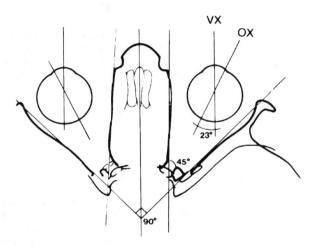

Fig. 1.2.   Line drawing of the geometry of the globe and orbit. OX, orbital axis; VX, visual axis. (With permission from ref. 23.)

Planes of the orbit

In computed tomography studies of the orbit, coronal and sagittal planes are usually with reference to the anatomic axis of the orbit (Figs 1.2, 1.3). The coronal planes of the orbit are perpendicular to the optic nerve. The sagittal planes of the orbit are parallel to the optic nerve (globe in primary gaze) and at an angle of 23 degrees from the sagittal planes of the head (Fig. 1.2). The sagittal plane of the orbital axis transects the globe, when in primary gaze anteriorly near to the lateral limbus and posteriorly at the point where the optic nerve enters the globe (Fig. 1.3).[22] The optic nerve enters the globe 3 mm to the nasal side of its posterior pole.

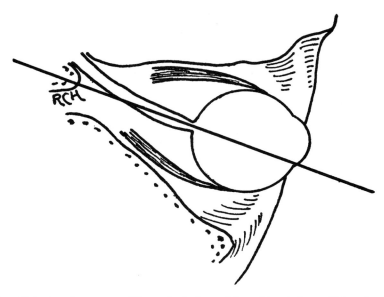

Fig. 1.3. Globe in primary gaze. The sagittal plane of the orbit axis is parallel to the distal and middle parts of the optic nerve and is rotated 23 degrees away from the sagittal plane of the head. Anteriorly this plane passes lateral to the eye lens, almost but not quite as far lateral as the lateral limbus. Posteriorly and near the orbital apex the optic nerve turns medially towards the optic canal. (With permission from Gimbel Educational Services.)

OSTEOLOGY

Geometry of the orbits

Paired orbital cavities are mirror-imaged, bilaterally symmetrical and located on each side of the mid-line sagittal plane of the skull. Each of the orbits is shaped like a truncated pear lying on its side (heavy end of pear sliced off) and is made up from seven bones: frontal, zygomatic, maxillary, sphenoid, ethmoid, lacrimal and palatine (Fig. 1.4).

The medial wall of each orbit is in the sagittal plane of the head and parallel to the contralateral medial orbit wall. The lateral wall of each orbit forms a 90-degree angle with the contralateral lateral orbit wall. The medial and lateral walls of each orbit make a 45-degree angle with each other (Fig. 1.2). Note that the apex including the optic foramen are in the same sagittal plane as the medial orbit wall. Thus the optic foramen is located both posteriorly and medially in the orbit (Figs 1.2, 1.5, 1.6). The globe occupies the front half of each orbit and projects anteriorly beyond it (Figs 1.2, 1.7). The visual axis (eye in primary gaze) is sagittal; the anatomic axis of each orbit diverges from the visual axis by 23 degrees (Fig. 1.2).

The facial, or anterior, aspect of the orbit is known as the orbit rim, which forms a protecting buttress for the vital structures held within, and comprises

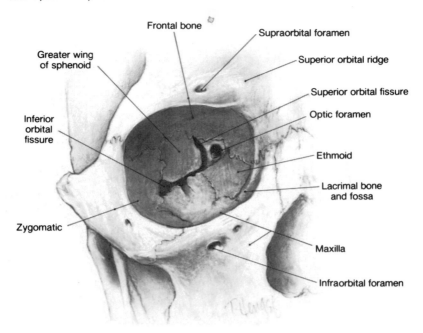

Fig. 1.4.   Frontal view of the orbit. The skull is rotated slightly to the left to visualize more clearly the orbital apex. (With permission from ref. 5.)

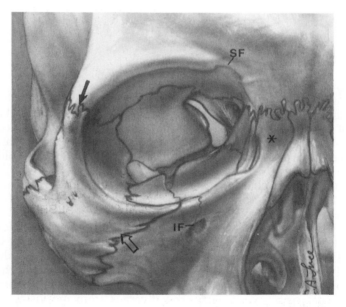

Fig. 1.5.   True frontal view of the orbit. The optic foramen is located medially at the apex. SF, supraorbital notch; IF, infraorbital foramen; *frontal process of the maxilla; open arrow, zygomaticomaxillary suture; solid arrow, zygomaticofrontal suture. (With permission from ref. 23.)

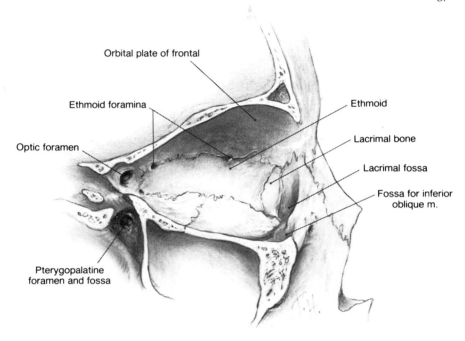

Orbital plate of frontal

Ethmoid foramina

Optic foramen

Pterygopalatine
foramen and fossa

Ethmoid

Lacrimal bone

Lacrimal fossa

Fossa for inferior
oblique m.

Fig. 1.6.   Medial orbital wall. (With permission from ref. 5.)

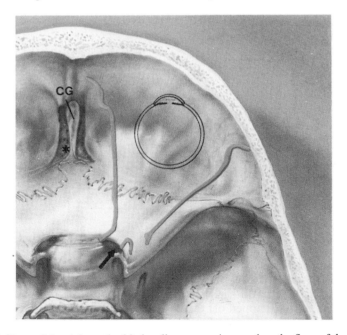

CG

Fig. 1.7. Outlines of the globe and orbital walls are superimposed on the floor of the anterior cranial fossa. CG, midline crista galli; *cribriform plate. (With permission from ref. 23.)

three robust bones: zygomatic, frontal and maxillary. Detailed knowledge of the surface anatomy of the orbit rim as palpated through its superficial periorbital coverings is the key to successful regional orbital anaesthesia (Figs 1.4, 1.8). The rim forms the rounded rectangular base of a pear-shaped pyramid which tapers posteriorly to form a tight apex, made up from the greater and lesser wings of the sphenoid bone. The greatest diameter of the orbit is that portion immediately inside the rim. The volume of the adult orbit is 30 ml, while that of an average-sized globe is 6.5 ml. The typical dimensions at the rim are 35 mm vertically and 40 mm horizontally. The depth of the orbit from inferior orbit rim to the optic foramen ranges from 42 to 54 mm.[11] The lateral orbit rim is set back 12–18 mm behind the cornea, allowing exposure of the globe to its equator (Fig. 1.9). The orbital margin breaks its continuity at the lacrimal fossa medially (Figs 1.8, 1.10).

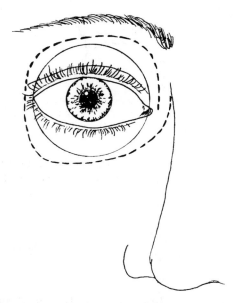

Fig. 1.8.   The outline of the globe is superimposed on a template of the orbital rim. (With permission from Gimbel Educational Services.)

Periorbita and orbital septum

The periosteum of the orbit is known as the periorbita. It blends with the facial bone periosteum and with the orbital septum circumferentially at the anterior orbital margin. Posteriorly at the orbital apex, the periorbita is continuous through the optic canal with the pericranium and with the dural sheath of the optic nerve. It is easily stripped off the underlying orbital bones.

The orbital septum is a weak membranous sheet attached to the anterior margin of the orbit in continuity with the facial periosteum and the periorbita. It defines the anatomical anterior border of the orbit and on the nasal side has

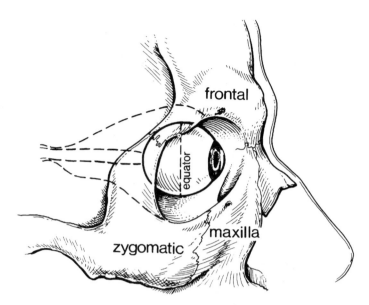

Fig. 1.9. The lateral orbital rim is set back in line with the globe equator. The orbit, in sagittal section, is C-shaped rather than U-shaped with a greater overhang superiorly. (With permission from ref. 24.)

attachments with both the anterior and posterior lacrimal crests. Its central attachments are in the upper and lower eyelids and it lies deep to the orbicularis oculi muscle (Fig. 1.11).

Orbit roof, walls and floor

The roof, walls and floor of the orbit are all triangular in shape.

Orbit roof

The roof of the orbit is predominantly formed by the frontal bone with a small contribution from the lesser wing of the sphenoid bone (Fig. 1.12). The fossa for the lacrimal gland is located anteriorly and laterally. The fovea trochlearis, for attachment of the cartilaginous trochlear pulley, which transmits the tendon of the superior oblique muscle, is a small dimple located 5 mm behind the rim on the medial side. The supraorbital foramen (25%) or notch (75%) for the nerve of the same name is found at the junction of the medial third with the lateral two-thirds of the rim. The zygomaticofrontal suture joins the roof with the lateral wall anteriorly; the roof and wall are separated by the superior orbital fissure posteriorly. The frontoethmoidal suture joins the roof to the medial orbit wall and has foramina for the anterior and posterior ethmoidal vessels and nerves (posterior ethmoidal nerve frequently absent). Superior to the roof of the orbit, the frontal lobe of the brain lies in the anterior cranial fossa separated by thin bone and the frontal sinus borders anteromedially.

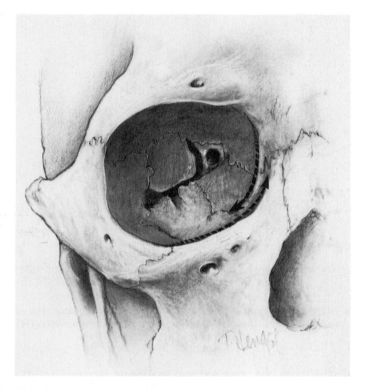

Fig. 1.10.   The discontinuity of the inferonasal orbital margin creates the fossa for the lacrimal sac. (With permission from ref. 5.)

Lateral wall of the orbit

The lateral wall of the orbit consists of the zygomatic and sphenoid (greater wing) bones (Fig. 1.13). The superior and inferior orbital fissures separate the posterior portion of the lateral wall from the roof and floor, respectively. The bone of the lateral wall is alternately thick, thin, thick again and thin again from anterior to posterior (Figs 1.12, 1.14). The two thin areas of the lateral wall respectively separate the orbit from the temporalis and middle cranial fossae, respectively. The lateral orbital tubercle for attachment of the lateral canthal tendon and lateral globe support ligaments is located 4 mm back from the rim and 10 mm inferior to the zygomaticofrontal suture. The zygomatic bone on the lateral wall has two minute foramina for the zygomaticofacial and zygomaticotemporal nerves on their way to innervate the facial skin.

Orbit floor

The floor of the orbit is made up from the zygomatic bone laterally and the maxillary bone medially with a small contribution from the palatine bone posteriorly (Fig. 1.14). Blunt large object trauma compressing the orbit contents frequently

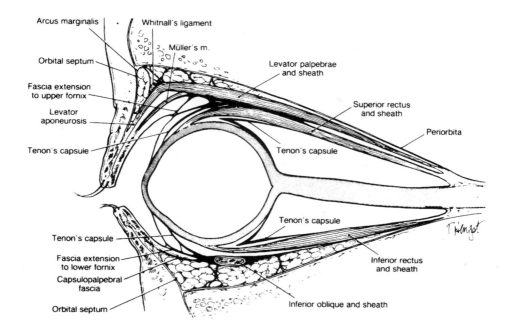

Fig. 1.11. Connective tissue systems of the orbit. Sagittal section of the orbit demonstrating the diffuse attachments of the extraocular muscles to the periorbita and Tenon's capsule. (With permission from ref. 5.)

causes blow-out fractures of the thin bony plate which separates the floor from the maxillary sinus. The infraorbital fissure (posteriorly) and canal (anteriorly) extend from the apex forward (Fig. 1.14). The canal, which transmits the infraorbital vessels and nerve, exits at the infraorbital foramen 1 cm inferior to the midpoint of the inferior orbit rim (Fig. 1.5). The nasolacrimal canal, 12 mm in length, lies in the maxillary bone and commences anteromedially from the orbit floor and passes vertically and slightly laterally to the nasal cavity; it transmits the nasolacrimal duct for drainage of tears to the inferior meatus of the nose. In the extreme anteromedial angle of the floor, just behind the inferior orbital margin and lateral to the nasolacrimal canal, lies the fossa of origin of the inferior oblique muscle.

Medial wall of the orbit

The medial wall of the orbit comprises four bones: most anteriorly the frontal process of the maxilla, followed by the lacrimal, ethmoid and lesser wing of the sphenoid in that order (Fig. 1.6). The lacrimal fossa which houses the lacrimal sac is formed between the lacrimal bone posteriorly and the frontal process of

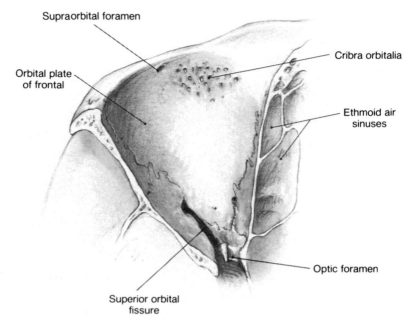

Supraorbital foramen

Cribra orbitalia

Orbital plate
of frontal

Ethmoid air
sinuses

Optic foramen

Superior orbital
fissure

Fig. 1.12.   The roof of the orbit. (With permission from ref. 5.)

the maxilla anteriorly. The fossa is bounded anteriorly and posteriorly by the anterior and posterior lacrimal crests, respectively. The anterior crest is in continuity with the inferior orbital rim, while the posterior crest extends superiorly to join with the superior rim (Fig. 1.10). The nasolacrimal canal, described above, commences from the inferior edge of the lacrimal fossa. The anterior and posterior ethmoid foramina, mentioned above, traverse the suture line between the ethmoid bone and orbital plate of the frontal bone. The ethmoid bone is thin, making this a part of the orbit also subject to blow-out fractures. Because of their close relationship on the medial side, infection from the paranasal sinuses may spread to involve the orbit by this route.

THE EYE

The eyeball or globe is suspended within the bony orbit by a complex matrix of connective tissues embedded in fat. Accessory structures – the extraocular muscles, eyebrows, eyelids, conjunctiva and lacrimal apparatus – are intimately associated with the globe, the whole arrangement serving to protect the vital organ of sight from damage. The globe is in the shape of a sphere about 23.5 mm in diameter (average size, but great variations exist, commonly ranging from 20 to 30 mm and more rarely outside these limits) with an anterior bulge of smaller radius of curvature (Fig. 1.15) The equator of the globe is situated at, or slightly in front of or behind, the lateral orbit rim (Fig. 1.9); in any one normal individual, globe position may vary up to more than 3 mm in the anteroposterior

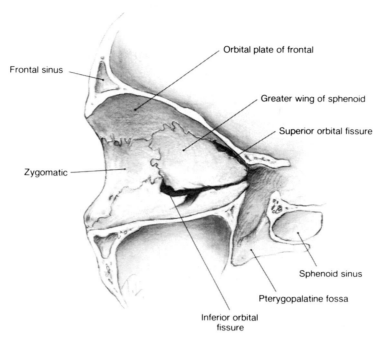

Orbital plate of frontal

Frontal sinus

Greater wing of sphenoid

Superior orbital fissure

Zygomatic

Sphenoid sinus

Pterygopalatine fossa

Inferior orbital
fissure

Fig. 1.13.   The lateral orbital wall. (With permission from ref. 5.)

dimension from one time to another.[3] Within the globe are the refracting media (aqueous humour, lens and vitreous humour); these are retained within a wall consisting of three coats.

THE COATS OF THE EYE

The three coats of the eye are an outer fibrous coat (the cornea and sclera), an intermediate vascular coat known as the uveal tract (choroid, ciliary body and iris) and the inner neural layer (the retina).

The cornea and sclera

The semi-rigid coat known as the sclera maintains the shape of the eye. It has a bulge anteriorly, the cornea, which has a smaller radius of curvature (Fig. 1.15) than the posterior part and is transparent. The corneoscleral junction separates the cornea from the rest of the sclera, the opaque posterior portion, which has a white glistening external surface and a brown grooved deep surface (grooves for the short ciliary nerves, see below). The conjunctival membrane is reflected from the deep surfaces of the eyelids on to the anterior part of the sclera, and becomes continuous with the corneal epithelium at the corneoscleral junction.

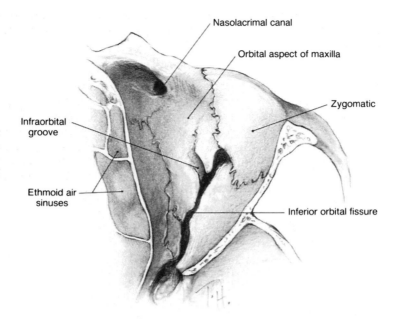

Nasolacrimal canal

Orbital aspect of maxilla

Zygomatic

Infraorbital
groove

Ethmoid air
sinuses

Inferior orbital fissure

Fig. 1.14.   The floor of the orbit. (With permission from ref. 5.)

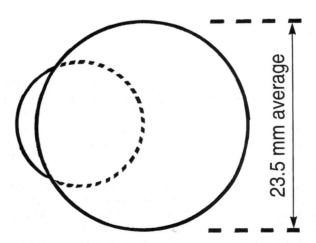

23.5 mm average

Fig. 1.15.   The eye is spherical in shape, with an average maximum diameter of 23.5 mm. The anterior segment has a radius of curvature smaller than that of the posterior segment. (With permission from Gimbel Educational Services.)

The sclera is pierced posteriorly by the optic nerve (its nerve bundles pass though multiple orifices in the sclera) and is continuous with the dural sheath covering that nerve.

The uveal tract

The uveal tract is the intermediate vascular coat of the globe consisting of the choroid, ciliary body and iris. The choroid coat is present in the posterior five-sixths of the eyeball and is juxtaposed to the sclera. It extends forward to the ora serrata of the retina (Fig. 1.16). Coloured chocolate brown, it is highly vascular, being fed by branches of the short posterior ciliary arteries and drained by a venous network ultimately converging into four or five vortex veins which

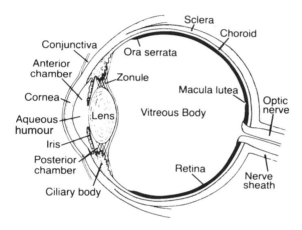

Fig 1.16. Diagram of ocular anatomy. (With permission from ref. 25.)

pierce the sclera 5–8 mm posterior to the globe equator.[10] One of these is located at the lateral border of the inferior rectus muscle belly, 5 mm posterior to the equator,[10,19] and may be the source of bleeding from inferotemporal needle placement; this can be avoided by such placement being nearer to the inferior border of the lateral rectus (see Chapter 7). The choroid is responsible for the nutrition of the outer layers of the retina (the inner layers of the retina receive their blood supply from the central retinal artery). The vascularity of the choroid layer increases with systemic venous congestion, arterial hypertension and hypercarbia. The sclera and choroid are loosely adherent, separated by the potential suprachoroidal space which may fill with blood during an expulsive or suprachoroidal haemorrhage, a dreaded surgical complication.

The ciliary body, anterior to the choroid, encircles the lens and is responsible for aqueous humour production. It consists of a posterior part, the pars plana, and a folded anterior part including the ciliary processes and the ciliaris muscle (chief agent in accommodation, i.e. ability to see near objects). Parasympathetic nerve fibres (by way of the oculomotor nerve) provide the motor supply to the ciliaris muscle. The ciliary muscle is exquisitely sensitive to stretching of the zonular fibres,[7] for which the sensory pathway is by way of the long ciliary nerves.

The iris is the most anterior of the uveal tract structures. It functions as a muscular diaphragm controlling the amount of light entering the eye by varying the diameter of its aperture, the pupil. Its circumferential sphincter muscle is controlled by parasympathetic fibres (by way of the oculomotor nerve), while its radial dilator muscle is supplied by cervical sympathetic fibres by way of the long ciliary nerves. It is also a highly sensitive intraocular structure,[7] with innervation through the long ciliary nerves. Its arterial supply is from the long posterior ciliary arteries (directly fed from the ophthalmic artery) and the anterior ciliary arteries (derived from muscular branches of the ophthalmic artery).

The retina

The retina, the innermost coat of the globe, is a ten-layered neurosensory membrane which is a transducer for conversion of light to neural impulses. As mentioned above, the nutrition of the retina depends on the choroid coat for its outer layer and the central retinal artery for its inner layer. The macula lutea near the centre of the posterior retina is its most sensitive portion; at its centre a small pit called the fovea centralis is required for finest vision discrimination (Fig. 1.16).

THE CONTENTS OF THE EYEBALL

The eyeball has two major compartments: the anterior segment representing about one-fifth of the globe volume and the posterior segment representing four-fifths. Separating the anterior and posterior segments is a diaphragm consisting of the crystalline lens and its supporting zonular fibres (passing from the ciliary body to the lens capsule). The action of the ciliary muscle is relayed to the lens through the zonules, enabling the lens to change shape and produce variable refraction of light entering the eye.

The iris divides the anterior segment into anterior and posterior chambers (Figs 1.16, 1.17), which communicate freely through the pupil. Aqueous humour, essential for the nutrition of the avascular crystalline lens and the corneal endothelium, is produced by the epithelium of the ciliary body at the perimeter of the posterior chamber and circulates anteriorly through the pupillary opening to leave the eye by filtration through the trabecular meshwork at the perimeter of the anterior chamber (Fig. 1.17). The aqueous humour filters through to the canal of Schlemm and by way of the episcleral venous system to the central venous pool (Fig. 1.17).

The posterior segment extending from the region immediately behind the crystalline lens to the retina contains the vitreous body enclosing a transparent jelly-like fluid called the vitreous humour within the delicate hyaloid membrane. The anterior face of the vitreous body is indented by the hyaloid fossa, into which the crystalline lens fits.

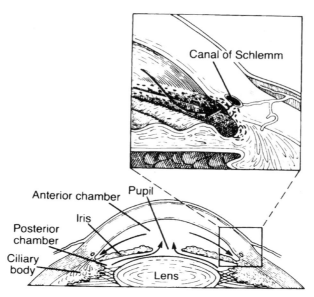

Fig. 1.17. Circulation of aqueous humour secreted by the ciliary body in the posterior chamber, passing through the pupil into the anterior chamber, and exiting through the trabecular meshwork into the canal of Schlemm. (With permission from ref. 25.)

ORBITAL CONNECTIVE TISSUES AND ADIPOSE TISSUE COMPARTMENTS

There are essentially three distinct connective tissue systems within the orbit: Tenon's capsule, an anterior globe-supporting system and the diffuse system of the posterior orbit.[5]

Tenon's capsule

The bulbar fascia (Tenon's capsule) invests the globe and the extraocular muscles in the anterior central orbit. Tenon's capsule extends from the corneal limbus anteriorly to the optic nerve posteriorly and is penetrated posterior to the equator of the globe by the four rectus muscles and by the two oblique muscles more anteriorly, prior to their insertion in the sclera. Each of the six muscles has a sleeve of the capsule reflected along it to allow unrestricted control of globe movement within the capsule (Figs 1.11, 1.18). The globe rotates around its centre point within the smooth inner lining of Tenon's capsule, this movement being made possible by the great mobility of the anterior part of the optic nerve.[15,18]

Anterior globe-supporting connective tissue system

A supporting connective tissue diaphragm extends from Tenon's capsule and globe out to periorbita just behind the orbit margin (Fig. 1.19).[12] Condensations

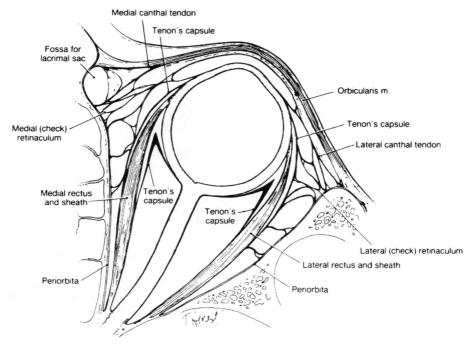

Fig.1.18. Connective tissue systems of the orbit. Schematic transverse section of the orbit demonstrating the diffuse attachments of the extraocular muscles to the periorbita and Tenon's capsule, and the formulation of the medial and lateral check ligaments and canthal tendons. (With permission from ref. 5.)

of these tissues above and below the globe, respectively named after Whitnall and Lockwood who first described them, form suspensory ligaments to support the globe and limit its displacement. The medial and lateral check ligaments, considered to act as a servo-mechanism of the eyeball, fan out in several sheets from the respective muscle sheaths to attach to periorbita at the sides of the orbit. Intermuscular septa between adjacent margins of the four rectus muscles are well developed in this, the anterior part of the orbit. They merge with Tenon's capsule in this area.

Diffuse connective tissue system of the posterior orbit

A diffuse connective tissue matrix in the posterior orbit derived from the fascial sheaths of the extraocular muscles radiates from their sheaths out to the periorbita and is vital to their efficient functioning (Fig. 1.18). Koornneef's extensive investigation of these orbital connective tissues demonstrated a septal framework with general structure having 'unquestionable inter-individual uniformity' and bilateral symmetry, and with adipose tissue compartments lying between the connective tissue septa.[13] The fat of the posterior orbit has a macro-arrangement into central and peripheral compartments, respectively, inside and outside the

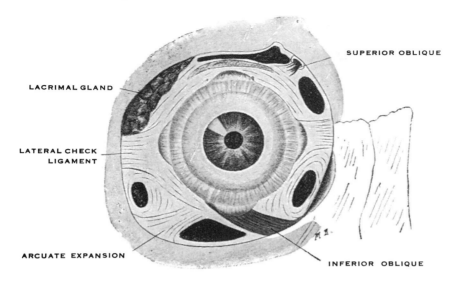

SUPERIOR OBLIQUE

LACRIMAL GLAND

LATERAL CHECK
LIGAMENT

ARCUATE EXPANSION

INFERIOR OBLIQUE

Fig. 1.19. The connective tissue diaphragm situated just anterior to the globe equator demonstrating 'hernial orifices' within it. The eyelids and orbital septum have been removed. (With permission from ref. 26.)

cone of rectus muscles. The architectural network of connective tissues permits the muscles to function, allows for movement of the optic nerve and ciliary vessels and nerves as the globe rotates, and transmits the motor, autonomic and sensory nerves and blood vessels from the orbit apex to the extraocular muscles and the globe. Koornneef's schematic drawings of the major connective tissues in coronal section at four differing orbital depths are reproduced in Fig. 1.20. Unlike in the anterior orbit, retrobulbarly the intermuscular septa are less well developed, particularly in the inferotemporal quadrant where none exists (Fig. 1.20b). Although there is anatomic continuity here between the central and peripheral retrobulbar fat compartments, structurally and functionally they differ. In the central or intracone compartment, the fat is arranged in large fusiform lobules held in loose alignment with and surrounding the optic nerve.[1] The peripheral or pericone compartment is composed of less mobile smaller lobules and is arranged into four lobes each communicating more or less directly with the intracone compartment through the gap between an adjacent pair of rectus muscles (Fig. 1.21).

Of the rectus muscles, only the medial is significantly separated from the adjacent bony orbit wall by an adipose tissue compartment. This compartment on the nasal side of the anterior part of the medial rectus muscle is of considerable interest to the ophthalmic anaesthetist. On the medial side of the orbit at its apex (Fig. 1.20a), the connective tissues around the medial rectus muscle exhibit connections to the orbital floor. Near the posterior pole of the globe on the medial side (Fig. 1.20b,c), there are also, in addition to these orbit floor connections, extensions to the orbit roof. At the level of the equator of the globe (Fig. 1.20d),

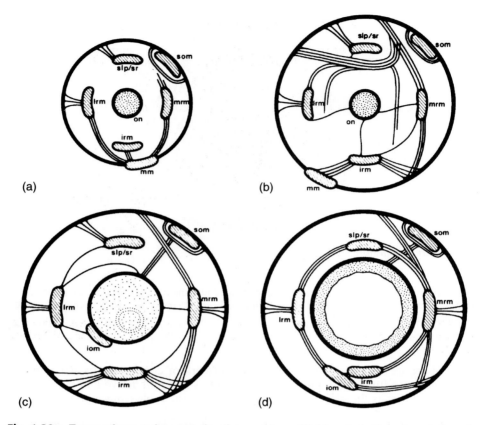

Fig. 1.20. Extraocular muscle connective tissue system. Highly schematic representation of coronal sections: (a) near the orbital apex; (b) near the posterior pole of the globe; (c) mid-way between the posterior pole and equator of the globe; (d) at the globe equator. slp/sr, levator palpebrae superioris/superior rectus complex; lrm, lateral rectus muscle; iom, inferior oblique muscle; irm, inferior rectus muscle; mm, Müller's muscle; mrm, medial rectus muscle; som, superior oblique muscle; on, optic nerve. (With permission from ref. 27.)

further to the roof and floor connections, a consolidation of connective tissue extending nasally to the medial orbit wall produces the medial check ligament. It can be seen that there is a discrete compartment posterior to the check ligament on the nasal side of the medial rectus muscle, which encloses the superior oblique muscle and communicates with fat compartments superiorly and inferiorly; bulk spread of local anaesthestic injected into this medial compartment occurs into these compartments and into the orbital apex posteriorly. However, the orbit roof and floor connective tissue attachments described above limit direct spread from the medial compartment laterally into the central cone fat compartment. Access of local anaesthetics to the motor nerve supply of the

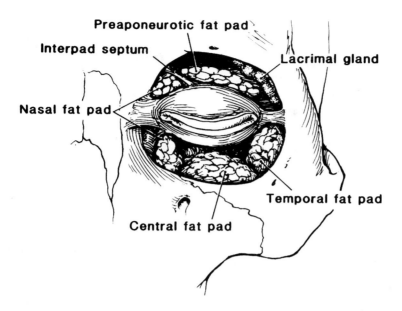

Fig. 1.21.   Orbital fat pads. Connective tissue systems of the orbit. Sagittal section of the orbit demonstrating the diffuse attachments of the extraocular muscles to the periorbita and Tenon's capsule. (With permission from ref. 5.)

superior oblique muscle and superior rectus/levator complex is facilitated. The medial compartment opens anteriorly, above and below the medial check ligament as two of the 'hernial orifices' in the connective tissue diaphragm that surrounds the globe just anterior to its equator (Fig. 1.19). Just as fat may herniate in the elderly through these 'hernial orifices' as connective tissues deteriorate with advancing age, likewise (and in any age group) local anaesthesia injectate deposited within the medial fat compartment will spread through these same areas and through the orbital septum into the upper and lower eyelids. This spread into the upper and lower eyelids is in a tissue plane on the deep surface of the orbicularis oculi muscle where the fine terminal motor branches of the seventh nerve are readily blocked.

The quality of connective tissues among different individuals varies;[14] orbital connective tissues deteriorate with increasing age. Because weaker connective tissues are more permeable to anaesthetics injected into the mid-orbit, critical muscle-blocking concentrations in the oculomotor nerves near the apex are more easily attained in elderly as compared with young adults. Likewise, orbital haemorrhage in the elderly, although resulting in a 'black eye' from anterior drainage, may be of less import than a similar bleed in younger patients in whom more sturdy tissues may trap blood and result in dramatic vision loss from un-relieved pressure build-up.

THE EYELIDS

The reflex blinking action of the eyelids protects the eye from foreign material, while their regular automatic action spreads the tear film across the cornea to keep it moist. Four tissue types make up the eyelids, from superficial to deep: the skin, a muscular layer, the cartilaginous tarsal plate and the conjunctiva. The skin contains sebaceous and sweat glands. Close to the eyelid margin, the muscle layer is composed of one muscle only, the orbicularis oculi, but is more complex nearer to the orbital rim. In the upper lid this takes the form of the aponeurotic extension of the levator palpebrae superioris muscle inserting on the front of the tarsal plate 3 mm from the lid margin. The non-striated Müller's muscle originates from the undersurface of the levator palpebrae superioris muscle and inserts in the superior border of the tarsal plate.

The upper eyelid crease, about 1 cm above the lid margin in occidental races, is created by slight bulging of the orbital fat superior to the fusion point of the orbital septum with the levator aponeurosis (Fig. 1.22). In oriental races, the orbital septum inserts lower on the aponeurosis to allow a more inferior extension of the orbital fat, resulting in the absence of an upper lid skin crease (Fig. 1.23). In the lower lid, the capsulopalpebral ligament, analogous to the levator aponeurosis of the upper lid, arises from the inferior Tenon's capsule and sheath of the inferior rectus muscle, splits to envelop the inferior oblique muscle and inserts in the inferior border of the tarsal plate (Fig. 7.15, p. 128).

The eyelash hair follicles are in the upper and lower tarsal plates. The elliptical space enclosed between the eyelid margins is known as the palpebral fissure. Its horizontal limits are the medial and lateral canthi, the skin overlying each of

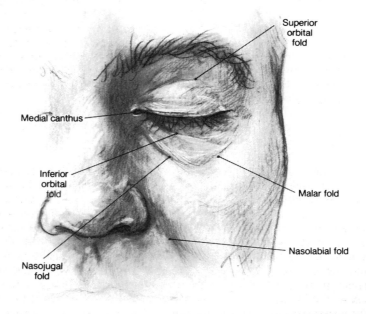

Fig. 1.22.   Schematic representation of the eyelid folds. (With permission from ref. 5.)

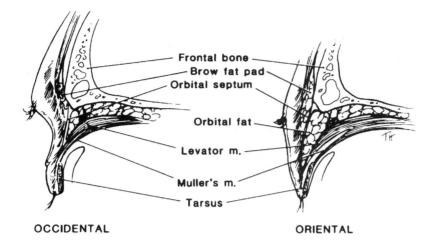

OCCIDENTAL   ORIENTAL

Fig. 1.23. Schematic representation of the differences between occidental and oriental eyelid anatomy. In the oriental eyelid the orbital septum fuses with the levator aponeurosis below the superior tarsal border. (With permission from ref. 5.)

these being known as the medial and lateral canthal folds. There is considerable variation in the width of the palpebral fissure between individuals. In a patient with a narrow palpebral fissure (with a wide lateral canthal fold), the usual amount of downward retracton of the lower lid may be difficult or impossible, making inferotemporal transconjunctival injection of local anaesthetics inadvisable. There is also a great range in the tightness of the lower eyelid margin between individuals. Eyelid laxity in the elderly results from stretching of the medial and lateral canthal tendons. In the presence of an excessively tight lower eyelid, inferotemporal transcutaneous injection of local anaesthesics may be the more prudent choice.

THE LACRIMAL APPARATUS

The lacrimal apparatus includes tear production, distribution and drainage.

The main lacrimal gland lies in a fossa carrying its name situated just posterior to the superotemporal orbit rim (Fig. 1.24). Short excretory ducts exit to the conjunctival sac. Smaller accessory glands complement the aqueous tear output from the main gland and other specialized glands add lipid and mucus components. Sensory innervation is from the lacrimal nerve; parasympathetic secretomotor innervation is by way of the zygomaticotemporal branch of the infraorbital nerve (Figs 1.24, 1.25, 1.26). Blinking distributes tears vertically, while collection is horizontally in the eyelid marginal meniscus towards the nasal side. At the junction of the medial one-sixth and the lateral five-sixths of each of the upper and lower eyelid margins is found the papilla lacrimalis and on its summit the punctum lacrimalis. At the nasal side of the palpebral fissure, the

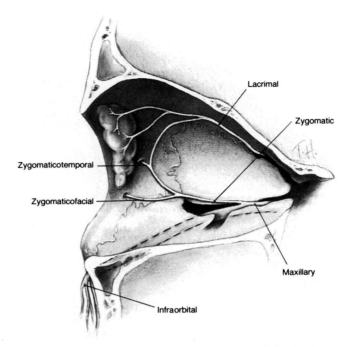

Labrimal

Zygomatic

Zygomaticotemporal

Zygomaticofacial

Maxillary

Infraorbital

Fig. 1.24. Communication between zygomaticotemporal and lacrimal nerves, supplying parasympathetic secretomotor innervation to the lacrimal gland. (With permission from ref. 5.)

medial canthal region, is found a specialized part of the conjunctiva called the caruncle with, lateral to it, the semilunar fold or plica semilunaris. This area functions as a collecting pool for tears about to be taken up by the tear duct drainage system. From the lacrimal puncta, canaliculi in the upper and lower lid margins direct tears by way of a common canaliculus to the lacrimal sac situated in the lacrimal fossa situated anteromedially in the orbit and from there in the nasolacrimal duct lying in the nasolacrimal canal to the nasal cavity (Fig. 1.27).

THE SKELETAL MUSCLES OF THE PERIORBIT AND ORBIT

Orbicularis oculi muscle

The orbicularis oculi muscle is intimately attached to the deep surface of the skin and is responsible for eyelid closure, including automatic and reflex blinking action. Innervation is by the upper branches of the facial nerve (VII cranial) entering on the deep surface of the muscle. It is comprised of three portions: the orbital (overlying the orbit rim), preseptal and pretarsal (Fig. 1.28). It intermixes with the brow musculature. The muscle surrounds the palpebral fissure and orbit

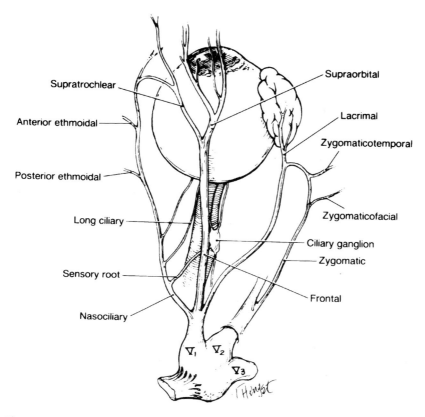

Supratrochlear

Anterior ethmoidal

Posterior ethmoidal

Long ciliary

Sensory root

Nasociliary

Supraorbital

Lacrimal

Zygomaticotemporal

Zygomaticofacial

Ciliary ganglion

Zygomatic

Frontal

V_1 V_2

V_3

Fig. 1.25. Trigeminal nerve; view from above. V_1, ophthalmic nerve; V_2, maxillary nerve; V_3, mandibular nerve. (With permission from ref. 5.)

in horseshoe fashion, with its origin from the medial orbit rim, including connections with the medial canthal tendon. The preseptal and pretarsal portions have specialized morphology pertaining to the tear-pump mechanism.

Extraocular muscles

Six extraocular muscles operate synergistically to produce rotational movements of the globe. The levator of the upper eyelid is usually considered along with them. The orbital connective tissues, discussed above, are vital to the normal functioning of these muscles and, if disrupted, as for example in a blow-out fracture of the orbit floor, it will have a profound adverse effect on their mechanical actions. Physiological movements of the globe are: elevation, depression, adduction, abduction intorsion and extorsion. There are four rectus muscles (the lateral rectus, despite its name, has a curved course) and two oblique muscles (Figs 1.29, 1.30, 1.31). Only the medial and lateral recti produce pure globe duction movements, adduction and abduction respectively. The others, because of the

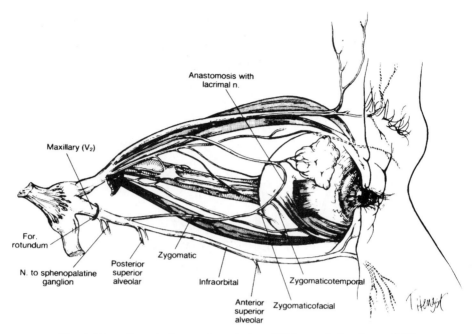

Fig. 1.26. Trigeminal nerve: lateral view. (With permission from ref. 5.)

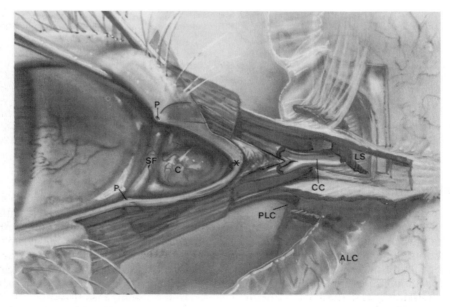

Fig. 1.27. The lacrimal drainage system. C, caruncle; P, punctum; SF, semilunar fold; CC, common canaliculus; LS, lacrimal sac; ALC, anterior lacrimal crest; PLC, posterior lacrimal crest; *medial canthus. (With permission from ref. 23.)

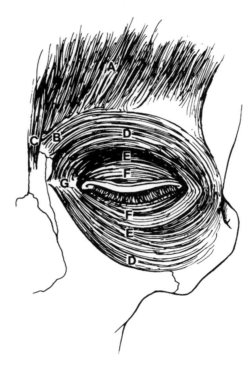

Fig. 1.28. Musculature of the brow and eyelids. A, frontalis; B, corrugator superciliaris; C, procerus; D, orbital orbicularis; E, preseptal orbicularis; F, pretarsal orbicularis; G, medial canthal tendon. (With permission from ref. 5.)

mechanical angle of their attachments to the globe, produce complex resultant movements. With upgaze, downgaze, abduction and adduction, the contracting rectus muscle thickens and the opponent rectus muscle thins with relaxation. With angled gazes, two adjacent muscles thicken with contraction as their opponents thin and relax.[15] For further reading on this complex topic, the reader is referred to a specialized text.[17]

Rectus muscles

The rectus muscles have their origin from a fibrous ring, the annulus of Zinn, which is attached to the sphenoid bone at the orbit apex (Fig. 1.32). The ring encircles the optic foramen and the medial end of the superior orbital fissure. The annulus is at the apex of the intracone space whose base is Tenon's capsule covering the posterior surface of the globe. Although no longer considered a closed compartment, nevertheless the intracone space, because of its intimate relationship with the optic, oculomotor, sensory and autonomic nerves, is important in understanding and mastering orbital regional anaesthesia. The rectus muscles average 40–42 mm in length (superior and inferior rectus muscles are slightly longer than the other two) and, after piercing Tenon's capsule, insert into the sclera posterior to the corneal limbus.

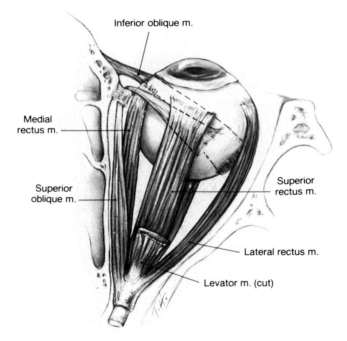

Inferior oblique m.

Medial
rectus m.

Superior
oblique m.

Superior
rectus m.

Lateral rectus m.

Levator m. (cut)

Fig. 1.29.   The orientation of the extraocular muscles in the orbit: view from above.   (With permission from ref. 5.)

Levator palpebrae superioris muscle

The levator palpebrae superioris muscle arises from the orbital apex just superior and slightly medial to the superior rectus muscle (Fig. 1.32). It passes forward, partially superimposed on the superior rectus (somewhat off to the medial side of it) and with fascial attachments to it. At Whitnall's ligament, the muscle is reoriented from an anterior–posterior to a superior–inferior direction (Fig. 1.11), fans out medially and laterally and gradually transforms into a wide aponeurosis with anterior and posterior lamellae. The former has diffuse terminal attachments, while the latter is the sympathetic muscle of Müller, which inserts on the superior border of the tarsal plate (Fig. 1.23).

Oblique muscles

The superior oblique muscle, averaging 40 mm in length, arises superior and medial to the annulus of Zinn (Fig. 1.32), passes forward at the junction of the orbit roof with its medial wall, and becomes tendinous anteriorly before passing through the cartilaginous trochlear ring. The reflected tendon, 2 cm in length, pierces Tenon's capsule and is directed backwards and temporally. It passes superior to the globe between it and the superior rectus muscle to insert as a flattened expansion on the temporal side of the posterior surface of the sclera (Fig. 1.29). The superior oblique muscle is innervated at its superolateral edge by the trochlear nerve.

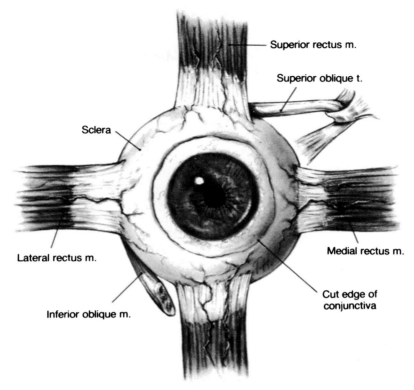

Fig. 1.30.   Insertions of the extraocular muscles on the globe. (With permission from ref. 5.)

The inferior oblique is the shortest of the extraocular muscles (37 mm average). It arises from a bony depression in the anteronasal orbit lateral to the commencement of the nasolacrimal duct, passes laterally and posteriorly while wrapping around the inferior rectus muscle, and, after piercing Tenon's capsule, inserts (while remaining muscular) on the posterior surface of the sclera (Fig. 1.29). It contributes to the ligamentous support diaphragm for the globe including Lockwood's ligament. The capsulopalpebral ligament, which passes between Tenon's capsule and the tarsal plate of the lower eyelid, encloses the belly of the inferior oblique muscle above and below. There are also important septal connections with the inferior rectus muscle. The motor nerve to the inferior oblique has a longer intraorbital course than any of the other oculomotor nerves.

THE NERVES OF THE EYE, ORBIT AND PERIORBIT

Cranial nerves II–VII inclusive are responsible for sight, motor function, sensation and autonomic control of the region. Fig. 1.33 is a schematic diagram of the orbital apex showing the fissures, vessels, muscle origins and nerves.

II optic

III occulomotor

IV trochlear

V trigeminal

VI abducent

VII facial

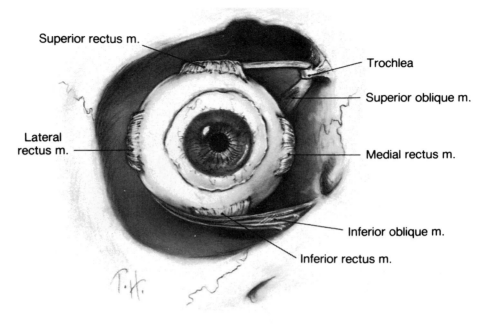

Fig. 1.31.   The orientation of the extraocular muscles in the orbit: frontal view. (With permission from ref. 5.)

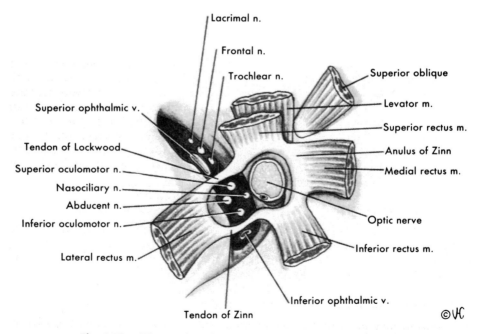

Fig. 1.32.   The annulus of Zinn. (With permission from ref. 28.)

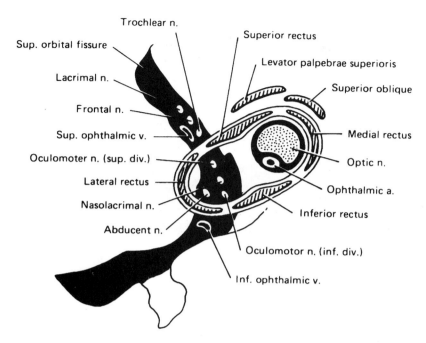

Fig. 1.33.   Schematic of orbital apex, fissures, vessels and nerves. (With permission from ref. 29.)

The optic nerve

The optic nerve, cranial nerve II, is strictly speaking not a cranial nerve but rather an extension of the brain and, unlike the other cranial nerves, carries with it, from the cranial cavity, meningeal coverings: an outer sheath derived from the dura and continuous anteriorly with the sclera, a thin and delicate middle sheath derived from anachnoid, and a vascular inner sheath derived from pia. Subdural and subarachnoid spaces separate the three sheaths. The optic nerve, on average 5 cm in length, extends from the optic chiasm to the retina, and has four anatomically distinguishable parts: intracranial, intracanalicular, intraorbital and intraocular.

The intracranial portion of the optic nerve

The intracranial portion is 1 cm in length (optic chiasm to cranial end of optic canal). The anterior cerebral artery and frontal lobe of the brain lie superiorly, the internal carotid artery laterally, as the optic nerve emerges from the cavernous sinus (Fig. 1.34).

The intracanalicular portion of the optic nerve

The intracanalicular section, 5–6 mm long, passes in an anterolateral and slightly downward direction through the optic canal[15] which it shares with the

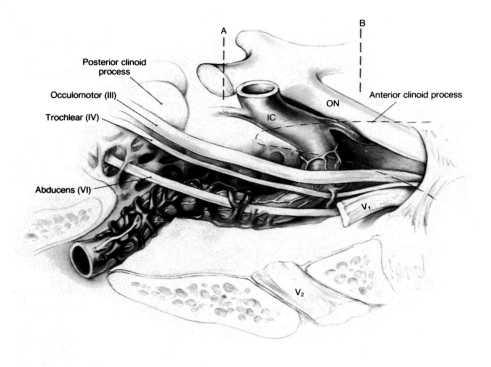

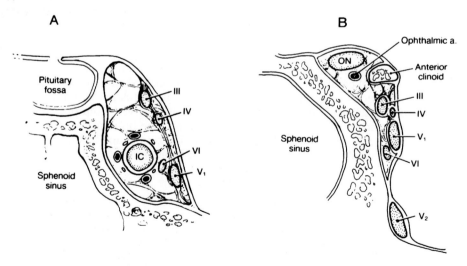

Fig. 1.34.   Anatomic relationships within the cavernous sinus. IC, internal carotid nerve; ON, optic nerve; V_1, ophthalmic nerve; V_2, maxillary nerve; A, coronal section at the level of the pituitary fossa; B, coronal section at the level of the anterior clinoid process. (With permission from ref. 5.)

ophthalmic artery (inferior and slightly lateral to it). This portion of the optic nerve should be regarded as completely rigid, since its sheath is tethered at both ends of the optic canal by a superior dural sling at its cerebral end and by the annulus of Zinn at its orbital end.[20] If the optic canal were extended in continuity with its anterolateral and slightly downward direction to the front of the orbit, it would emerge slightly below the mid-point of the lateral orbit rim.

The intraorbital portion of the optic nerve

The intraorbital part of the optic nerve is about 4 mm in diameter, averages slightly more than 3 cm in length and has a winding course across the 2.5-cm gap between the optic foramen and the hind surface of the globe; within the orbit, therefore, the nerve has about 7 mm of 'excess play'. The dural covering of the nerve fuses with the sclera anteriorly and with the periorbita posteriorly at the optic foramen. Cerebrospinal fluid flows freely within the dura surrounding the nerve and is in continuity with the cerebrospinal fluid surrounding the mid-brain. The transverse plane at the level of the optic foramen is mid-way between the transverse planes of the upper and lower orbital rims (Figs 1.3, 1.6). The orbit apex is thus medial to the globe and not behind it (Fig. 1.7). The optic foramen is the most superior and medial structure in the apex of the orbit.[6]

In primary gaze the intraorbital portion of the optic nerve is closer to the medial than the lateral rectus muscle and assumes a sinuous course between the posterior pole of the globe and the optic foramen (Figs 1.35, 1.36).[15] This sinuosity of the nerve accommodates the approximately 7 mm of 'excess play' resulting from the nerve being that much longer than the distance it has to traverse and permits free movement of the nerve in all globe positions without detriment to its function. As the globe moves in all directions of gaze away

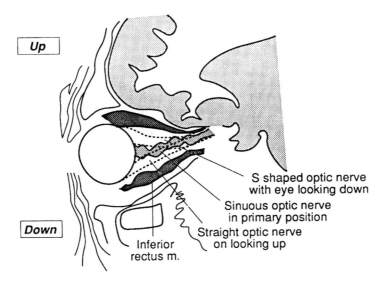

Fig. 1.35. Composite schematic illustration of MRI scans in the mid-sagittal plane of the orbit in primary position, upgaze and downgaze. (With permission from ref. 15.)

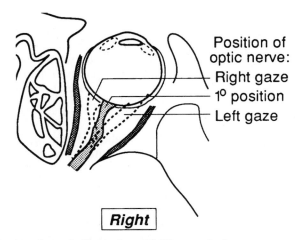

Position of
optic nerve:
Right gaze
1° position
Left gaze

Right

Fig. 1.36.   Composite schematic illustration of MRI scans in the transverse plane of the right orbit in primary position, right gaze (abduction) and left gaze (adduction). (Modified with permission from ref. 15.)

from primary, the intracanalicular portion of the optic nerve assumes a variety of positions between its 'anchor' at the orbit apex and its 'wandering' connection to the globe 3 mm on the nasal side of its posterior pole. The anterior portion of the nerve moves in the opposite direction from that of any particluar direction of gaze.[15] In adduction and upgaze the optic nerve straightens out; on the other hand, in abduction and downgaze the optic nerve takes on an S-shaped curve.[15] The plane of the optic canal is forward, slightly downward and 35 degrees lateral.[15] In adduction and upgaze the nerve moves closer to the plane of the optic canal and therefore is straight. Mainly because the optic nerve has a certain rigidity and the orbital contents are closely packed at the apex, in abduction and downgaze the nerve cannot turn sharply and is forced to bend in the reverse direction from the plane of the optic canal to assume an S-shaped configuration.[15] With the globe in primary gaze position the nerve lies totally on the nasal side of the mid-sagittal plane (visual axis) running in the transverse plane towards the optic foramen (Fig. 1.37). The sagittal plane of the orbital axis is longitudinally through the greater part of the intraorbital portion of the optic nerve and through the lateral limbus anteriorly (Fig.1.3).[22] It is essential for the anaesthetist to have a clear three-dimensional image of the location of the orbital portion of the optic nerve.

The intraocular portion of the optic nerve

The intraocular section of the nerve is 1 mm long, representing the thickness of the sclera where the nerve enters near the posterior pole of the globe.

Motor nerves to the extraocular muscles

There are three cranial nerves that supply motor function to the extraocular muscles: the oculomotor (III) the trochlear (IV) and the abducens (VI). The latter two

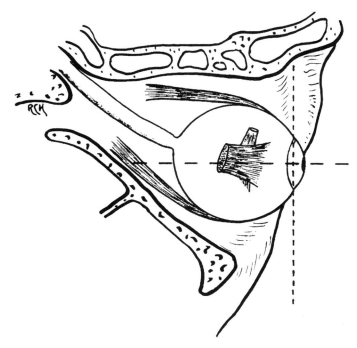

Fig. 1.37.   Globe in primary gaze. Fine dashed line indicates the plane of the iris (useful in gauging depth of needle advancement); coarse dashed line indicates the mid-sagittal plane of the eye and the visual axis through the centre of the pupil. The optic nerve lies on the nasal side of the mid-sagittal plane of the eye. (With permission from Gimbel Educational Services.)

nerves supply one muscle each – the superior oblique (IV) and the lateral rectus (VI), respectively. The oculomotor nerve innervates the remaining four extraocular muscles plus the levator palpebrae superioris, and carries parasympathetic fibres destined for the sphincter muscle of the iris and the ciliary muscle. The motor nerves to the four rectus muscles and the inferior oblique access their respective muscle bellies from within the muscle cone, whereas the trochlear nerve remains outside the cone and enters its muscle, the superior oblique, at its superolateral edge. This anatomic difference explains the delayed onset of akinesia following small volume intracone local anaesthetic injection (see Chapter 7).

Oculomotor nerve

The oculomotor nerve (cranial nerve III) emerges from the interpeduncular sulcus on the ventral surface of the brainstem as a leash of fibres which quickly coalesce into a single trunk. It passes between the posterior cerebral and superior cerebellar arteries, runs forward on the lateral side of the posterior communicating artery, traverses the upper lateral wall of the cavernous sinus above the trochlear nerve (Fig. 1.34), and divides into superior and inferior branches before entering, through the inferomedial end of the superior orbital fissure (within the annulus of Zinn), into the intracone space of the orbit. The superior branch rises within the intracone space lateral to the optic nerve to enter the conal surface of the belly of the superior rectus 1.25 cm from its origin (Fig. 1.38). Part of the nerve passes through or around the superior rectus to supply the superimposed levator palpebrae superioris muscle. The inferior branch of the oculomotor nerve divides into three: one which passes under the optic nerve to enter the conal surface of the belly of the medial rectus muscle 1.25 cm from its origin; one which supplies the inferior rectus muscle by entering its belly from the conal surface also 1.25 cm from its origin; and one which runs a long course close to the floor of the orbit, on the lateral side of the inferior rectus muscle, before supplying the inferior oblique muscle by entering its posterior surface at its mid-point (Fig. 1.38). This nerve to the inferior oblique may be traumatized by needles entering from the inferotemporal quadrant of the orbit rim (see Chapters 7 and 8). Near the apex of the orbit, the third division of the inferior branch of the oculomotor nerve gives off a fine ramus which rises to join the ciliary ganglion (Fig. 1.39). It carries preganglionic parasympathetic fibres to the ganglion.

Trochlear nerve

The trochlear nerve (cranial nerve IV) exits from the dorsum of the brainstem, then winds around it and traverses the upper lateral wall of the cavernous sinus (Fig. 1.33) inferior to the oculomotor nerve before entering the orbit outside the annulus of Zinn (Figs 1.32, 1.38). Its long intracranial course renders it vulnera-

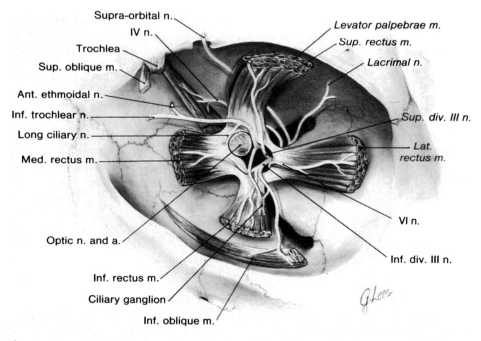

Fig. 1.38. The extraocular muscles are innervated from their conal surface except for the superior oblique muscle which is innervated at its superolateral edge.

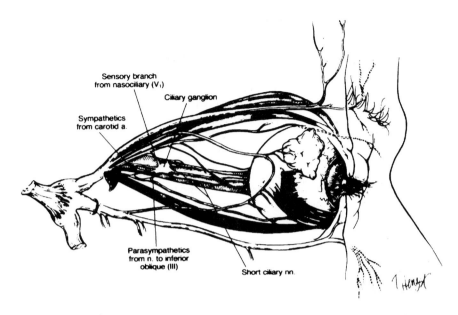

Fig. 1.39.   Anatomy of the ciliary ganglion. (With permission from ref. 5.)

ble to contrecoup injury. In the orbit it passes forward near the roof and enters the superior oblique muscle at its superolateral edge at the junction of the posterior one-third and anterior two-thirds of its belly. Because its motor nerve supply is outside the cone of rectus muscles, there may be retained activity of the superior oblique muscle (intortion) following small volume intracone local anaesthetic injections.

Abducens nerve

The abducens nerve (cranial nerve VI), motor nerve to the lateral rectus muscle, emerges from the groove between the medulla and the pons, ascends on the brainstem, makes a sharp bend over the petrous temporal bone, and enters the posterior cavernous sinus where it lies between the internal carotid artery medially and the trigeminal ganglion laterally. Passing forward in the cavernous sinus inferior to the oculomotor and trochlear nerves (Fig. 1.34), and then by way of the superior orbital fissure within the annulus of Zinn (Fig. 1.32) to the intracone space, it finally enters the belly of the lateral rectus muscle on its conal surface 1.25 cm from its origin (Fig. 1.38).

Ciliary ganglion

The ciliary ganglion is situated in the posterior intracone space at a distance of 1 cm from the orbital apex and 1.5 cm posterior to the globe. It lies between the optic nerve and ophthalmic artery (medially) and the lateral rectus muscle (laterally). It measures 2×1 mm in size and is of a reddish-grey colour. It is a peripheral ganglion of the parasympathetic nervous system. From its anterior surface, 8–10 branches called the short ciliary nerves arise; they subdivide into 15–20 smaller branches which penetrate the sclera in a circle close to the optic nerve. The ciliary ganglion has three roots which connect to it posteriorly: motor or parasympathetic, sensory and sympathetic (Fig. 1.39).

The motor root, from the nerve to the inferior oblique, contains preganlionic fibres which synapse in the ganglion to send postganglionic motor fibres (by way of the short ciliary nerves) to the sphincter pupillae and ciliary muscles. The sensory root is from the nasociliary nerve (see below) and transmits sensory fibres from the globe (also by way of the short ciliary nerves) which have passed through the ciliary ganglion without interruption. The sympathetic root has postganglionic fibres from the superior cervical ganglion which travel in the plexus surrounding the internal carotid artery and thence to the orbit in periarterial sheaths. They also travel uninterrupted through the ciliary ganglion and the short ciliary nerves, and are destined for control of the blood vessels of the globe.

Trigeminal nerve

The trigeminal nerve attaches by a small motor root and a much larger sensory root to the ventral surface of the pons near its upper border. The motor branch supplies the muscles of mastication; the larger root carries the sensory fibres for the skin of the face and scalp, the teeth, and the mucous membranes of the mouth and nasal cavities. The nerve cell bodies for the sensory fibres are in the trigeminal ganglion, measuring 1×2 cm, situated lateral to the internal carotid artery and the posterior part of the cavernous sinus. The peripheral nerve fibres arising from cells of the trigeminal ganglion divide into three trunks: the ophthalmic nerve, the maxillary nerve and the sensory portion of the mandibular nerve (combines with the motor root to form the mandibular nerve). The anatomy of the mandibular nerve is not directly relevant for the ophthalmic anaesthetist and will not be discussed further in this chapter.

Ophthalmic nerve

The ophthalmic nerve, the smallest division of the trigeminal nerve, emerges from the anteromedial aspect of the trigeminal ganglion and passes foward to enter the lateral wall of the cavernous sinus inferior to the oculomotor and trochlear nerves (Fig. 1.33). Towards the front of the cavernous sinus, the nerve splits into three branches – lacrimal, frontal and nasociliary (Fig. 1.25) – which pass separately through the superior orbital fissure, the former two branches being outside and the latter inside the annulus of Zinn (Fig. 1.32).

The lacrimal nerve, which is smaller than the other two branches of the ophthalmic nerve, courses anteriorly (and aligned with the superior border of the lateral rectus muscle) to enter the posterior border of the lacrimal gland lying in a bony fossa just behind the superotemporal margin of the orbit; it also innervates the most lateral skin of the upper eyelid and adjacent conjunctiva.

The frontal, which is larger than the other two branches of the ophthalmic nerve (Fig. 1.25), courses anteriorly close to the periorbita of the orbital roof, between it and the levator palpebrae superioris muscle, before splitting unequally into the smaller supratrochlear nerve on the medial side and the larger supraorbital which continues forward to emerge from the front of the orbit either through the supraorbital foramen (20%) or notch (80%). The supratrochlear innervates the central forehead skin, the skin of the upper medial eyelid and the medial conjunctiva. The supraorbital nerve provides sensation to the rest of the forehead, the anterior two-thirds of the scalp, and the skin of the upper central eyelid and adjacent conjunctiva (Fig. 1.40). Because peripheral conjunctival sensation is mediated via the lacrimal and frontal nerves, both of which do not course through the intracone space, incomplete conjunctival anaethesia may result from small volume intracone local anaesthetic injection.

The nasociliary branch of the ophthalmic nerve (Fig. 1.25) passes through the annulus of Zinn (Figs 1.32, 1.38) to enter the intracone space and sends a communicating ramus to the ciliary ganglion. As it passes over the optic nerve, the long ciliary nerves (two or three in number) are given off. They accompany the short ciliary nerves and pierce the sclera close to the optic nerve. In addition to afferent sensation from the iris, ciliary body, cornea and central bulbar conjunctiva, these nerves carry sympathetic motor fibres to the dilator pupillae muscle. Whereas the retina is devoid of pain fibres, the sclera is innervated by free nerve endings, which explains the analgesic requirement of patients following scleral buckling procedures.[4] Continuing to the medial orbital wall in close relationship with the ophthalmic artery, the nasociliary nerve gives off anterior and posterior ethmoidal branches (posterior often absent) which pass through their respective foramina on the medial orbital wall and supply the mucosa of the ethmoid sinuses and nasal cavity. The most anterior division of the nasociliary nerve is

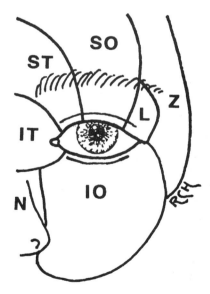

Fig. 1.40.   The cutaneous nerve supply to the periorbital region. IT, infratrochlear nerve; ST, supratrochlear nerve; SO, supraorbital nerve; L, lacrimal nerve; Z, zygomaticotemporal and zygomaticofacial nerves; IO, infraorbital nerve; N, nasal nerve. (With permission from Gimbel Educational Services.)

the infratrochlear nerve; it runs along the superior border of the medial rectus muscle and penetrates the orbital septum to innervate the skin of the side of the nose, the medial skin of the lower eyelid and adjacent conjunctiva, and the lacrimal sac (Fig. 1.40).

Maxillary nerve

The maxillary nerve, the second division of the trigeminal nerve, is the sensory nerve for the midface, anterior temporal region, lower eyelid and upper lip. In addition, it supplies sensation for the upper gums and teeth, mucous membranes of the upper mouth, nasopharynx and maxillary sinuses. It emerges from the anterior and central aspects of the trigeminal ganglion and passes forward through the lower lateral part of the cavernous sinus. It exits from the cranial cavity through the foramen rotundum, crosses the pterygopalatine fossa and enters the orbit through the inferior orbital fissure as the infraorbital nerve. Passing anteriorly, this nerve next lies in the infraorbital groove and descends with the infraorbital canal to reach the front of the face at the infraorbital foramen 1 cm below the mid-point of the inferior orbital rim (Figs 1.5, 1.24). In the subcutaneous tissues of the cheek, it breaks up into branches which innervate the skin of the lower eyelid, nose, upper lip and central face (Fig. 1.40). In the pterygopalatine fossa, the maxillary nerve gives off its zygomatic branch which ascends to the orbit through the infraorbital fissure and divides into zygomaticofacial and zygomaticotemporal nerves. The former exits a foramen bearing the same name to supply skin sensation overlying the malar bone. The latter travels a short distance along the lateral orbital wall and exits a foramen bearing its name to innervate the skin of the anterior temporal region (Figs 1.24, 1.44). Parasympathetic secretomotor fibres to the lacrimal gland, whose preganglionic fibres emerge from the brainstem with the facial nerve and transfer to the trigeminal nerve by a complex pathway, travel in the maxillary nerve and relay in another peripheral ganglion of the parasympathetic system, the sphenopalatine ganglion, which lies in the pterygopalatine fossa. Postganglionic fibres reach the lacrimal gland via interconnections between the zygomaticotemporal and lacrimal nerves (Figs 1.24, 1.25, 1.26).

The anatomic proximity of the central and peripheral orbital nerves and their shared investing adipose tissue compartments explain easily the widespread area of peripheral sensory anaesthesia associated with major intraorbital regional anaesthetic blocks. Spread to the frontal nerve complex in the superior orbit, and to the maxillary nerve complex in the inferior orbit, regularly results in unilateral loss of sensation extending from near the occiput to the upper lip, and from the mid-line of the nose to the anterior temporal region, including anaesthesia of the mucosa of the upper mouth and teeth and the nasal cavity (patients may experience unilateral nasal stuffiness or feel that their nose is 'running').

Facial nerve

The facial nerve (cranial nerve VII) has large motor and small sensory/parasympathetic components. The former is the part of main interest to the ophthalmic anaesthetist because motor innervation of the facial musculature, especially that of the periorbital muscles, is thus mediated; however, it should be noted that secretomotor fibres to the lacrimal gland originate in the smaller portion (see above). The anatomy of this complex nerve will be discussed only in its peripheral distribution.

The facial nerve originates in the pons and exits the base of the skull at the stylomastoid foramen in close proximity to the glossopharyngeal, vagus and spinal accessory nerves emerging from the jugular foramen (Fig. 1.41). Block techniques at this location result in complete hemifacial akinesia; spread of local anaesthetic injectate to the adjacent major cranial nerves may occur (see Chapters 7 and 8, respectively). The nerve at its exit from the stylomastoid foramen is 2 cm deep to the middle of the anterior border of the mastoid process. It next crosses the styloid process of the temporal bone, passes under the external auditory meatus and enters the substance of the parotid, inside which it divides first into two divisions but subsequently into several branches (Fig. 1.42). The pattern of the break-up and distribution of the facial nerve branches varies greatly between individuals. As it passes through the parotid tissues, there are close relationships to the ramus and head of the mandible (these are important landmarks in certain block techniques). The upper branches (temporal and zygomatic) of the facial nerve innervate the forehead and brow musculature, and the three components of the orbicularis oculi (see above). It is most important to

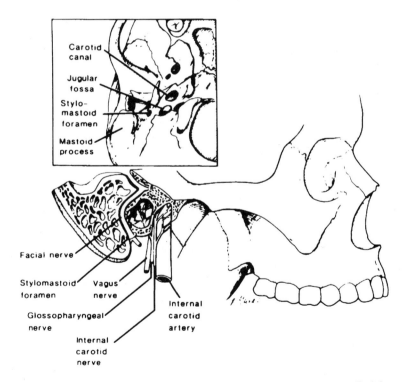

Fig. 1.41.   Anatomic depiction of the proximity of the stylomastoid foramen (facial nerve) to the jugular foramen (vagus, glossopharyngeal and spinal accessory nerves). The latter is not shown. (With permission from ref. 31.)

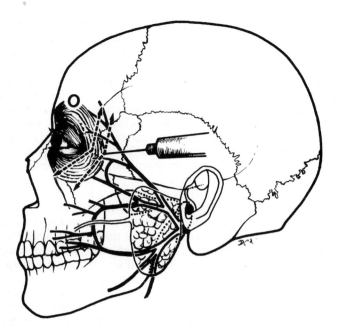

Fig. 1.42.   Extracranial path of the facial nerve. Detail of van Lint block technique is shown. O, orbicularis muscle. (With permission from ref. 32.)

note that all of the facial muscles are innervated on their deep surface; block techniques in the peripheral distribution of the facial nerve depend on the blockade of fine terminal fibres. Local anaesthetics injected superficial to the facial muscles often do not spread effectively to their deep surface; this frequently results in poor abolition of muscle action. The zygomatic arch and orbital rim are the bony landmarks used in these peripheral facial nerve blocks (see Chapter 7).

BLOOD VESSELS OF THE EYE AND ORBIT

Unlike in most of the rest of the body where arteries and veins travel together to and from a given tissue, orbital arterial and venous channels behave differently from one another in their anatomic distribution. The veins of the orbit do not accompany the arterial system, but rather take their own course and direction.[8] Arteries have considerable inter-individual variation in their layout. Arteries of the orbit radiate towards their target organs and perforate connective tissue septa in passing from one compartment to the next. The veins, however, run circularly and are confined to the connective tissue septa. Radiologists are most aware of the differences in variability between the arterial and venous systems. They consider topographical information obtained from phlebograms more dependable than that obtained from arteriograms.[2] In particular, the superior ophthalmic vein, the largest orbital venous channel, presents a constant course making it a major reference point for interpretations of orbital space occupying lesions.[2, 22]

Viewing the orbit in general, arteries are located centrally in the intracone space near the orbit apex and superiorly in the anterior orbit, whereas veins are located peripherally, mainly outside the central intracone area.[2] The rear of the intracone space is an area of high arterial density with, in addition, the venous drainage system of the retina. With clinical intervention this far back in the orbit (e.g. by needle placement), damage to the system, either directly or resulting from pressure build-up of haematoma, is more likely than in any other part of the orbit. Considering arteries and veins as a common entity, the posterior orbit on the lateral side has the greatest vascular constellation, while in the anterior orbit the reverse is true. Here most vessels are found medially.[2]

Arterial

Because there is so much variability between individuals in the anatomic layout of the orbital arterial system, authors have abandoned the concept of a 'normal' pattern and come to recognize that there is at most a 'usual' pattern.[2] The orbital arterial system is fed predominantly from the ophthalmic artery, a branch of the internal carotid artery. There are minor contributions from the external carotid artery.

The ophthalmic artery, typical of the orbital arteries in general, does not have a pattern that can be regarded as 'normal'.[9] In 80% of individuals the ophthalmic artery crosses superior to the optic nerve and in 20% lies underneath the nerve in a more vulnerable position for needles directed towards the orbital apex. The origin of the ophthalmic artery from the internal carotid artery siphon (S-shaped configuration), and their relationship within the cavernous sinus to the ocular motor and ophthalmic nerves, are best appreciated from a good illustration (Fig. 1.34). After this short intracranial path, the ophthalmic artery traverses the optic canal, lying inferior to the optic nerve and slightly to the temporal side. On entering the intracone space, the artery (Figs 1.43, 1.44) runs temporally and superiorly between the optic nerve and the ciliary ganglion and gives off its first branch, the central retinal artery, which pierces the dural sheath of the optic nerve, usually from its inferomedial aspect, 1.25 cm posterior to the globe, to reach the centre of the optic nerve. This tiny vital artery then runs forward in the core of the optic nerve to emerge at the optic nerve head, where it divides into the retinal arteries which supply the retina. The lacrimal artery is the next branch (which has many sub-branches before supplying the lacrimal gland and terminating as the superior and inferior lateral palpebral arteries). The main vessel then turns nasally and passes above (usually) the optic nerve where muscular slips to the rectus muscles and then the long and short posterior ciliary arteries arise. These enter the globe in association with the long and short ciliary nerves, close to the optic nerve. The long posterior ciliary arteries, usually two in number, course forward within the globe deep to the sclera to supply the anterior part of the uveal tract. Multiple short posterior ciliary arteries pierce the sclera and supply the choroid coat of the eye and the ciliary body. The anterior ciliary arteries arise from the muscular arteries (mentioned above) and enter the globe close to the limbus to supply the anterior parts of the uveal tract. At this point the supra-orbital branch, which courses forward with the nerve of the same name, is given off prior to the posterior and anterior ethmoidal arteries (these vessels, as they exit their respective foramina, anchor the ophthalmic artery to the medial orbit

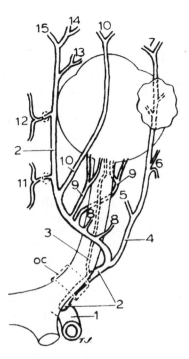

Fig. 1.43. Arterial supply to the orbit. 1, internal carotid artery; 2, ophthalmic artery; 3, central artery of the retina; 4, lacrimal artery; 5, muscular branch of lacrimal artery; 6, zygomatic branches of lacrimal artery; 7, lateral palpebral arteries; 8, muscular branches of ophthalmic artery; 9, long and short posterior ciliary arteries; 10, supraorbital artery; 11, posterior ethmoidal artery; 12, anterior ethmoidal artery; 13, medial palpebral arteries; 14, supratrochlear artery; 15, dorsal nasal artery; OC, optic canal. (With permission from ref. 29.)

wall). Continuing in the superonasal quadrant of the orbit, superior and inferior medial palpebral arteries are given off next and, finally, the end arteries of the ophthalmic artery system, namely the dorsal nasal and supratrochlear (sometimes called frontal) arteries. Arterial cascades in the eyelids are fed from the upper and lower medial and lateral palpebral arteries with communications from the supraorbital artery and facial vessels, part of the external carotid distribution.

Regional anaesthesia needles should not be introduced into the posterior 1.5 cm of the orbit because large vessels, the potential sources of vision-threatening bleeding, are located there and also because the vital structures (optic nerve and extraocular muscle origins) are tightly packed and subject to serious damage (see Chapter 8). There are, however, three adipose tissue compartments in the anterior and mid-orbit which are relatively avascular and the preferred sites of local anaesthetic injection (see Chapter 7): inferotemporal, superotemporal (sagittal plane of the lateral limbus and close to the orbit roof extending back from the orbit rim for 3 cm) and medial (needle entry point at the extreme medial end of the palpebral fissure on the nasal side of the caruncle, needle directed a maxi-

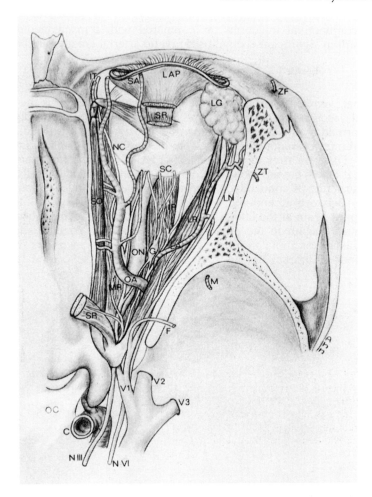

Fig. 1.44.   Superior view of orbital contents. C, internal carotid artery; OC, optic chiasm; N III, oculomotor nerve; N VI, abducens nerve; V1, ophthalmic nerve; V2, maxillary nerve; V3, mandibular nerve; F, frontal nerve; SR, superior rectus muscle; MR, medial rectus muscle; OA, ophthalmic artery; M, communicating branch with middle meningeal artery; ON, optic nerve; G, ciliary ganglion; LA, lacrimal artery; LR, lateral rectus muscle; IR, inferior rectus muscle; SO, superior oblique muscle; T, trochlea; LN, lacrimal nerve; SC, short posterior ciliary nerves; NC, nasociliary nerve; SA, supraorbital artery; LAP, levator aponeurosis; LG, lacrimal gland; ZT, zygomaticotemporal artery; ZF, zygomaticofacial artery; IT, infratrochlear neurovascular bundle. (With permission from ref. 33.)

mum distance of 25 mm in the transverse plane and 5 degrees medial to the direct sagittal plane). The superonasal quadrant, containing as it does the end arteries of the ophthalmic artery and the large venous connections between the facial angular vein and the superior orbital vein, not to mention the trochlear mechanism of the superior oblique muscle, should be avoided as an injection site. Transconjunctival injections, as compared with transcutaneous, are less likely to result in significant ecchymoses (eyelid arterial arcades are bypassed).

Venous

The principal vein of the orbit, the superior ophthalmic, which is the most constant orbital vascular structure (referring to inter-individual morphology differences), is formed by the confluence, near the anterior rim of the medial orbit, of superior and inferior major tributaries from the supraorbital vein and the angular facial vein. The vein runs to the medial border of the superior rectus muscle, from where it enters the intracone space to run backwards and laterally in a hammock-like structure of connective tissue septa suspended under the superior rectus muscle, between it and the optic nerve (Figs 1.45, 1.46),[12] to exit the intracone space again at the lateral border of the superior rectus muscle. Here it turns backwards again in the direction of the superior orbital fissure through which it gains access above the annulus (Fig. 1.32) to the cavernous sinus. There are up to four additional venous systems (Fig. 1.46): the central retinal vein

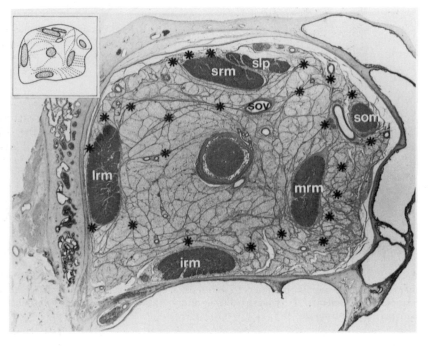

Fig. 1.45.   Cross-section of the orbit 2.6 mm posterior to the hind surface of the globe showing the connective tissue hammock carrying the superior ophthalmic vein (sov) diagonally across the superior orbit from anteronasal to posterotemporal. slp, levator palpebrae superioris muscle; srm, superior rectus muscle; som, superior oblique muscle; lrm, lateral rectus muscle; irm, inferior rectus muscle; mrm, medial rectus muscle; *connective tissue septa. (With permission from ref. 24.)

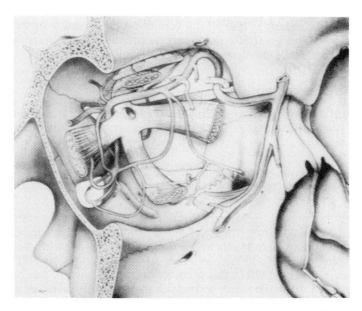

Fig. 1.46. Drawing of the venous system of the human orbit. Note in particular the superior ophthalmic vein communicating anteriorly with the angular vein of the face, and crossing diagonally in the superior orbit from the superonasal to posterotemporal side. (With permission from ref. 2.)

which accompanies the central retinal artery and usually drains directly to the cavernous sinus; the inferior orbital vein formed from an inferior venous network in the intracone space and running laterally and posteriorly on the orbit floor either to join the superior vein at the superior orbital fissure, or drain directly into the cavernous sinus below the annulus at the medial end of the superior orbital fissure; a posterior muscular vein described by Henry in 1959;[2] and the medial ophthalmic vein running along the medial wall of the orbit and connecting either the upper or lower root tributary of the superior orbital vein with the cavernous sinus. The latter two systems are less constant in their morphology. Venous blood from the globe and other orbital contents drains to finer tributaries of the major venous systems. The most constant of these are the four or five vortex veins, the muscle collateral veins and the lacrimal vein.

The orbital venous system has direct communication with extraorbital vein systems for drainage purposes. The most important of these is by way of the superior orbital fissure via the posterior end of the superior orbital vein to the cavernous sinus. Also, the inferior ophthalmic vein communicates via the inferior orbital fissure with the pterygoid plexus. To the front the orbit venous system has major communication with the facial venous system (the anterior end of the superior ophthalmic vein with the angular vein; Fig. 1.46). Other sites of drainage include through the lateral wall with the zygomaticotemporal vein and through the medial wall to the veins of the nasal cavity via the ethmoidal veins. The direction of venous blood flow in the orbit is pressure gradient dependent in a system that is devoid of valves. Although a controversial topic throughout the centuries, current thinking is that orbital venous blood normally flows from ante-rior to posterior.[2] The level of central venous pressure, deep breathing and eye movements all influence the flow.

Lymphatics of the globe

The orbit itself contains no lymphatic vessels or lymph nodes; however, the eye-lids have a lymphatic drainage system to nodes situated in the submandibular and parotid regions.

ORBITAL AND OCULAR IMAGING

Until recently, diagnostic techniques for evaluating ocular and orbital diseases, such as conventional X-ray films, orbital arteriography and venography, and radionuclide scanning, left much to be desired. However, with the advent of ultrasonography, both A- and B-scan, computerized tomography (CT) and mag-netic resonance imaging (MRI), this relatively inaccessible area has been opened up allowing diagnoses to be made with much greater ease and accuracy.

Ultrasonography

The A-scan provides a one-dimensional view of the orbit, whereas the B-scan provides a two-dimensional or cross-sectional display. The advantages of orbital ultrasound are its low cost, relative ease of performance, lack of radiation, and usefulness in differentiating soft tissue masses, for example solid from cystic tumours and vascular from avascular lesions. Its disadvantages are its limited usefulness in assessing orbital foreign bodies and lesions of the orbital apex, paranasal sinuses and intracranial cavity. It has no role in the evaluation of orbital fractures. As a consequence of these drawbacks, it has been largely sup-planted by CT and MRI, which offer better and more precise anatomic detail of the whole orbit. In recent years, the two-dimensional B-scan has been combined with colour flow Doppler technology to determine orbital blood flow.

A-scan ultrasonography is regularly employed in the assessment of ocular dimensions prior to cataract surgery. B-scan ultrasonography is an effective means of investigating ocular pathology when the media are insufficiently clear for definitive ophthalmoscopy.

Computerized tomography

In many respects, CT and MRI are complementary diagnostic tools, although the former remains the most available and the most cost-effective means of assess-ing orbital pathology.[22] It is able to demonstrate a number of parameters con-cerning orbital masses, both inflammatory and neoplastic, such as location, shape, consistency and effect on surrounding structures. Characterization of bone pathology, such as orbital fractures and bone destruction, and tissue calcifi-cation cannot be matched by MRI. Metallic and non-metallic foreign bodies can usually be readily visualized, although this does not hold true for organic foreign matter such as wood, where MRI has the clear advantage. Intravenous contrast enhancement may be used to investigate the vascularity of a lesion.

Magnetic resonance imaging

Unlike CT, MRI does not employ ionizing radiation.[15,18] Other advantages over CT include the ability to display information in multiple planes without repositioning the patient, better soft tissue differentiation, and better assessment of tissues in the orbital apex and periorbital spaces. It, too, can be combined with intravenous contrast material to enhance vascular lesions. The drawbacks of this diagnostic modality include its high cost, lengthy examination time with the attendant problems of motion artifacts, patient anxiety, claustrophobia, and contraindications to its use in patients with ferromagnetic bodies and aneurysm clips, and in patients with cardiac pacemakers.

REFERENCES

1. Atkinson WS. Local anesthesia in ophthalmology. *Am J Ophthalmol* 1948; **31:** 1607.
2. Bergen MP. *Vascular Architecture in the Human Orbit.* Swets and Zeitlinger: Lisse, 1982: 149.
3. Bogren HG, Franti CE, Wilmarth SS. Normal variations of the position of the eye in the orbit. *Ophthalmology* 1986; **93:** 1072.
4. Cannon CS, Gross JG, Abramson I *et al.* Evaluation of outpatient experience with vitreoretinal surgery. *Br J Ophthalmol* 1992; **76:** 68.
5. Doxanas MT, Anderson RL. *Clinical Orbital Anatomy.* Williams and Wilkins: Baltimore, MD, 1984: 232.
6. Goldberg RA, Hannani K, Toga AW. Microanatomy of the orbital apex: Computed tomography and microplaning of soft and hard tissue. *Ophthalmology* 1992; **99:** 1447.
7. Grabow HB. Topical anesthesia for cataract surgery. *Eur J Implant Ref Surg* 1993; **5:** 20.
8. Gurwitsch M. Ueber die Anastomosen zwischen den Gesichts- und Orbitalvenen. *Albrecht von Graefes Arch Klin Ophthalmol* 1883; **29:** 31.
9. Hayreh SS. The ophthalmic artery. III. Branches. *Br J Ophthalmol* 1962; **46:** 212.
10. Hogan MJ, Alvarado JA, Weddell JE. *Histology of the Human Eye: An Atlas and Textbook.* W.B. Saunders: Philadelphia, PA, 1971: 687.
11. Katsev DA, Drews RC, Rose BT. An anatomic study of retrobulbar needle path length. *Ophthalmology* 1989; **96:** 1221.
12. Koornneef L. Details of the orbital connective tissue system in the adult. *Acta Morphol Neerl-Scand* 1977; **15:** 1.
13. Koornneef L. The architecture of the musculo-fibrous apparatus in the human orbit. *Acta Morphol Neerl-Scand* 1977; **15:** 35.
14. Koornneef L. Eyelid and orbital fascial attachments and their clinical significance. *Eye* 1988; **2:** 130.
15. Liu C, Youl B, Moseley I. Magnetic resonance imaging of the optic nerve in extremes of gaze: Implications for the positioning of the globe for retrobulbar anaesthesia. *Br J Ophthalmol* 1992; **76:** 728–733.
16. O'Brien CS. Local anesthesia in ophthalmic surgery. *JAMA* 1928; **90:** 8.
17. Parks MM. Ocular motility and strabismus. In *Clinical Ophthalmology* (edited by Duane TD). Harper and Row: New York, 1975: 185.

18. Smiddy WE, Michels RG, Kumar AJ. Magnetic resonance imaging of retrobulbar changes in optic nerve position with eye movement. *Am J Ophthalmol* 1989; **107:** 82.
19. Stevens JD. A new local anaesthesia technique for cataract extraction by one quadrant sub-Tenon's infiltration. *Br J Ophthalmol* 1992; **76:** 670.
20. Unsöld R, Seeger W, DeGroot J. A narrow passage – anatomic considerations. In *Compressive Optic Nerve Lesions at the Optic Canal* (edited by Unsöld R, Seeger W). Springer-Verlag: Berlin, 1989: 3–14.
21. Wong DHW. Review article: Regional anaesthesia for intraocular surgery. *Can J Anaesth* 1993; **40:** 635.
22. Zonneveld FW. *Computed Tomography of the Temporal Bone and Orbit.* Urban and Schwarzenberg: Munich, 1987: 202.
23. Zide BM, Jelkes GW. *Surgical Anatomy of the Orbit.* Raven Press: New York, 1985: 75.
24. Grizzard WS. Ophthalmic anesthesia. In *Ophthalmology Annual* (edited by Reinecke RD). Raven Press: New York, 1989: 265–294.
25. McGoldrick KE. *Anesthesia for Ophthalmic and Otolaryngologic Surgery.* W.B. Saunders: Philadelphia, PA, 1992: 318.
26. Warwick R. The extraocular muscles. In *Eugene Wolff's Anatomy of the Eye and Orbit,* 7th edn. W.B. Saunders: Philadelphia, PA, 1976: 273.
27. Koornneef L. Orbital septa: Anatomy and function. *Ophthalmology* 1979; **86:** 876.
28. Smith BC. *Ophthalmic Plastic and Reconstructive Surgery,* Vol. 1. CV Mosby: St Louis, MO, 1987: 54.
29. McCord CD. *Oculoplastic Surgery.* Raven Press: New York, 1987.
30. Miller NR. *Walsh and Hoyt's Clinical Neuro-ophthalmology,* 4th edn, Vol. 1. Williams and Wilkins: Baltimore, MD, 1982.
31. Lindquist TD *et al.* Complications of Nadbath facial nerve block and a review of the literature. *Ophthalmic Surg* 1988; **19:** 271–273.
32. Zahl K. Blockade of the orbicularis oculi. *Ophthalmol Clin North Am* 1990; **3:** 93–100.
33. Krupin T, Waltman SR (eds). *Complications in Ophthalmic Surgery.* J.B. Lippincott: Philadelphia, PA, 1984.

CHAPTER 2

The physiology of the eye of interest to anaesthetists

G BARRY SMITH

Although anaesthetists have an easy familiarity with many fields of physiology, that of the special senses is often neglected. The eye has been intensively studied by ophthalmologists and a great deal is now known about its structure and function in health and disease. It is only recently that interest has been taken in its response to anaesthetic agents. This account has been deliberately simplified and only passing reference is made here to the primary object of the eye – its visual function.

THE STRUCTURE AND DIMENSIONS OF THE GLOBE

In form, the globe is formed by parts of two spheres joined together. The smaller sphere has a radius of 8 mm and forms the transparent cornea which has a diameter of about 11 mm; it is 0.5 mm thick centrally and is 1 mm thick peripherally. The curvature of the cornea is the major refracting power of the eye, producing a convergence of 45 diopters, while the lens only has a convergent power of 17 diopters. These allow an image to be formed on the light-sensitive retina in the normal eye that is 24 mm long.

The large sphere is formed by the opaque white sclera of varying thickness but mostly about 1 mm thick, except when it is thinned in myopia or scleromalacia. The volume of the globe is about 6.5 ml, a useful statistic when the surgeon replaces the contents with air, gas or silicone oil.

Both the cornea and the sclera consist of interlocking lamellae of collagen, with some elastic fibres and ground substance which are designed to withstand an internal pressure. The wavy collagen fibres may initially straighten and allow an increase in volume, but this slack is soon absorbed and a small increase in the contents then leads to a sharp increase in pressure. There are more elastic fibres than collagen round the area of the optic disc and the stretching of these by chronically raised pressure leads to the clinical observation of a 'cupped disc'.

THE CORNEA

The cornea is normally exposed to the air but is moistened by the action of blinking every 30 s. In the unconscious or anaesthetized patient, the cornea may become chronically exposed and may eventually ulcerate and even perforate or keratinize.

As a protection, the cornea lies beneath a complex tear film whose outer part is oily and sebaceous and whose deeper part is aqueous and contains dissolved proteins. Deeper still is a mucoid layer secreted by goblet cells in the conjunctiva. The tear film not only cleans and protects the cornea, it is also the pathway for dissolved oxygen and nutrients destined for the cornea and endothelium. It serves an important visual service by smoothing the surface of the cornea.

Beneath the tear film lies the epithelium, a layer six cells deep which is resistant to some chemicals and to bacteria. When the epithelium is intact it does not stain with fluorescein, but painful corneal abrasions, resulting from trauma, stain deeply. The epithelium has remarkable powers of regeneration and may be completely replaced in a week, for instance, following corneal grafting. This regeneration may be slowed in chemical burns, for example following exposure to mustard gas. The basement membrane of the epithelium is called Bowman's membrane, which is continuous with the corneal stroma. The transparent embryonic collagen fibrils forming this layer do not replicate if injured but form scar tissue or are covered by epithelial downgrowth.

Beneath the stroma is the highly specialized basement membrane of the endothelium, Descemet's membrane, which is mechanically strong and resistant to inflammation and vascularization. The endothelium is a single layer of cells lying on the internal surface of Descemet's membrane. These form the anterior border of the anterior chamber. These cells, which do not proliferate after birth, number about 2000 cells/mm^2. They are metabolically extremely active as they extract water from the ground substance of the cornea, thereby maintaining its transparency. The healthy cornea contains no blood vessels in its central part and all the oxygen and nutrients for the endothelial activity have to pass through the cornea or from the aqueous humour. The wearing of contact lenses appreciably diminishes the oxygen available for the endothelial layer.

The endothelial cells are very delicate and are easily poisoned by acid or alkalis. They are also easily dislodged by surgery. The cells spontaneously diminish in number with ageing.

The corneoscleral junction is marked by a grey line called the limbus, which is of great importance to surgeons and anaesthetists as it overlies the principal drainage area for aqueous humour, which lies in the anterior chamber at this point.

THE AQUEOUS HUMOUR

Aqueous resembles an ultra filtrate of plasma which is nearly devoid of protein. This appearance is misleading, as it is almost certainly actively secreted by the ciliary body from whence it passes forward through the pupil and then flows centrifugally to the angle of the anterior chamber where it passes through the trabecular meshwork into the canal of Schlemm. A number of ducts connect this to the episcleral veins.

In Table 2.1 it should be noted that there are higher values for bicarbonate, phosphate, lactate, urea and ascorbate in aqueous than would be found in a plasma dialysate. These values tend to vary as the aqueous flows forward owing to metabolic exchanges with the lens and endothelium and passive resorption by veins in the iris.

Table 2.1   The composition of aqueous humour

	Aqueous humour (mm)	*Plasma (mm)*
Na	143.5	151.5
K	5.25	5.5
Ca	1.7	2.6
Mg	0.78	1.0
Cl	109.5	108.0
HCO_3	33.6	27.4
Pyruvate	0.66	0.22
Ascorbate	0.96	0.02
Urea	7.0	9.1
Glucose	6.9	8.3
Protein	10–15 mg/100 ml	7 g/100 ml

From ref. 4.

THE CILIARY BODY AND AQUEOUS HUMOUR

The ciliary body lies behind the root of the iris and consists of two parts: posterior and anterior. The posterior muscular part with a smooth internal surface is called the pars plana. This muscle has three important actions, the most important of which is to relax the suspensory ligament of the lens which thus becomes more spherical and allows accommodation of the vision for near objects. As a secondary action, it exerts tension on the scleral spur, which widens the spaces in the trabecular meshwork and facilitates drainage of aqueous. A minor action of the muscle is as a dilator of the iris. The pars plana is the favoured site for the insertion of instruments into the eye through sclerotomies during vitreoretinal surgery.

The anterior part of the ciliary body is thrown into about 70 folds and is called the pars plicata, and it is from these folds that the aqueous humour is secreted. The stroma here is richly supplied with blood vessels and fenestrated capillaries extend into each fold. These capillaries are quite permeable to the plasma proteins which build up in the stroma. On the surface is a double layer of epithelium, an inner layer of pigmented cells and a superficial layer of clear vacuolated cells. These cells form a complete barrier to protein in normal circumstances but, in response to injury and possibly neuronal influences, prostaglandin E is produced which allows free passage of protein.

Aqueous humour is produced at a rate of about 2 µl/min, which is just over 1% of the volume of the anterior chamber. Although there is some diffusion of solutes posteriorly into the vitreous, the main flow of aqueous is centrally over the surface of the lens and then forward through the pupil. Finally, it passes laterally towards the angle of the anterior chamber (see Fig. 1.17, page 15).

DRAINAGE OF AQUEOUS

The principal drainage system of the eye is situated in the iridocorneal angle of the anterior chamber. Here the aqueous passes through the spaces of the trabecular meshwork, which abuts onto the canal of Schlemm from which aqueous veins run back to join episcleral veins, and the aqueous flows alongside venous blood until it mixes with it. There are subsidiary drainage routes for about a third of the aqueous which passes directly into the iris veins and the suprachoroidal space.

Control of intraocular pressure has been extensively studied in health and disease. In health, it remains fairly constant at about 15 mmHg throughout life. It fluctuates slightly according to posture and time of day.[6] There is some response to changes in blood pressure but these are slow. There are rapid rises on coughing, straining and other types of Valsalva manoeuvre. In response to trauma and inflammation, there is a rapid rise in intraocular pressure resulting from the increased permeability of the pars plicata epithelium.

The balance between secretion and drainage is complex and in the healthy state finely adjusted. This balance can be disturbed by mechanical, hormonal, nervous and therapeutic effects. Mechanical blockage of the drainage angle by iris root is a cause of acute glaucoma. This may result from a blockage of the pupil, causing the iris to be distended forwards in the form of iris bombé. A high dosage of glucocorticoids raises the pressure, whereas progesterone may cause a slight fall. There are obvious nervous influences controlling the pressure and parasympathetic nerves are conspicuous in the trabecular meshwork. There is no surprise that parasympathomimetic agents such as pilocarpine and eserine lower the pressure, perhaps by a direct mechanical action on the iris root and possibly by a more subtle effect on the meshwork itself. What is more surprising is that sympathomimetic agents such as adrenaline (epinephrine), beta-adrenergic agents such as timoptol and adrenergic neurone blockers such as guanethidine also have a pressure-lowering effect. The postulated pharmacological actions of these drugs have not been completely elucidated. It is significant that only one group of drugs seems to block secretion by the ciliary body effectively. Acetazolamide, a carbonic anhydrase inhibitor, and related drugs are very effective when given systemically, but not topically, in reducing the secretion of aqueous. It is not clear whether normal secretion depends on carbonic anhydrase and whether this is another physiological mechanism controlling secretion.

THE MUSCLES OF THE EYE: ANATOMY

The true extraocular muscles consist of the four rectus muscles and the two obliques. Their function is to rotate the globe of the eye in three planes so as to align the visual axes of the two eyes in all directions of gaze. Focused images simultaneously formed at each fovea are perceived as one in a process known as fusion, of fundamental importance for binocular single vision and stereopsis. This is more thoroughly dealt with in Chapter 11 on strabismus.

The medial, superior and inferior rectus muscles are supplied by the oculomotor nerve (III), the lateral rectus is innervated by the abducens nerve (VI) and the superior oblique receives its nerve supply by the trochlear nerve (IV). All these nerves arise from nuclei in the mid-brain at the level of the corpora quadrigema and leave it ventrally between the posterior cerebral artery and the superior cerebellar artery. The exception is the abducens nerve, which arises from the nucleus of the contralateral side and then leaves the mid-brain dorsally through the superior medullary velum and runs forward to enter the inferior petrosal sinus and through this enters the cavernous sinus. The oculomotor and abducens nerves invaginate the superior surface of the cavernous sinus. All three nerves enter the orbit through the superior orbital fissure.

There are a number of other muscles which influence the eye and orbit. The levator of the upper lid is probably a true ocular muscle which arises from the tendinous ring at the superior orbital fissure and is innervated by a branch from the oculomotor nerve. Its function is to raise the upper lid through several attachments to the tarsal plate, superior fornix and skin of the eyelid.

The muscles of facial expression close the eyelids by the orbicularis oculi, elevate the eyebrows and exert traction on the lacrimal sac. Closure of the eyes by the palpebral part of the muscle does not alter the orbital pressure, whereas forcibly screwing up the eyes causes a sharp rise in orbital pressure and may cause a long surgical section with inadequate suturing to break down. The orbicularis is innervated from the upper division of the facial nerve (VII) which runs deep to the muscle.

The orbit contains a diffuse meshwork of smooth muscle innervated by the sympathetic nerve system. There is a condensation of this muscle beneath the levator, which is inserted into the upper margin of the tarsal plate. This is Müller's muscle, which is innervated from the superior cervical ganglion. Paralysis of this muscle accounts for the slight ptosis seen in Horner's Syndrome, while its overaction is seen in thyroid eye disease or when sympathomimetic drugs such as phenylephrine are instilled into the conjunctival sac.

THE PHYSIOLOGY OF THE EXTRAOCULAR MUSCLES

At rest or in the deeply anaesthetized patient, the eyes are fixed and central. In sleep or during light anaesthesia without muscle relaxation, the eye tends to rotate upwards under the upper lid. This is Bell's phenomenon and is a normal protective action which varies somewhat from person to person. This movement is inconvenient for the ophthalmologist, as he or she usually wishes to operate on the upper part of the eye. It is blocked by local anaesthesia, although the superior rectus muscle is the last muscle to achieve akinesia.

Under general anaesthesia, the surgeon can control the eye by placing a traction stitch beneath the tendon of the superior rectus or the anaesthetist can induce neuromuscular blockade or deepen the plane of anaesthesia. Strong traction on the superior rectus may put that muscle into spasm or may provoke an oculocardiac reflex.

Eye movements are controlled by a complex neuronal pathway with coordinating centres in the occipital cortex and the superior colliculi. The neurones in these centres fire at 100 impulses per second but this can rise to over 300. Each axon of the nerve supplies a motor unit of only six muscle fibres (compared with over 100 in a typical skeletal muscle).

In 1963, Hess and Pilar[5] described two types of muscle fibres in the extraocular muscles of the cat – twitch fibres and tonic fibres. This finding has since been confirmed in man by Katz and Eakins.[7] The fast, white, twitch fibres have a pattern of regularly arranged fibrils which on electron microscopy form complex, regular longitudinal and transverse arrangements called triads, which are presumed to permit the rapid transmission of impulses throughout the fibre. Such a fibre can respond to 350 impulses per second for short periods without tetany, but shows rapid fatigue to 30% of the original tension. The axons supplying impulses to these fibres are large and have a high rate of conduction. Their terminations are described as 'en plaque' or 'sole plate' single nerve endings.

The slow, red, tonic fibres produce a sustained contraction when stimulated at rates above 20 impulses per second. They have irregularly arranged fibrils in clumps and owe their red colour to the presence of myoglobin inside the fibre. They have plentiful mitochondria. The nerve endings on this type of fibre are multiple, distributed along its length and described as 'en grappe'. They are supplied by thinner nerve fibres.

Like skeletal muscle, the extraocular muscles contain muscle spindles and about 50 have been identified near the tendon in a single, superior rectus muscle. Nerve impulses passing along the gamma efferent nerves cause contraction and increase sensitivity to stretch. Stretching stimuli are registered by 'annulospiral' or 'flowerspray' endings, and impulses are conveyed by large Group 1 fibres to the trigeminal ganglion and on up the proximal axon to the reticular formation and the cervical spinal cord.

THE OCULOCARDIAC REFLEX

In 1908, Aschner[1] observed that application of pressure to the eyeball caused a reduction in the pulse rate.

Mechanism

Afferent impulses arise from stretch and pressure receptors throughout the globe and orbit, passing through the long and short ciliary nerves and along the ophthalmic division of the trigeminal nerve, and synapsing in the main sensory nucleus of the trigeminal nerve near the fourth ventricle. Efferent impulses pass down the vagus.

Recently, attention has been drawn to the effects of stimuli on the depth and rate of respiration. These have been named 'oculo respiratory' reflexes.[2] They probably have the same mechanisms as the cardiac reflex and may result from radiation of impulses in the brainstem. There have been no reports of serious clinical effects. As might be expected, anticholinergics do not block this response and their main significance could be to lead the anaesthetist to assume that the spontaneously breathing patient was too lightly anaesthetized. The management of these reflexes has not been determined.[3]

It is sometimes forgotten that rises in intraocular pressure (IOP) are a potent stimulus and that the symptoms of acute glaucoma are themselves initiated by pressure and demonstrated through visceral vagal effects. Inflammatory responses in the eye lead to a rise in pressure. Surgery may be the cause of this inflammation and smaller surgical sections and more accurate suturing may increase the risks of postoperative rises in pressure, which may be partly or completely controlled by anti-inflammatory drugs such as steroids or prostaglandin inhibitors, while aqueous secretion is inhibited by acetazolamide. Vitreous replacement by air, gas or silicone oil and scleral buckling procedures may also cause a rise in IOP that persists. Vagal effects may occur not only during surgery but also during the postoperative period. Even in the absence of the globe, pressure in the orbit from haematoma may initiate a response resembling myocardial infarction and this may occur following enucleation.

It is interesting to contrast the depressant effects of these reflexes with the stimulatory reflexes which follow laryngoscopy and intubation, which are nearly always associated with tachycardia and a pressor response and are blocked by analgesics and beta-blockade.

Extraocular muscles

Traction on the extraocular muscles almost invariably causes some slowing of the pulse rate. This is most likely to arise during the insertion of a superior rectus suture to fixate and rotate the globe before cataract or glaucoma surgery. During vitreoretinal surgery, the movements of the eye are controlled by 'bridle' sutures underrunning the rectus muscles and the eye may be forcibly rotated to obtain access to the posterior sclera.

It is during strabismus surgery that the most pronounced reflexes occur. These occur in most patients who have not received an anticholinergic drug. Traction on the medial rectus produces more marked effects than traction on other muscles. The reflex seems to be most active in children.[8]

Results of the oculocardiac reflex

The primary result is a sinus bradycardia which is sometimes so severe that periods of asystole lasting up to 30 s occur. It is rare for the asystole to persist. Total cardiac arrest is prevented by escape rhythms such as idioventricular beats. Deaths from oculocardiac reflex in young patients are so uncommon that other causes such as anoxia should be sought. Prolonged bradycardia may depress cardiac output to such an extent that severe hypotension may be recorded, and in a few elderly patients cardiac failure and pulmonary oedema may occur.

Although bradycardia is the most common cardiac irregularity, other disturbances of rhythm may occur and may be alarming. These include atrio ventricular block, bigeminy and junctional rhythm. The visceral effects of the reflex are uncomfortable for the patient and include nausea, vomiting, abdominal pain, vasoconstriction, sweating and salivation.

Management

Routine prophylaxis with anticholinergic drugs such as atropine, hyoscine or glycopyrollate reduces the incidence and the severity of the reflex. Unfortunately, used as premedication, these drugs cause some discomfort from drying of the mouth and it may be preferable to give them at the time of induction. A wide variety of drugs have some anticholinergic side-effects, particularly the antihistamines and the tricyclic antidepressants. Cataract patients may derive some protection from dilating drops such as cyclopentolate, which are absorbed mainly through the nasal mucosa. Gallamine triethiodide is a muscle relaxant with strong anticholinergic effects. It should only be used with tracheal intubation and mechanical ventilation of the lungs.

Retrobulbar and peribulbar block with local anaesthetic agents totally prevent the reflex, and other mechanisms must be sought to explain bradycardias in patients having local anaesthesia.

TREATMENT

Monitoring of the heart rate, ECG and blood pressure are mandatory during all eye surgery. This should be both visible and audible so that both surgeon and anaesthetist can detect changes in heart rate.

If the heart rate falls more than 20%, the surgeon should release traction immediately, and if he does not do so the anaesthetist should instruct him to stop. This should restore the cardiac output and buy time for the anaesthetist to administer an anticholinergic. It is good practice during eye surgery to have an anticholinergic available for instant injection.

The doses of anticholinergics usually recommended produce only partial vagal block but are usually sufficient to control the reflex.

REFERENCES

1. Aschner B. Uber einer Bisher noch nicht beschriebenen Refex von Auge auf Drieslauf und Atmung: Verschinden des Radialispulses bei Druk auf das Auge. *Weinen Klinisches Wochenschrift* 1908; **21:** 1529.
2. Blanc VF, Jacob JL, Milot J, Cryenne L. The oculo respiratory reflex revisited. *Can J Anaesth* 1988; **35:** 468.
3. Cunningham AJ, Barry P. Intraocular pressure physiology and implications for anaesthetic management. *Can Anaesth Soc J* 1986; **33:** 195.
4. Davson H. *The Physiology of the Eye*, 4th edn. Churchill Livingstone: Edinburgh, 1980.
5. Hess A, Pilar G. Slow fibres in the extraocular muscles of the cat. *J Physiol* 1963; **169:** 780.
6. Hvidberg A, Kessing SVV, Fernandez A. Effect of changes in pCO_2 and body positions on intraocular pressure during general anaesthesia. *Acta Ophthalmol* 1981; **59:** 465.
7. Katz RL, Eakins. *Proc Roy Soc Med* 1969; **62:** 1217.
8. Smith RB, Douglas H, Petruscak J. The oculocardiac reflex and sinoatrial arrest. *Can Anaesth Soc J* 1972; **19:** 138.

CHAPTER 3

The action of drugs on the eye

G BARRY SMITH

TOPICAL

Many substances are capable of penetrating the cornea and this is a common method of administering local anaesthetics, antibiotics, steroids, catecholamines, alkaloids and beta-blockers. Many of the results of subconjunctival injections are obtained by leakage back along the injection track to the conjunctival sac and subsequent absorption through the cornea. Noxious substances such as acids, alkalis and ammonia also pass freely but cause destruction of the endothelium with oedema, scarring and vascularization. Ophthalmic solutions for instillation into the conjunctival sac should be sterile and buffered to a physiological pH. Many solutions contain a preservative such as benzalkonium chloride or phenylmercuric nitrate. Local allergy to the drug or to the preservative is a major problem with repeated administration of drugs by this route. Excess medication tends to drain into the nose where it is rapidly absorbed to produce systemic and unwanted side-effects.[1, 5, 10, 11, 13, 18]

MYDRIATICS

Before vitreo retinal or cataract surgery, the pupil needs to be well dilated to provide a good view, provide access for instruments, aid the removal of the old lens and the introduction of the implant. Patients are usually prepared with an anticholinergic drug supported by a sympathomimetic drug. In patients with very dark brown irides, dilation may be poor and the eye may need to be irrigated internally with adrenaline 1:500 000.

Phenylephrine

Phenylephrine 10% dilates the pupil more rapidly than any other drug. It may be used with homatropine or cyclopentolate. Locally it causes contraction of Müller's muscle so that the upper lid is elevated. It is absorbed systemically and may produce a rise in blood pressure and ventricular ectopics.[3, 8, 10, 19] It should not be given to patients who are having antidepressant treatment with monoamine oxidase inhibitors. Weak solutions (2.5–5%) should be used in children, hypertensives and patients with cardiac disease. There is no effect on the power of accommodation.

Atropine

Atropine 0.25–2% as a solution or atropine 0.5–1% as an ointment is a slow-acting mydriatic of long duration. A large pupil may persist for weeks after the end of treatment. It enables the ophthalmologist to relax and rest the pupil in painful conditions such as uveitis. It relaxes the ciliary body and paralyses the power of accommodation. For this reason, ointment is often given daily to babies prior to refraction by retinoscopy (in which a beam of light is passed through a lens and focused on the retina). There is some risk that with repeated doses the child will develop the signs of atropine poisoning with tachycardia, pyrexia, restlessness, thirst and a scarlet erythematous rash peripherally on the face with a hot, dry skin.[9] It is important to stop the atropine, as convulsions and a dangerous pyrexia may occur. General anaesthesia may proceed with temperature monitoring and cooling if necessary.

Hyoscine

Hyoscine 0.25% may be used as an alternative to atropine, particularly when there is an allergic reaction to the latter. It has the advantage of producing a more rapid cycloplegic effect but may have central effects on the elderly, causing confusion.[7]

Other mydriatics

Homatropine 1–5%, cyclopentolate 0.5–1% and tropicamide 0.5–1% are all used as cycloplegics for refraction and as mydriatics prior to cataract extraction. They have the advantage of being rapid in onset and recovery occurs in a few hours.

Homatropine has a longer effect than the others. All mydriatics may precipitate an attack of acute closed angle glaucoma in patients who have shallow anterior chambers.

MIOTICS

The pupil is reduced in size by the constriction of the sphincter of the iris, which is controlled by cholinergic fibres from the parasympathetic system whose cell bodies lie in the ciliary ganglion. Miotics belong to the group of drugs which are either cholinergic agonists or which block the actions of enzymes which break down endogenously produced acetylcholine. Pilocarpine 1–4% falls into the former category and carbachol 3% into the latter. They throw the ciliary muscle into spasm, which may be painful; by so doing, they open the drainage angle and the trabecular meshwork and are used in the treatment of glaucoma.

Patients endure these drops which block visual accommodation; this is a major handicap, particularly in myopia and young people. The small pupil that is created makes night vision poor. Miosis is useful when a posterior chamber lens has been placed behind the iris, before refractive keratoplasty to protect the lens and to shield the retina from the microscope light, in glaucoma and to counteract the effects of mydriatic drugs. Following cataract extraction or after lens implantation, the surgeon may inject acetylcholine directly into the anterior chamber during surgery. This constricts the pupil and supports the lens implant. This has no systemic effect and only persists for a few minutes.

Pilocarpine

This historic drug is still a major treatment for glaucoma. It acts rapidly and puts the iris into rather painful spasm. It may cause bradycardia and hypotension.[12]

Eserine (physostigmine)

A similar drug to pilocarpine, but not often used.

Neostigmine

This is a cholinesterase inhibitor and allows endogenous acetylcholine to accumulate. It may be used in a concentration of 2.5–5%.[17]

Ecothiopate (phospholine iodide)

This drug is very powerful. It belongs to the same organophosphorus group as the nerve gases. It depletes serum anticholinesterase to very low levels, which may persist for as long as 3 weeks post-treatment. Its side-effects include salivation, diarrhoea and vomiting. It may reduce the effect of non-depolarizing (curare-like) muscle relaxants and prolong the paralysing effect of suxamethonium. Treatment with this drug and similar drugs has been discontinued for general use in the UK and in some other countries.

NON-MIOTIC DRUGS USED IN GLAUCOMA

Adrenergic drugs

Ophthalmic surgeons sometimes enhance the effect of pilocarpine with sympathomimetic drugs. These are predominantly adrenaline (epinephrine) up to 1% and propine (dipivefrine) 0.1%. The effect of these drops is to moderately dilate the pupil, to vasoconstrict the vessels in the ciliary body which are producing aqueous humour and to improve drainage. They have a place in patients who have cataracts associated with glaucoma. The massive dose of adrenaline administered seldom produces systemic effects and the only side-effect is the congested appearance of the conjunctiva.

Beta-blockers

Timolol, betaxolol and levobunolol (Betagan) are increasingly being used in the treatment of chronic glaucoma. They are expensive but do not alter pupil size. The beta-2 effect of timolol and betaxolol frequently exacerbates bronchial asthma.[4, 16] The beta-1 effect of betagan makes this less of a problem. All these drugs tend to cause bradycardia and may increase cardiac failure.[14, 15] Some of the previously used drugs in this group unexpectedly stopped lacrimal secretions permanently and gave patients dry eyes.

OTHER LOCALLY ADMINISTERED DRUGS

Fluorescein

This dye is not much taken up by intact cornea or conjunctival epithelium and is used in the diagnosis of corneal abrasions and ulcers as it fluoresces in ultraviolet light. There is enough staining of normal epithelium for corneal flattening to be identified during applanation tonometry. The solution must not be stored, as it is a culture medium for *Pseudomonas* species. It is conveniently supplied absorbed on to dry filter papers, which can be dipped into the tear film to stain the cornea.

Anti-inflammatory drops

Surgeons use a number of glucosteroid drops to reduce ocular inflammation, particularly after surgery in which implants have been used or after keratoplasty. Ocular inflammation may also require antibacterials, antivirals and drugs to lower the pressure in the eye. There is some risk that steroids may mask severe infections, make perforations of the cornea more likely, delay healing and, if used over a very long period, induce cataract or open angle glaucoma. Prescription of steroids should be for a specific reason and for as short a period as possible.

Non-steroidal anti-inflammatory drugs

Recent work has emphasized the value of other anti-inflammatory drugs such as indomethacin, which is a potent inhibitor of prostaglandin E. Despite their action on platelet stickiness mediated by blocking the cyclo-oxygenase pathway, it is unusual to encounter gross bleeding in or around the eye. Because of this, many surgeons use indomethacin locally, rectally or orally to reduce the inflammatory response. It is believed to assist in maintaining the membrane of the ciliary body by blocking the action of prostaglandin E. It is not at present clear whether these drugs interfere with wound healing.

ORAL MEDICATION WITH SPECIFIC EFFECTS ON THE EYE

Acetazolamide

This carbonic anhydrase inhibitor may be administered by mouth or intravenously in doses up to 1000 mg/day. It is an irritant to the gut and may upset some patients or cause paraesthesia in others.

Although acetazolamide was originally introduced as a diuretic, it is principally given to reduce the secretion of aqueous humour by the ciliary body and is highly effective. It is useful in the preparation of patients for glaucoma surgery and has been used for retinal detachment surgery in which a scleral indent was required by a surgeon who did not wish to drain subretinal fluid.

As it is related to the sulphonamides, it may produce depression of the bone marrow, rashes, urinary colic and crystalluria.

Opiates

Both diamorphine and morphine produce meiosis by stimulating the pretectal nucleus in the mid-brain. A similar action occurs with methadone in high dosage. Pethidine, fentanyl and alfentanyl seem to have little activity in this respect.

Steroids

Steroids have been used for many years in the treatment of inflammations of the eye when no infecting agent is present. They have a part to play in the management of the granuloma called pseudotumour of the orbit and may have some effect in reducing the signs of thyroid eye disease.

Local steroids have little effect on adrenal function, but parenteral steroids over a period lead to a reduced secretion of corticosteroids in response to the stress of surgery. In the high doses which are sometimes used, the complications of glycosuria, hypertension, cataract, peptic ulcer, osteoporosis and silent reactivation of old tuberculous lesions may occur.

Dehydrating agents

Acute glaucoma is treated by intensive local miotics, acetazolamide and dehydrating agents. This regime is so effective that temporary relief of pain is achieved in most patients and acute glaucoma only very rarely needs urgent surgery. Some types of chronic glaucoma, particularly those described as rubeotic in which the iris becomes highly vascularized, have a consistent high pressure which does not respond to medical treatment. Surgery may cause a sudden fall in intraocular pressure, which may precipitate an expulsive suprachoroidal haemorrhage. Such patients are prepared as far as possible with osmotic agents.

Glycerol 50%

This is given by mouth. Because it draws water into the stomach, it should not be given prior to general anaesthesia, particularly if opiates have slowed gastric emptying. If it has been used during the previous 8 h, then consideration should be given to passing a nasogastric tube to empty the stomach, administering metoclopramide and performing a 'crash induction' with preoxygenation and cricoid pressure.

This very potent agent causes severe generalized dehydration and electrolyte imbalance, particularly in the elderly who may require energetic parenteral rehydration with Ringer-lactate or Hartmann's solution at the end of surgery.

Mannitol 20%

Given as an intravenous infusion in a dose of 1 g/kg body weight, this inert sugar draws intracellular water into the extracellular compartment and then causes a brisk diuresis. Its main effect is on highly vascular tissues such as the brain; it has a lesser effect on the eye, which is partially set off by a degree of congestion of the choroid, although the overall effect is to reduce intraocular pressure. The increase in blood volume promotes operative bleeding. It is used to prepare glaucoma patients for surgery and is given rapidly 30 min prior to operation. Some patients may need to be catheterized to avoid acute retention.

SIDE-EFFECTS FROM THE TOPICAL APPLICATION OF DRUGS

Any drug given into the conjunctival sac tends to be poorly absorbed unless it passes into the nose. Ophthalmologists use high concentrations of drugs to achieve effects on the eye and anaesthetists note the results of significant doses absorbed rapidly through the nasal mucosa. There are many reports of single complications to individual drugs in patients and while rare cases cannot be ignored, it is important to consider the general principles and common complications which are seen in many patients.[1, 3]

Atropine, cyclopentolate and hyoscine (scopolamine) are all very long-acting cumulative drugs which have effects on all the systems of the body and there are considerable differences in patient responsiveness. Young adults and children respond with tachycardia and hypertension; older patients may develop urinary retention. The most serious effects are those of mental confusion and sedation in elderly patients, a factor which is often ignored when investigating the results of cataract extraction. The drying of secretions seems to be benign with early ambulation; postoperative respiratory complications are rare in this group of patients. I am not aware of any work on gastric emptying or the risks of reflux after the use of these drugs.

Adrenalin, phenylephrine, dipivefrine and cocaine cause tachycardia, hypertension and ventricular arrhythmias in patients with ischaemic heart disease, pre-existing hypertension, hyperthyroidism or whose hearts have been sensitized to catecholamines by volatile agents such as halothane.[5, 6]

Beta-blockers such as timolol and Betagan have significant bronchoconstrictor effects and unreliable results may be obtained from finger pulse oximetry because of reduced cardiac output and peripheral vasoconstriction. However, the effects on the heart overshadow those on the lungs owing to the bradycardia, hypotension and occasional cardiac failure which occur. Significant conduction defects such as bundle branch block may show on the ECG with ST depression.

It is rare for the minute doses of very dilute drugs such as adrenaline and acetylcholine, which may be infused inside the eye, to have any effects other than local by dilating or constricting the pupil. Adverse effects have been reported, but these may have been wrongly attributed and caused by other factors.[2]

REFERENCES

1. Awan KJ. Systemic toxicity of cyclopentolate hydrochloride in adults following topical ocular instillation. *Ann Ophthalmol* 1976; **8:** 803.
2. Brinkley JR Jr, Hendrick A. Vascular hypotension and bradycardia following intraocular injection of acetylcholine during cataract surgery. *Am J Ophthalmol* 1984; **97:** 40.
3. Brown MM, Brown GC, Spaeth GL. Lack of side effects from topically administered 10 per cent phenylephrine eye drops. *Arch Ophthalmol* 1980; **98:** 487.
4. Charan NB, Lakshminarayan S. Pulmonary effects of topical timolol. *Arch Intern Med* 1980; **140:** 843.
5. Chung B, Naraghi M, Adriani J. Sympathomimetic effects of cocaine and their influence on halothane and enflurane anesthesia. *Anesthesiol Rev* 1978; **50:** 16.
6. El–Din Asmak, Mostafa SM. Severe hypertension during anaesthesia for dacryocystorhinostomy. *Anaesthesia* 1985; **40:** 787.
7. Freund M, Merin S. Toxic effects of scopolamine eye drops. *Am J Ophthalmol* 1970; **70:** 637.
8. Fraunfelder FT, Scafidi AF. Possible adverse effects from topical ocular 10 per cent phenylephrine. *Am J Ophthalmol* 1978; **85:** 447.
9. Hoefnagel D. Toxic effects of atropine and homatropine eye drops in children. *New Engl J Med* 1961; **264:** 168.
10. Janssen ML, Cook FR. A case of ventricular fibrillation during halothane anaesthesia caused by eye drops. *Acta Anaesthesiol Belg* 1979; **4:** 225.
11. McGoldrick KE. Ocular drugs and anesthesia. *Int Anesthesiol Clin* 1990; **28:** 72.
12. Mishra P. Pilocarpine and timolol eye drops: Bradycardia and hypotension. *Br J Anaesth* 1983; **55:** 897.
13. Polak BCP. Drugs used in ocular treatment. *Side Effects of Drugs* 1980; **4:** 449.
14. Ros FE, Dake CL. Cardiovascular effects of timolol eye drops. *Documenta Ophthalmol* 1980; **48:** 283.
15. Samuels SI, Maze M. Beta receptor blockade following the use of eye drops. *Anesthesiology* 1980; **52:** 369.
16. Schoene RB, Martin TR, Charan NB *et al*. Timolol induced bronchospasm in asthmatic bronchitis. *JAMA* 1980; **245:** 1460.
17. Schwartz H, Apt H. Mydriatic effects of anticholinergic drugs used during reversal of non-depolarizing muscle relaxants. *Am J Ophthalmol* 1979; **88:** 609.
18. Selvin BL. Systemic effects of topical ophthalmic medications. *Southern Med J (Rev)* 1983; **76:** 349.
19. Solosko D, Smith RB. Hypertension following 10 per cent phenylephrine ophthalmic. *Anesthesiology* 1972; **36:** 187.

CHAPTER 4

Diabetes and medical conditions commonly found in eye patients

G BARRY SMITH

Patients presenting for ophthalmic surgery with either cataracts or retinal disease frequently have a history of diabetes or are diagnosed at the time of the surgery. The diabetic physician is concerned with the initial diagnosis and long-term management of the patient with this disease; however during the preoperative period, the anaesthetist must understand the many facets of this fascinating disease and its interaction with anaesthesia.[4, 10]

Diabetes mellitus is caused by an absence of, or a diminished secretion of, the polypeptide hormone insulin by the beta cells of the islets of Langerhans in the pancreas. This shortage of insulin may be associated with a tissue resistance to its actions. Insulin regulates the level of glucose in the blood by promoting its storage as glycogen in the liver and muscles and inhibiting secondary pathways for the production of energy by the metabolism of fat and other substrates. Insulin does not work in isolation but in conjunction with corticosteroids, growth hormone, thyroid hormone, glucagon and the sex hormones.

It is convenient to divide diabetic patients into three types with different characteristics and management:

1. Insulin dependent diabetes mellitus (IDDM) or Type 1.
2. Non-insulin dependent diabetes mellitus (NIDDM) or Type 2.
3. Diabetes secondary to other endocrines or drugs.

INSULIN DEPENDENT DIABETES MELLITUS

There is almost a total absence of insulin in this condition, but antibodies to the beta cells are found in the weeks following onset. The anaesthetist seldom sees the early stages, which are characteristically sudden in children, adolescents and young adults. There are inherited factors such as certain subgroup antigens of the HLA series which make the individual more susceptible, but the precipitating incident often follows a virus infection. It seems to be most common in Scandinavia and is rare among the Chinese. In Britain and North America, about 25% of diabetics belong to this group.[5]

A severe catabolic disorder develops with the classical symptoms of thirst, polyuria, weight loss proceeding to ketoacidosis, nausea and vomiting, dehydration and coma. Diagnosis is confirmed by blood sugar estimation and treatment is by energetic resuscitation with intravenous insulin, normal saline and potassium. This resuscitation must be closely monitored by attention to the vital signs, blood sugar, pH, osmolality and serum potassium. Management of the airways, decompression of the dilated stomach and a search for (and treatment of) any infection are the main principles and the details can be found in texts of internal medicine.

The anaesthetist is normally presented with a patient who has been more or less stabilized on insulin and whose life has been regulated to provide regular meals and adequate exercise. The insulin is usually given two or three times a day by subcutaneous injection. A base level is provided by a long-acting insoluble insulin of the lente or protamine (NPH) types, with additional doses of short-acting soluble or regular insulin to coincide with the peaks of blood sugar occurring at meals. Various insulin pens and indwelling devices help to provide this short-acting insulin in a convenient and acceptable way.

Adequacy of control over the previous month can be estimated from the measurement of glycosylated haemoglobin (HbAlC) in a small sample of blood. During a period of hyperglycaemia, glucose combines irreversibly with a number of proteins and HbAlC is a good measure of previous periods of hyperglycaemia. Many young diabetics resent their disease and the limitations it imposes on their lifestyle, and this group provide a number of 'brittle' diabetics whose disease is very unstable.

The reduction of physical activity in hospital, associated with the stress or excitement of preoperative tests, and a hospital diet which may contain more carbohydrate and less fibre, usually induces a sharp rise in blood sugar and this should be counterbalanced by an upward adjustment in insulin dosage.

Local anaesthesia should always be considered for a diabetic patient, as it allows the patient to follow his or her normal insulin and dietary regime and produces minimal disturbance. Heavy sedation should not be used with a full stomach.

General anaesthesia may be required to assist surgery or to make the procedure acceptable to the patient. The operation may be minimal (such as prophylactic laser therapy), but the anaesthetist must take every precaution to ensure a successful outcome. The preoperative assessment must demonstrate any abnormalities in the electrocardiogram and any tendency to renal failure. The stomach must be empty at the time of induction. Insulin and glucose must be administered intravenously as the subcutaneous route is slow and uncertain.[2] Potassium supplements may be required but only after confirming that potassium levels are low.

Alberti and co-workers provide 10 units of insulin, 1000 ml glucose 10% and potassium 10 mEq mixed in an infusion bag and administered over a period of ~ 4 h, adjusting the rate with hourly monitoring.[1] This rather pragmatic approach is not suitable for all ophthalmic patients, particularly those with a degree of renal failure and, at Moorfields, the formula is modified to provide 2–3 units of insulin per hour with 5% glucose. Potassium is added if there is evidence of low levels or there is evidence of dehydration.

This intravenous infusion of glucose and insulin is continued into the postoperative period and the patient can return to his or her normal regime. Frequent monitoring of blood glucose is used and the aim is to provide a blood level similar to the preoperative level, probably aiming at a level between 6 and 10 mM to avoid the risks of cerebral damage associated with hypoglycaemia.

The diabetic patient should have priority on the operating list to assist with the timing of preoperative food and insulin. Preferably, the patient should be first on the list, as this avoids the possibility that the anaesthetist may be called from the operating theatre to set up an infusion because the patient has unexpectedly become hypoglycaemic.

The blood sugar should be estimated soon after admission to hospital and shortly before going to the operating theatre, for example when the premedication is administered. The preoperative insulin dose is omitted and an infusion of glucose 5% containing a short-acting insulin is set up. This is run at a rate so that the patient receives 2–3 units of insulin per hour. The anaesthetist should monitor the blood glucose at induction and not less than hourly into the recovery period.

Complications of IDDM usually occur after 20 years or more. They take the form of cataracts, microvascular disease of the retina and kidney, neurological disease such as polyneuritis and autonomic dysfunction and atheromatous arterial disease. It is controversial whether very accurate control of blood sugar delays the onset of complications. There is much evidence to suggest that avoidance of tobacco and close control of the blood pressure reduces vascular complications.

Cataracts in diabetes seem to be related to the accumulation of sorbitol in the lens during periods of intense hyperglycaemia. The sorbitol is formed when the normal glycolytic pathway to glucose-6-phosphate is blocked by a shortage of insulin, and glucose is metabolized to sorbitol and fructose by aldose reductase.

NON-INSULIN DEPENDENT DIABETES MELLITUS

More than two-thirds of diabetic patients needing eye surgery suffer from NIDDM. In this disease, there is a relative inadequacy of production of insulin and an associated resistance to its action on the tissues. The raised blood sugar causes an osmotic polyuria which is occasionally sufficiently severe for it to lead to such a loss of water and electrolytes that hyperosmolar coma occurs. This is rare and all degrees of hyperglycaemia can occur, but ketoacidosis does not occur.

This disease is genetically determined but it is only revealed later in life when there is a rising incidence with increasing age. There is little or no weight loss and there is an association with obesity. The onset may be hastened by environmental factors such as diet, but such factors have not yet been clearly elucidated. The disease appears insidiously and may have been present for years prior to diagnosis and frequently presents with such complications as cataract, microvascular disease of the retina or hypertension. The glycosuria or hyperglycaemia may be picked up on routine preoperative screening, which may present the anaesthetist with a dilemma, particularly when a procedure is planned under general anaesthesia. Generally, when hyperglycaemia is mild and there is no ketosis or dehydration and the electrolytes are within normal limits, it is safe to proceed.

Non-insulin dependent diabetes mellitus is associated with disturbed lipid metabolism and many patients have arterial atheroma, cardiac ischaemia and renal-induced hypertension. Dysautonomia also occurs as part of the diabetic polyneuritis and may cause a resting tachycardia and an unstable blood pressure during anaesthesia.

General anaesthesia presents a hazard to these patients and should only be undertaken after full preoperative assessment and with adequate monitoring. Severe cases of NIDDM are, in fact, treated with insulin and, because of tissue resistance to its action, may require higher doses than in IDDM. The anaesthetic management is to administer an infusion of glucose and insulin as with the other types of diabetes, unless the operation is done under local anaesthesia.

Patients with milder forms of NIDDM are treated with a diet that is low in sugar but high in starch and fibre. A reduction in body weight towards the ideal helps to reduce the blood sugar, but not all patients are able to achieve this. Physical exercise aids in the reduction of blood sugar by improving utilization.

DIABETES SECONDARY TO OTHER ENDOCRINES OR DRUGS

Oral treatment with sulphonyl ureas is the mainstay for many diabetic patients. These drugs stimulate the production of insulin from the beta cells of the pancreas and over a period of time seem to improve the responsiveness of the tissues to endogenous insulin. Sulphonyl ureas can produce severe hypoglycaemia in the fasted patient. Chlorpropamide (Diabinese) has a particularly long half-life of 36 h and should be stopped for at least 24 h before induction of general anaesthesia. Careful monitoring of the blood sugar with stick tests and reflectance meters is a guide to management, although these tests are only 80% accurate in 10–20% of estimations. When the blood sugar approaches 150 mgm/100ml it is a safe precaution to start an infusion of glucose 5%.

In the UK, but not in North America, the biguanide metformin (Glucophage), may be added as a single agent or in addition to insulin or a sulphonyl urea. This drug is useful in obese diabetics, as it delays the absorption of glucose from the gut, decreases gluconeogenesis by the liver and increases peripheral utilization. It does not cause hypoglycaemia when used alone. Unfortunately, it is a dangerous drug in the presence of cardiac, pulmonary or renal failure and in shock or hypoxaemia. Fatal lactic acidosis is rare in these circumstances but has been reported.

In summary, NIDDM should be managed by the withdrawal of routine therapy before preoperative fasting commences. Frequent estimation of the blood sugar and the use of intravenous glucose and insulin infusions may be required until recovery is completed. Many patients do not need any infusion, as fasting controls the blood sugar adequately.

OTHER CONDITIONS TO MONITOR CLOSELY

Cardiac disease

Anaesthetists must frequently be their own judge of a patient's fitness for anaesthesia. Cardiology departments are not always co-located with eye hospitals, nor are cardiologists very familiar with the effects of anaesthesia.[3,13,14]

The criteria an anaesthetist should use to judge the effectiveness of the heart as a pump include cardiac output, conduction defects and resistance to outflow which is measured as blood pressure.[15] A well perfused patient with warm extremities, an easily palpable radial pulse and a reasonable exercise tolerance presents no problems.

Cardiac ischaemia

Many elderly patients have Q waves or inverted T waves on their ECG indicating previous myocardial damage and suggesting that more myocardial damage could occur at any time. The presence of good exercise tolerance indicates satisfactory compensation and minimal injury. Restricted activity, breathlessness, an inability to lie flat, congested neck veins and oedema imply decompensation and a high risk. Such patients should have treatment with diuretics, digitalis glycosides and angiotension converting enzyme inhibitors and be stabilized and brought to peak condition before being offered surgery.

Angina pectoris

Angina at rest or angina with increasing severity or frequency should be referred to a physician, as a coronary artery bypass graft or angioplasty should probably take precedence over ophthalmic surgery. In some patients, the administration of aspirin daily may stabilize the situation. Calcium channel blockers may be given.

Stable angina occurring occasionally on exercise does not contraindicate anaesthesia. It is my impression that general anaesthesia may be less stressful (and thus less productive of catecholamines) in some patients than local anaesthesia. There are some advantages in protecting the patient against these hormones and any associated rise in blood pressure or arrhythmia by the administration of a beta-blocker, provided that there is no chronic obstructive airways disease or cardiac failure.[8]

Conduction defects

Atrial fibrillation, right bundle branch block and first degree atrioventricular block are common in elderly patients. They have no significance if the heart rate is within normal limits and the aim of therapy is to avoid gross tachycardia or bradycardia which will alter cardiac output. Left bundle branch block tends to be unstable and if possible general anaesthesia should be avoided.

Variable blocks of any sort, particularly those causing severe bradycardia or arrest, such as the sick sinus syndrome, Stokes-Adams syncope or those producing gross tachycardia or atrial flutter, should be referred to a cardiologist for insertion of a pacemaker or other treatment.

Ectopic beats

Irregular beats which are infrequent are of no significance. When they occur with every beat (in bigeminy), then cardiological opinion should be sought.

Hypertension

This is common in the elderly population. It is difficult to quantify the extent of any increased risk for a particular anaesthetic and the value of attempted temporary reduction. Most general anaesthetic agents are minor vasodilators but laryngeal intubation and painful stimuli are potent hypertensive stimuli. It is very uncommon to encounter stroke in association with an ophthalmic anaesthetic. The main risks appear to be those of cardiac ischaemia and left ventricular failure with pulmonary oedema during the recovery period.

There is a strong case for reducing and stabilizing blood pressure to a systolic pressure below 160 mmHg and a diastolic pressure below 110 mmHg for some time before surgery. It is important to continue medication up to the time of surgery and to take account of this, particularly at the time of induction when instability may occur with either hypertension or hypotension.

With all cardiac conditions, the margins of safety are reduced and it is vital to inject drugs slowly in minimal dosage and ensure that oxygen saturation does not fall during the procedure – this is just as true of local anaesthesia as it is of general anaesthesia.

Postoperative pulmonary oedema

Regularly, but infrequently, a patient's condition may deteriorate on being taken off the ventilator. The oxygen saturation falls, the pulse rises and the blood pressure may rise initially.

It is important to consider the differential diagnosis of pulmonary aspiration and left ventricular failure. Unfortunately, the physical signs are similar in both conditions, with poor air entry at the base of the lungs and multiple moist sounds on auscultation. The management is to give intravenous frusemide and ventilate with 100% oxygen. It is then possible to take stock of the situation and consider measures to reduce afterload by injecting small doses of hydralazine or other vasodilators.

Chronic obstructive airways disease

Bronchospasm, cough, sputum and poor gaseous exchange present a problem for the anaesthetist, whether the operation is to be done under local or general anaesthesia.[23] When these conditions are severe, the anaesthetist needs time to evaluate the situation so that the patient is in the best possible condition for surgery. Under local anaesthesia, the patient may be unable to lie flat and paroxysms of cough may endanger the eye. General anaesthesia may lead to postoperative respiratory failure, sputum retention and bronchopneumonia. More alarmingly, acute exacerbations of bronchospasm during anaesthesia may render inflation of the lungs extremely difficult and the high pressures used may precipitate a pneumothorax.

Assessment of ophthalmic patients is the same as that for general surgical patients and depends on history, examination and investigation. The differential diagnosis of left ventricular failure, carcinoma of the lung and tuberculosis should be considered, particularly with progression or change of symptoms, and chest X-ray is mandatory in these circumstances. Recent weight loss would also suggest immunodeficiency, tuberculosis or *Pneumocystis carinii* infection.

The effects of exercise and recumbency are a good guide to respiratory function and peak flow is an excellent guide to bronchospasm and the response to bronchodilators. If patients are thought to require blood gases or more sophisticated tests of pulmonary function, then they should be referred to a respiratory physician.

To get patients to peak condition probably requires a period of up to 2 weeks before operation. The regime should consist of the withdrawal of cigarettes and the use of a nebulized bronchodilator such as salbutamol, a beta-2 adrenergic receptor agonist which is profoundly effective at relieving acute bronchospasm.[7,9] Reduction in the inflammatory response of the bronchial mucosa can be achieved over a period with nebulized steroids, and this can be reinforced by a 5-day course of prednisolone 40 mg immediately before surgery. Intravenous steroids at the time of surgery take 6–8 h to produce a maximum effect.

Breathing exercises and postural drainage with percussion may assist in patients who have sputum. Appropriate antibiotics may be given after bacterial culture and sensitivity.

Histamine-releasing drugs should be avoided in the anaesthetic sequence. Etomidate has advantages over thiopentone and propofol. Curare, vecuronium and atracurium may all release histamine in some individuals but alternative agents are numerous. Inhalational agents are potent bronchodilators. Halothane, isoflurane and enflurane (in descending order of potency) are useful to treat established bronchospasm. Under local anaesthesia, cough depressants such as codeine phosphate or diamorphine may make the operation safer. Hypoxaemia is avoided by continuous pulse oximetry both during and after an operation.[6]

GENETIC DISEASES ASSOCIATED WITH EYE DISEASE IN THE ADULT

In children, a large number of genetic diseases have now been identified which cause cataract, retinal or optic nerve disease. These are discussed in those chapters devoted to anaesthesia for children. In adults, a few genetic defects express themselves with some frequency, although only sickle-cell trait is very common.

Dystrophia myotonica

Patients with this condition tend to develop cataracts in early middle age and there may be a family history. A number of different clinical syndromes are described. The myotonia is characterized by slow relaxation of striated muscle after contraction and a tendency to tonic muscle spasm which is enhanced by depolarizing muscle relaxants and neostigmine. There is generalized muscle weakness and wasting which may be associated with poor respiratory function. Some patients have hormonal and gonadal hypofunction. There is an increased response to central nervous system depressants, possibly due to a severe reduction in lean body mass.[11,18] The association of central depression and weak muscles may lead to respiratory failure, pulmonary collapse or retention of secretions.

General anaesthesia should aim at minimal depression, succinylcholine must be avoided, non-depolarizing relaxants should be used sparingly and neostigmine should be avoided. A short-acting muscle relaxant, such as atracurium, is suitable.[22] Even with these precautions, some patients will require a period of ventilation postoperatively.

MESODERMAL GENETIC DEFECTS

Marfan's syndome, Stickler syndrome and Ehlers–Danlos syndrome are diseases in which dislocation of the lens and retinal detachment cause loss of vision requiring surgery.

Marfan's syndrome

This syndrome is characterized by tallness, arachnodactyly, joint hyperextensibility, kyphoscoliosis, pectus excavatum and a high arched palate. Lung cysts are common. Valvular disease of the heart – in particular mitral valve prolapse, and less commonly pulmonary and aortic incompetence – is often found. Dissecting aneurysm of the aorta may be a terminal event. The anaesthetist should address these three problems and then anaesthesia is usually straightforward.[18] The high arched palate with a long neck and mandible means that a longer blade will be required on the laryngoscope and the jaw will appear heavy. It may be necessary to use a longer tube than usual. Inflation should be gentle to avoid rupturing a lung cyst and thereby causing a pneumothorax. Vasopressor responses on induction should be damped to avoid stressing the aorta.

Stickler syndrome

This syndrome is also linked with the names of Wagner and Marshall. The non-ocular features include sensineural deafness, high arched or cleft palate, maxillary hypoplasia and micrognathia. Patients may also have arachnodactyly and kyphoscoliosis. Forty-five percent of patients have mitral prolapse.[19, 24] The facies is characteristic in a typical case, but many patients have a forme-fruste and have only some of the features. These patients come for vitreoretinal surgery but may also require glaucoma or squint surgery. The major problem for the anaesthetist is intubation.

Ehlers–Danlos syndrome

This is a complex series of diseases characterized by hyperextensible joints and fragile skin. Valvular incompetence of the heart and conduction defects are the usual problems encountered.[12, 18] One rare variety tends to bleed after minor trauma, which adds to the problems of laryngoscopy. These patients may present for corneal grafting of their keratoconus, or they may have subluxation of the lens or retinal detachment.

Homocystinuria

This is a genetically determined enzyme deficiency disease in which abnormal collagen is formed. While the skeletal features may resemble Marfan's syndrome, there is often some mental retardation. The additional hazard for the anaesthetist lies in the increased adhesiveness of the platelets and the greatly increased risk of thromboembolism. These patients secrete excessive quantities of insulin and, during the period of fasting, hypoglycaemia may occur.[17, 20, 21] It is recommended that surgery be preceded by treatment with cystine and pyridoxine. Elastic stockings, a ripple mattress and early ambulation reduce the risks of thrombosis. Aspirin, heparin and dextran-40 have all been recommended for use with these patients.[25]

Sickle cell disease and trait[16]

Trait (HbAS) is found in about 10% of black patients of Afro-Caribbean ethnic origin, and the disease (HbSS, HbSC, HbSThall) in about 0.5%. Because haemoglobin C has a more deleterious effect on the microvasculature than haemoglobin S, haemoglobin C is represented more frequently than expected in eye hospitals. In the absence of major stress, hypoxia or infection, trait presents no major problem. The anaesthetist should be most punctilious and provide preinduction oxygenation and postoperative oxygen supplementation. Due regard should be given to preventing tissue hypoxia by keeping the patient reasonably warm, hydrated and not prolonging excessively the period of inflation of the sphygmomanometer cuff.

Sickle cell disease is a dangerous condition, and when possible, the advice of a haematologist should be sought. The patient who has HbSS disease is usually small, anaemic, may have had splenic infarcts and may have pulmonary fibrosis or poor renal function. On the other hand, patients with HbSC are often of normal size and not anaemic, but they may still have pulmonary or renal disease. Some haematologists recommend partial exchange transfusion a few days before surgery to provide 40–50% adult haemoglobin. Against this are the hazards, cost and inconvenience of a major blood transfusion. Whatever course is chosen, stagnation and hypoxia must be rigorously avoided. The vitreoretinal operations required by these patients are often long and precautions need to be taken against progressive aveolar and pulmonary collapse during anaesthesia.

ACQUIRED IMMUNE DEFICIENCY SYNDROME

The prolongation of life in patients with immunosuppression means that an increased number with cytomegalovirus infection of the retina leading to vitreous opacity and retinal detachment are seen by the eye surgeon.[26] Many of these patients are seriously ill, with anaemia and with residual respiratory insufficiency resulting from previous episodes of *Pneumocystis* pneumonia. They have sustained major weight loss and are maintained on many medications, some of which are given from reservoirs attached to indwelling catheters. These patients require the back-up which is not always easily available in specialized eye units detached from general hospitals. The basis of anaesthesia does not differ from that in other patients, but the doses of drugs can usually be reduced. Special precautions are indicated to avoid pressure sores.

REFERENCES

1. Alberti KGMM, Thomas DJB. The management of diabetes during surgery. *Br J Anaesth* 1979; **51**: 693.
2. Bowen DJ, Nance Kievill ML, Proctor EA, Norman J. Perioperative management of insulin dependent diabetic patients. *Anaesthesia* 1982; **37**: 852.
3. Branthwaite MA. Assessment of cardiac risks and complications for patients requiring non-cardiac surgery. *Anaesthesia Review* 3. Churchill Livingstone: Edinburgh, 1985.
4. Milaskiewicz RM, Hall GM. Diabetes and anaesthesia: The past decade. *Br J Anaesth* 1992; **68**: 198.
5. Eisenbarth GS. Type 1 diabetes mellitus: A chronic auto-immune disease. *New Engl J Med* 1986; **314**: 1360.
6. Moller JT, Jensen PF, Johannessen J, Espersen K. Hypoxaemia is reduced by pulse oximetry monitoring in the operating theatre and in the recovery room. *Br J Anaesth* 1992; **68**: 146.
7. Newhouse MT, Dolovich MB. Current concepts: Control of asthma by aerosols. *New Engl J Med* 1986; **315**: 870.
8. Patakas D, Argiropoulou V, Louridas G, Tsara V. Betablockers in bronchial asthma: Effect of propanalol and pinolol on large and small airways. *Thorax* 1983; **38**: 108.
9. Reed CE. Aerosols in chronic airway obstruction. *New Engl J Med* 1986; **315**: 888.
10. Thomson J, Husband DJ, Thai AC, Alberti KGMM. Metabolic changes in the NIDDM patient undergoing minor surgery: Effect of glucose:insulin:potassium infusion. *Br J Surg* 1986; **73**: 301.
11. Bourke TD, Zuck D. Thiopentone in dystrophia myotonia. *Br J Anaesth* 1957; **29**: 35.
12. Brandt KD, Sumner RD, Ryan TJ *et al.* Herniation of mitral leaflets in the Ehlers–Danlos syndrome. *Am J Cardiol* 1975; **36**: 524.
13. Derrington MC, Smith G. A review of the studies of anaesthetic risk, morbidity and mortality. *Br J Anaesth* 1987; **59**: 815.
14. Gilvarry A, Eustace P. The medical profile of cataract patients. *Trans Ophthalmol Soc UK* 1982; **102**: 502.
15. Goldman L. Assessment of the patient with known or suspected heart disease for non-cardiac surgery. *Br J Anaesth* 1988; **61**: 38.
16. Gibson JR. Anesthetic implication of sickle cell disease and other haemoglobinopathies. *ASA Refresher Course Lectures* 1986; **14**: 139.
17. Holmgren G, Falkmer S, Hambraeus L. Plasma insulin content and glucose tolerance in homocysteinuria. *Uppsala J Med Sci* 1975; **78**: 215.
18. Katz J, Benumof JL, Kadis LB. *Anesthesia and Uncommon Diseases*. W.B. Saunders: Philadelphia, PA, 1990.
19. Liberfarb RM, Goldblatt A. Prevalence of mitral valve prolapse in the Stickler syndrome. *Am J Med Genet* 1986; **24**: 387.
20. McDonald L, Bray C, Love F *et al.* Homocysteinuria, thrombosis and the blood platelets. *Lancet* 1964; **1**: 745.
21. McGoldrick KE. Anesthetic management of homocysteinuria. *Anesthet Rev* 1981; **8**: 42.
22. Nightingale P, Healy TEJ, McGuiness K. Dystrophia myotonica and atracurium. *Br J Anaesth* 1985; **57**: 1131.
23. Nunn JF, Milledge JS, Chen D, Dore C. Respiratory criteria for surgery and anaesthesia. *Anaesthesia* 1988; **43**: 543.

24. Opitz JM, France T, Hermann J *et al.* The Stickler syndrome. *New Engl J Med* 1972; **286:** 546.
25. Parris WCV, Quinby CW. Anesthetic considerations for the patient with homocystein-uria. *Anesthesia and Analgesia* 1982; **61:** 708.
26. Skolruk PR, Pomerantz RJ, de la Monte SM *et al.* Dual infection of the retina with human immunodeficiency virus Type 1 and cytomegalovirus. *Am J Ophthalmol* 1989; **107:** 361.

CHAPTER 5

Regional versus general anaesthesia

ROBERT C HAMILTON

INTRODUCTION

Historically, regional anaesthesia held sway over general anaesthesia for the first part of the century. In the 1950s and 1960s, a swing back to general anaesthesia occurred as improved drugs and techniques became available.[42] Over the past two decades, commencing in North America and later spreading to the UK, regional anaesthesia has again been supplanting general anaesthesia for many ophthalmic surgical procedures.[23,43,48] With modern high-technology equipment, the average surgery time for cataract extraction has markedly decreased; this, in combination with efficient scheduling and the predominant use of outpatient surgical facilities, has made possible high volume patient turnover. This form of practice lends itself to regional anaesthesia techniques.

STRESS AND ANAESTHESIA

Stress associated with release of catecholamines, glucose and cortisol into the circulation, and evidenced by typical signs of tachycardia and hypertension, is common in the perioperative period. Kehlet showed that epidural anaesthesia, by eliminating nociceptive input from the periphery, resulted in a reduction in the stress response.[31] Donlon and Moss found that the plasma level of catecholamines in patients having regional anaesthesia for cataract surgery resulted primarily from endogenous sources and secondarily and less importantly from exogenous adrenaline, injected with the local anaesthetics.[11] Up to 12 ml of local anaesthesia solution containing 1:200 000 adrenaline caused no untoward clinical effects. Moss and his colleagues further investigated the stress response to regional anaesthesia for cataract surgery and found that the more significant stressor was the entry of the patient into the operating theatre for the block to be administered, rather than the performance of the block itself, and emphasized that the management of the first meeting with the patient is extremely important in successful attenuation of stress.[39] Adams *et al.* found that the stress response to regional anaesthesia for cataract surgery could be reduced successfully by the judicious use of intravenous midazolam.[2] Barker *et al.* compared hormonal and metabolic responses in a group of patients having cataract surgery under general anaesthesia with a similar group under regional anaesthesia;[3] whereas plasma cortisol levels in the regional anaesthesia group failed to rise, that level more than doubled in the general anaesthesia group.[4] Although not a new idea,[29] many patients appreciate music as a distraction during surgery under regional anaesthesia.[51,59] The simple act of having a staff member hold the hand of the patient during surgery under regional block has a considerable calming effect.[20]

ANAESTHETICS AND THE IMMUNE DEFENCE

From early in the history of anaesthesia, surgeons and anaesthetists have been concerned about possible suppression of host defence against infection by anaesthetics.[53] Stanley *et al.* reported that spinal/epidural anaesthesia, unlike certain general anaesthetics, permitted the continuing migratory ability of leukocytes during surgery.[54,55] Similarly, the mononuclear phagocyte system of cells maintain their function better under epidural anaesthesia than general anaesthesia.[24] Reseach on the effects of the two types of anaesthesia on lymphocyte function are more equivocal. Whether there is any advantage of regional techniques, other than spinal/epidural methods, over general anaesthesia (including ophthalmic regional anaesthesia) has not been studied.

NATIONAL DIFFERENCES

The drive behind the current popularity of regional anaesthesia has been the mandation by funding agencies or government jurisdictions (particularly true in North America) to the effect that all ophthalmic surgeries shall be performed in an outpatient setting (same day admission and discharge) unless there is a justifiable reason to the contrary. For instance, in the USA, 1.3 million outpatient cataract extraction procedures were performed in 1990.[26] In the UK, a dramatic change in favour of regional anaesthesia is taking place.[23] There still remain great differences on opposite sides of the Atlantic. Whereas in the USA in two recent surveys involving 1625 and 1574 cataract surgery practices, respectively, only 1% of procedures were done under general anaesthesia,[34,35,48] in the UK two recent surveys indicated that the majority of surgeons preferred to operate under general anaesthesia.[6,23]

Using regional anaesthesia postoperative recovery time is shorter than with general anaesthesia, resulting in savings related to building space, equipment and staffing.[60] In the ambulatory setting preoperative sedative medications should be used to a minimum or not at all, which allows for patients to be discharged promptly after completion of surgery.

STANDARDS OF CARE COMMON TO BOTH FORMS OF ANAESTHESIA

Most geriatric patients have associated systemic disease, such as hypertension, coronary artery disease, chronic obstructive pulmonary disease, diabetes and obesity;[15,41,47] these present additional challenges to the operating team. A prospective survey of 198 000 anaesthetics demonstrated that the complications rate correlates with the number of associated diseases rather than the age of the patient.[58]

All patients require preoperative preparation and assessment with open communication of risks and potential complications that are based on a thorough history and physical examination. This requires cooperation among patients, their family doctors or internists and the surgeon/anaesthetist teams. A list of medications currently taken is required to ensure that essential therapy is continued through the time of surgery and that potential drug interactions can be anticipated. Laboratory and radiologic investigations should be ordered only when indicated and appropriate to the management of the case.[47] Whichever method of anaesthesia is used, every effort should be made to have patients in the best possible condition prior to surgery.[49] Most ophthalmic surgery is non-urgent, and therefore the date of surgery can usually be postponed until the status of each patient is optimal.

MORBIDITY AND MORTALITY

In the preface to their book, *Local Anaesthesia and Regional Blockade,* Löfström and Sjöstrand comment: 'today there is a widespread opinion that patients do better under regional blocks than under general anaesthesia. Scientifically, however, this has been hard to prove and only in some specific areas'.[36] Mortality and morbidity following both forms of anaesthesia have been studied in major retrospective and prospective non-randomized investigations.[10,13,17,25,45,57] These all failed to favour one method of anaesthesia over the other. Cataract surgery is more frequently performed on elderly patients than on younger adults; the more senior a patient is, the higher the intrinsic risk of death and this must be added to the risk of death associated with the clinical intervention. The average age of these elderly patient populations is on the increase. In the USA, 11% of the population in 1980 were 65 years of age or older; by 2020 this group will constitute 16% of the population.[32]

PSYCHOLOGICAL ASPECTS OF CHOICE BETWEEN REGIONAL AND GENERAL ANAESTHESIA

Time spent establishing a good rapport with the patient is more effective in allaying anxiety than to resort to pharmacologic methods.[14] On the other hand, there are practices in which surgeons prefer to operate on non-responsive patients for all of their procedures. The surgeon who does not believe in local anaesthesia, or who is not prepared to wait for the local anaesthetic to act, or expects conditions to be as perfect as under the oblivion of general anaesthesia, should not attempt to operate on the conscious patient.[5] Frequent inquiries as to whether the patient 'feels pain' or ponderous attempts at reassurance such as 'just let me know if you feel pain', are absolutely guaranteed to sap the confidence of the patient and lead to the interpretation of touch as pain.[50] In performing regional anaesthesia, anaesthetists must have the personality traits and communiction skills that will enable them rapidly to gain their patients' trust and educate them regarding the experiences they are about to have. Treated and prepared thus, patients will have minimal anxiety and have a low incidence of complications in the perioperative period.[61] If such skills are absent or not attainable (not all practitioners have the necessary prerequisites!), a decision in favour of general anaesthesia may be indicated.

THE CHOICE – REGIONAL VERSUS GENERAL

The decision as to whether general or regional anaesthesia is to be used must be based on consensus among the team members involved, and also the patient.[42,47,61] The choice of technique within a particular surgeon/anaesthetist team may be predicated by what that team knows they do best. The skill of application of a technique, whether regional or general, for a given operation is more important for the patient's well-being than any academic discussion of the merits of one or other modality. High standards of perioperative monitoring must be maintained for both forms of anaesthesia.[47,48] Knill and others reported a significant problem with long-term cognitive impairment in the elderly following general anaesthesia for procedures more major than cataract surgery.[33] In a prospective study of 169 elderly cataract surgery patients who were randomized to receive either local or general anaesthesia, there was no long-term evidence of postoperative cognitive dysfunction nor of performance differences between the groups.[7] There was a suggestion that the general anaesthesia group had a measurable cognitive function deficit in comparison with the local

Table 5.1   Respective advantages of regional and general anaesthesia

Regional anaesthesia	General anaesthesia
Simple technique (minimal equipment)[a]	Complete control of patient
Less postoperative nausea and vomiting	No risk of retrobulbar haemorrhage
Faster recovery	No risk of globe perforation
Postoperative analgesia superior	No risk of myotoxicity
Blockade of oculocardiac reflex	Applicable to all ages
Absence of respiratory depression	Preferable for teaching of surgery
Less physiological trespass	
Full mental status retained[b]	
No loss of 'control' for patient	
Potential for reduced stress	
No risk of toxic hepatitis	
Avoids trace gas exposure for staff	
Less expensive	
Not contraindicated with low serum K+	
No risk of malignant hyperthermia	
Easily applicable at high altitude	

[a] However, basic cardiopulmonary resuscitative equipment should be available.
[b] Enhanced ability to communicate intra- and postoperatively.[40]

anaesthesia group at 24 h. In the study, urinary retention problems were precipitated in a significant number of men in the general anaesthesia group and was a cause for some concern. General anaesthesia has been shown to increase the incidence of unplanned hospital admission after outpatient cataract extraction surgery.[30]

The advantages and contraindications for general and regional anaesthesia in a given patient are dependent on multiple factors which are elucidated in Tables 5.1 and 5.2, respectively. Of note are the amelioraton of the stress response,[4,40] the virtual absence of nausea and vomiting (provided narcotic drugs are not used) and superior postoperative pain control with regional anaesthesia. The

Table 5.2 Contraindications to regional and general anaesthesia (decreasing order of significance from absolute at top of table)

Regional anaesthesia	*General anaesthesia*
Reversible medical condition, uncorrected	Reversible medical condition, uncorrected
Informed patient refusal of RA	Informed patient refusal of GA
Anaesthetist inexperience	History of serious adverse effect from GA
True allergy to RA (very rare)	History of difficult airway
Surgeon preference for GA	Known problems or disease states:
Emergency surgery (open eye wound)	• malignant hyperthermia history
Prolonged surgery (more than 2 h)	• muscle diseases: dystrophia myotonica,
Children up to age of early teens	myasthenia gravis
Unsuitable psychological status:	• haemoglobinopathies
• behavioural or psychiatric disorder	• chronic obstructive pulmonary disease
• agitated, or phobic patient	• diabetes mellitus
• uncooperative patient	Caution with:
Mental retardation	• history of porphyria
Senile dementia	• atypical pseudocholinesterase
Head movements or tremors:	• patients on MAO inhibitors
• Parkinson's disease	• interactions with regular medications
• tardive dyskinesia	• patients on anticoagulants
Inability to lie flat (from cardiac or respiratory disease)	
Intractable cough	
Communication barrier:	
• language	
• deafness	
Moderate to severe arthritis	
Neurological disease	
Needle phobia	
Claustrophobia	
Complication from RA in same patient on an earlier occasion	
Patients with high myopia[a]	
Caution with patients on anticoagulants[b]	

[a] Suggestion by Duker *et al.*[12]
[b] See chapter on complications.
RA, regional anaesthesia; GA, genaral anaesthesia.

ability, with regional anaesthesia used in the elderly, to maintain mental alertness and enhanced effectiveness of staff to patient communication is one of its great assets.[9,40] General anaesthesia or heavy sedation can easily add to any pre-existing mental confusion.[8] Regional anaesthesia, unlike general anaesthesia, avoids further depression of pre-existing cardiac and respiratory malfunction, often present in the elderly.[15,41] Although it is still common practice to select patients for regional anaesthesia because they are unfit for general anaesthesia,[23] it should be seen as an alternative to general anaesthesia for the more fit and healthy and not as a means of operating on unfit patients.[48] The elderly require less pharmacologic support of anxiety than do young patients, and can cope more easily with minor discomforts. For a small percentage of elderly patients who benefit from preoperative sedation, fine judgement is required to select the correct drug dosage to produce a calm patient who remains alert and cooperative without respiratory depression.[22,61] The advantages of regional anaesthesia can be negated rapidly with excessive use of sedation; the combination of regional anaesthesia with heavy sedation may produce a less satisfactory outcome than either method on its own.[1,42,43,52] In the management of mild to moderate degrees of senile dementia or mental retardation, the author frequently asks a family member to 'hold hands' with the patient and give verbal support in the operating room. Likewise, in the presence of a language communication barrier, family members are often recruited to interpret. Parkinsonian head tremors can be controlled effectively with titrated doses of intravenous sedative drug. Incomplete regional anaesthesia is best managed with block supplementation until complete; to operate in the presence of obvious block failure is to subject the patient to an unpleasant and stressful experience; use of intravenous sedation to cover gross block inadequacy is hazardous and inappropriate. There is, however, a real place for the judicious combination of light general anaesthesia with complete regional anaesthesia in certain cases (e.g. prolonged retinal or vitrectomy surgery).[27]

WHO DOES THE BLOCK?

Whereas general anaesthesia was the traditional domain of the anaesthetist and local anaesthesia that of the ophthalmologist, a change has been underway for more than two decades. In a 1990 survey involving 1625 members of the American Society of Cataract and Refractive Surgeons, 79% of the ophthalmologists performed the regional anaesthetic block on their own patients; in 56% of high volume practices (more than 50 cataract procedures per month), the block was delegated to anaesthesia personnel.[35] There is often considerable reluctance on the part of ophthalmologists to permit anaesthetists to perform orbital regional anaesthesia blocks because they have felt that only physicians in their own discipline can have the necessary anatomic and technical knowledge to avoid serious complications.[37] In Britain, measures to improve patient care by increasing the involvement of anaesthetists, ideally including administration of the anaesthetic block, have been given official sanction.[46,56]

The various commonly used methods of ophthalmic regional anaesthesia are essentially blind procedures,[44] irrespective of the medical discipline of the block administrator, and serious sequelae have been reported following regional anaesthesia carried out by both disciplines.[12,18,21] There are obvious disadvantages to the surgeon acting as both operator and anaesthetist,[48] especially in the absence of a specialist anaesthetist for continuous perioperative monitoring. An anaesthetist can give undivided attention to the patient's complete welfare.[48] In circumstances where the ophthalmologist is doing both the block and the surgery, a convincing case can be made for the routine presence of an anaesthetist.[28,38] In the event of serious cardiopulmonary complications, anaesthetists are more familiar with resuscitative measures than their surgical colleagues. The author has heard of two deaths in the UK, one in 1991 and one in 1992, and more recently of a death in America, none of which was reported in the literature, all three related to delayed recognition of respiratory failure following intraconal local anaesthetic injection; in these cases, the surgeon had been both operator and block administrator, without the participation of a specialist anaesthetist until the patient was found to be in trouble.[16] There is no inherent reason why a non-ophthalmologist should not become proficient at orbital block techniques. Ideally, practitioners of whatever medical discipline who are performing eye blocks should have special knowledge acquired from attending formal courses in orbit anatomy (including cadaver dissection), pertinent pharmacology and physiology, and the recognition and management of potential complications.[19]

SUMMARY

In summary, for a mainly elderly population, the advantages of regional anaesthesia surpass those of general anaesthesia in the attainment of an effective, safe and comfortable surgical outcome against a setting of economic practice efficiency; specific contraindications to its use have been discussed.

REFERENCES

1. Adams AK, Jones RM. Anaesthesia for eye surgery: General considerations. *Br J Anaesth* 1980; **52:** 663.
2. Adams HA, Hessemer V, Hempelmann G, Jacobi KW. Endocrine stress response during cataract operations with local anesthesia. *Klin Monatsbl Augenheilkd* 1992; **200:** 273.
3. Barker JP, Robinson PN, Vafidis GC *et al.* Local analgesia prevents the cortisol and glycaemic responses to cataract surgery. *Br J Anaesth* 1990; **64:** 442.
4. Barker JP, Vafidis GC, Robinson PN *et al.* The metabolic and hormonal response to cataract surgery. *Anaesthesia* 1993; **48:** 488.
5. Boulton TB. Local anaesthesia in difficult environments. In *Local Anaesthesia and Regional Blockade* (edited by Löfström JB, Sjöstrand U). Elsevier: Amsterdam, 1988: 279–300.
6. Campbell DN, Spalton DJ. A national survey of the use of local anaesthesia for cataract surgery. *Eur J Implant Ref Surg* 1992; **4:** 213.
7. Campbell DNC, Lim M, Kerr-Muir M *et al.* Forum: A prospective randomised study of local versus general anaesthesia for cataract surgery. *Anaesthesia* 1993; **48:** 422.
8. Chung F, Lavelle PA, McDonald S *et al.* Cognitive impairment after neuroleptanalgesia in cataract surgery. *Anesth Analg* 1989; **68:** 614.
9. Chung F. Which is the best anaesthesia technique? *Can J Anaesth* 1991; **38:** 882.
10. Cohen MM, Duncan PG, Tate RB. Does anesthesia contribute to operative mortality? *JAMA* 1988; **260:** 2859.

11. Donlon JV, Moss J. Plasma catecholamine levels during local anaesthesia for cataract operations. *Anethesiology* 1979; **51:** 471.
12. Duker JS, Belmont JB, Benson WE *et al.* Inadvertent globe perforation during retrobulbar and peribulbar anesthesia: Patient characteristics, surgical management, and visual outcome. *Ophthalmology* 1991; **98:** 519.
13. Duncalf D, Gartner S, Carol B. Mortality in association with ophthalmic surgery. *Am J Ophthalmol* 1970; **69:** 610.
14. Egbert LD, Battit GE, Turndorf H *et al.* The value of the preoperative visit by an anaesthetist. *JAMA* 1963; **185:** 553.
15. Fisher SJ, Cunningham RD. The medical profile of cataract patients. *Geriatric Clin N Amer* 1985; **1:** 339.
16. Fletcher SJ, O'Sullivan G. Grand mal seizure after retrobulbar block. *Anaesthesia* 1990; **45:** 696.
17. Goldman L, Caldera DL, Southwick F *et al.* Cardiac risk factors and complications in non-cardiac surgery. *Medicine* 1978; **57:** 357.
18. Grizzard WS, Kirk NM, Payan PR *et al.* Perforating ocular injuries caused by anesthesia personnel. *Ophthalmology* 1991; **98:** 1011.
19. Hamilton RC. Non-ophthalmologists and orbital regional anesthesia (Letter). *Ophthalmology* 1992; **99:** 169.
20. Havener WH. Hand-holding anesthesia (Letter). *Ophthalmic Surg* 1990; **21:** 375.
21. Hay A, Flynn HW Jr, Hoffman JI, Rivera AH. Needle penetration of the globe during retrobulbar and peribulbar injections. *Ophthalmology* 1991; **98:** 1017.
22. Heyworth PLO, Seward HC. Local anaesthesia – The ophthalmologist's view. *Eur J Implant Ref Surg* 1993; **5:** 12.
23. Hodgkins PR, Luff AJ, Morrell AJ *et al.* Current practice of cataract extraction and anaesthesia. *Br J Ophthalmol* 1992; **76:** 323.
24. Hole A, Unsgaard G, Breivik H. Monocyte functions are depressed during and after surgery under general anaesthesia but not under epidural anaesthesia. *Acta Anaesthesiol Scand* 1982; **26:** 301.
25. Hosking MP, Warner MA, Lobdell CM *et al.* Outcomes of surgery in patients 90 years of age and older. *JAMA* 1989; **261:** 1909.
26. Hustead RF, Hamilton RC. Pharmacology. In *Ophthalmic Anesthesia* (edited by Gills JP, Hustead RF, Sanders DR). Slack Inc.: Thorofare, NJ, 1993: 69–102.
27. Hustead RF, Hamilton RC. Techniques. In *Ophthalmic Anesthesia* (edited by Gills JP, Hustead RF, Sanders DR). Slack Inc.: Thorofare, NJ, 1993: 103–186.
28. Jackson PW. In support of general anaesthesia for cataract surgery. *Eur J Implant Ref Surg* 1993; **5:** 17.
29. Kane EO. Phonograph in the operating room. *JAMA* 1914; **63:** 1829.
30. Kareti RKP, Callahan H, Draper GA. Factors leading to hospital admission of elderly patients following outpatient eye surgery: A medical dilemma. *Anesth Analg* 1989; **68:** S144.
31. Kehlet H. Epidural analgesia and the endocrine-metabolic response to surgery: Update and perspectives. *Acta Anaesthesiol Scand* 1984. **28:** 25.
32. Kline D, Sekular R, Dismukes K. Social issues, human needs, and opportunities for research on the effects of age on vision: an overview. In *Aging and Human Visual Function* (edited by Sekuler R, Kline D, Dismukes K). Alan R. Liss: New York, 1982: 3–6.
33. Knill RL. Clinical research in anaesthesia. Past accomplishments and a future horizon (Editorial). *Anaesthesia* 1990; **45:** 271.
34. Leaming DV. Practice styles and preferences of ASCRS members – 1990 survey. *J Cataract Refract Surg* 1991; **17:** 495.
35. Leaming DV. Practice styles and preferences of ASCRS members – 1991 survey. *J Cataract Refract Surg* 1992; **18:** 460.
36. Löfström JB, Sjöstrand U. Preface. In *Local Anaesthesia and Regional Blockade* (edited by Löfström JB, Sjöstrand U). Elsevier: Amsterdam, 1988: xi.

37. Lichter PR. The relative value of quality care (Editorial). *Ophthalmology* 1991; **98:** 1151.
38. Morgan GE. Retrobulbar apnea syndrome: A case for the routine presence of an anesthesiologist (Letter). *Regional Anesth* 1990; **15:** 107.
39. Moss J, Donlon JV, McGoldrick KE. Stress response to local anesthesia for cataract surgery (Abstract). *Anesthesiology* 1987; **67:** A67.
40. Mulroy MF. Regional anesthesia for adult outpatients. In *Outpatient Anesthesia* (edited by White PF). Churchill Livingstone: New York, 1990: 293.
41. Neima D, Ramsey MS. Systemic illnesses in cataract patients: 1. Incidence. 2. Prevalence. *Can J Ophthalmol* 1987; **22:** 165
42. O'Brien HD. Anesthesia for cataract surgery. *Am J Ophthalmol* 1964; **57:** 751.
43. Pearce JL. General and local anaesthesia in eye surgery. *Trans Ophthalmol Soc* (UK) 1982; **102:** 31.
44. Petersen WC, Yanoff M. Complications of local ocular anesthesia. *Int Ophthalmol Clin* 1992; **32:** 23.
45. Quigley HA. Mortality associated with ophthalmic surgery. *Am J Ophthalmol* 1974; **77:** 517.
46. Report of the Joint Working Party on Anaesthesia in Ophthalmic Surgery. College of Ophthalmologists, Royal College of Anaesthetists, March 1993.
47. Rosen E. Editorial review: Anaesthesia for cataract surgery. *Eur J Implant Ref Surg* 1993; **5:** 1.
48. Rubin AP. Anaesthesia for cataract surgery – time for change? (Editorial). *Anaesthesia* 1990; **45:** 717.
49. Rubin AP. Local anaesthesia for ophthalmic surgery: An anaesthetist's view. *Eur J Implant Ref Surg* 1993; **5:** 8.
50. Scott DL. Sedation for local analgesia. Distraction and diazepam. *Anaesthesia* 1975; 30: 471.
51. Sjöstrand U. Psychological aspects of regional analgesia. In *Local Anaesthesia and Regional Blockade* (edited by Löfström JB, Sjöstrand U). Elsevier: Amsterdam. 1988: 273–278.
52. Smith DC, Crul JF. Oxygen desaturation following sedation for regional analgesia. *Br J Anaesth* 1989; **62:** 206.
53. Snel JJ. Immunität und narkose. *Berl Klin Wochenschr* 1903; **10:** 1.
54. Stanley TH, Hill GE, Portas MR *et al*. Neutrophil chemotaxis during and after general anesthesia and operation. *Anesth Analg* 1976; **55:** 668.
55. Stanley TH, Hill GE, Hill HR. The influence of spinal and epidural anesthesia on neutrophil chemotaxis in man. *Anesth Analg* 1978; **57:** 567.
56. Steele ADMcG. Cataract management. (Editorial). *Br J Ophthalmol* 1992; **76:** 321.
57. Steen PA, Tinker JH, Tarhan S. Myocardial reinfarction after anesthesia and surgery. *JAMA* 1978; **239:** 2566.
58. Tiret L, Desmond JM, Hatton F *et al*. Complications associated with anaesthesia – A prospective survey in France. *Can J Anaesth* 1986; **33:** 336.
59. Walther-Larsen S, Diemar V, Valentin N. Music during regional anesthesia: A reduced need for sedatives. *Reg Anesth* 1988; **13:** 69.
60. Watts MT, Pearce JL. Day case cataract surgery. *Br J Ophthalmol* 1988; **72:** 897.
61. Wilson RP. Complications associated with local and general ophthalmic anesthesia. *Int Ophthalmol Clin* 1992; **32:** 1.

CHAPTER 6

The local anaesthetics and adjuvant drugs

ROBERT C HAMILTON

INTRODUCTION

The successful practitioner of regional anaesthesia for ophthalmologic surgery must be conversant, not only with anatomic knowledge and the necessary dexterity of needle placement, but also with the pharmacology of the local anaesthetics and adjuvant drugs.

THE LOCAL ANAESTHETICS

Local anaesthetics all bear the suffix -caine. Nerve axons exposed to local anaesthetics in sufficient concentration exhibit temporary interruption of neural transmission. The term 'regional anaesthesia' signifies conduction block in a region by having gained access to a specific nerve or nerves, rather than using the term 'local anaesthesia' which should be restricted to the technique of infiltration of a specific tissue resulting in blockade of its nerve endings. Topical anaesthesia, of great importance in ophthalmology, implies action of a local anaesthesia agent when applied on the surface of epithelial tissues. Table 6.1 provides information about the local anaesthetics with which the ophthalmic anaesthetist should be familiar, including details of some of their biological and physicochemical properties. A brief summary of the chief properties of the individual local anaesthetics can be found at the end of the chapter.

CHEMICAL STRUCTURE

Local anaesthesia drugs possess in common certain molecular structural similarities:

Aromatic Lipophilic Pole		Intermediate Linking Chain		Amine Hydrophilic Pole
	-----------		----------	

The intermediate chain may be an ester-link (—COO—) or an amide-link (—NHCO—); this difference not only categorizes the local anaesthetics into two main groups (Table 6.1), but also is of considerable clinical importance. The amide-linked agents are more stable than the ester-linked ones, have a longer shelf life, and are much less likely to evoke allergic reactions (see below). Because of their relatively unstable ester-linkage such agents may not be sterilized by heat, and because of their rapid metabolism are too short acting for routine ophthalmologic use. In current practice, the chief remaining use of the ester-linked drugs, including cocaine, is for topical anaesthesia (see below). Nevertheless, historically they were important in the commencement of regional anaesthesia as an alternative to general anaesthesia and in the development of early ophthalmic regional techniques.[36]

Local anaesthetics are weak bases and are relatively insoluble in water. In this base form, they cannot be clinically effective and are therefore prepared commercially for clinical use as the water soluble salts of hydrochloric acid:

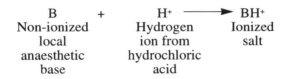

In this clinically used form, a partial dissociation of the salt takes place at body pH, back into the relatively insoluble base form:

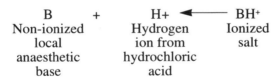

An equilibrium is set up between the un-ionized and ionized forms, the balance between the two being dependent on the prevailing tissue pH (capable of variation) and on the dissociation constant (fixed) of the drug being used:

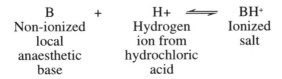

The dissociation constant (pKa) may be regarded as the pH at which equal amounts of cationic and basic form co-exist. If the tissue pH is low (acidic), the balance is in favour of the ionized form. For higher pKa agents at tissue pH 7.4,

Table 6.1 Local anaesthetics commonly used in ophthalmic regional anaesthesia

Biological properties	Ester-linked agents		Amide-linked agents			
	Cocaine	Procaine	Lignocaine	Mepivacaine	Bupivacaine	Etidocaine
Year introduced	1884	1905	1944	1957	1963	1972
Other names		Novocaine	Lidocaine, Xylocaine	Carbocaine	Marcaine, Sensorcaine	Duranest
Site of metabolism	Plasma and liver	Plasma ester hydrolysis	Liver amide hydrolysis	Liver amide hydrolysis	Liver amide hydrolysis	Liver amide hydrolysis
Onset	Slow	Slow	Fast	Fast	Intermediate	Fast
Duration (min)	Short (30–60)	Short (60–90)	Intermediate (75–150)	Intermediate (120–240)	Long (180–600)	Long (180–600)
Equieffective anaesthetic concentration	Not in clinical use	2% (low potency)	1% (intermediate potency)	1% (intermediate potency)	0.25% (high potency)	0.5% (high potency)
Other information	From coca leaf, cardiotoxic, addicting, vasoconstrictor	Potential for allergic reaction	Anti-arrhythmic, mild vasodilator	Lesser degree of vasodilation	Less motor block has potential for cardiotoxicity	Profound motor block

Physicochemical properties

	Ester-linked agents		Amide-linked agents			
	Cocaine	Procaine	Lignocaine	Mepivacaine	Bupivacaine	Etidocaine
Protein binding (duration of action)	Not available	6% (short)	65% (intermediate)	75% (intermediate)	95% (long)	95% (long)
Dissociation constant (pKa) (onset time, tissue penetrance)	Not available	8.9 (slow onset, poor penetrance)	7.7 (fast onset, good penetrance)	7.6 (fast onset, good penetrance)	8.1 (intermediate onset and penetrance)	7.7 (fast onset, good penetrance)
% Base (at pH of 7.4)	Not available	2%	35%	35%	20%	35%
Lipid/water partition coefficient (anaesthesia potency)	Not available	0.6 (low potency)	2.9 (intermediate potency)	0.8 (intermediate potency)	27.5 (high potency)	141 (high potency)

Dosage guidelines

	Cocaine	Procaine	Lignocaine	Mepivacaine	Bupivacaine	Etidocaine
Maximum single dose (plain solution)	1 mg/kg topical use only	800 mg	250 mg	300 mg	150 mg	300 mg
Maximum single dose (with adrenaline)	Unsafe when combined with adrenaline	1000 mg	500 mg	500 mg	225 mg	400 mg
Toxic dose (if given i.v.)	Most toxic! Do not use by injection	Not available	250 mg	300 mg	80 mg	180 mg

the balance will also favour the ionized form when compared with lower pKa drugs. In the clinical situation, when the balance is to the un-ionized basic side, this promotes fast blockade onset time and good tissue penetrance. These variations in degrees of dissociation between drugs explain in large part the superiority of lignocaine, mepivacaine and etidocaine over the others.

The un-ionized basic form favours penetration of the outer layers of a nerve and the nerve membrane. Once inside the nerve membrane, the more acidic tissue pH favours dissociation into the ionized form, which readily enters sodium channels to block conductance.[70] The site of action of local anaesthetics on myelinated nerves is at the nodes of Ranvier where the myelin sheath is interrupted. For clinical blockade of a myelinated nerve to be evident, a segment of at least 6.0 mm and preferably 10.0 mm of a nerve length, representing two to three nodes of Ranvier, must be exposed to the anaesthetic to deter impulses from 'skipping' over the blocked segment, a process known as saltatory conduction.[23,54,76] Motor nerves have greater internode distances than do sensory nerves,[23] which may account for differential block favouring sensory more than motor fibres in certain circumstances. Because the length of motor fibre available at the apex of the orbit for exposure to local anaesthetics may be as short as 10–12.5 mm (see Chapter 1), a decision to use higher concentrations of agent may be necessary in order to achieve akinesia, whereas if longer sections of motor nerve were available, less potentially toxic concentrations would suffice.[75] A certain minimum concentration of local anaesthetic is necessary to block a nerve fibre of given type. The clinical emphasis should always be on using the least effective concentration in smallest volume that produces the desired degree of blockade. Motor and proprioceptive nerves require higher minimum concentrations of agent for effective block than do other modalities such as pain and temperature. Hence if the achievement of motor akinesia is used as the yardstick of block effectiveness, pain will not be experienced; touch and tissue movement appreciation (proprioceptive mediation) are occasionally experienced, which, in the nervous patient, may be interpreted as discomfort.

PHYSICOCHEMICAL PROPERTIES

Certain physicochemical properties control important biological properties of the local anaesthetics. Table 6.1 lists the most important of these. Affinity for protein (protein binding) is the predominant property that governs duration of action. Agents with high protein affinity occupy active binding sites for longer times and therefore have a prolonged duration of activity (bupivacaine, etidocaine). Drugs with somewhat lesser affinity have an intermediate period of effective blockade (lignocaine, mepivacaine), whereas procaine, which is poorly protein bound, is short acting. Dissociation balance between the basic and ionized forms is largely responsible for speed of onset and tissue penetration ability of the drugs, those being more highly present in the ionized form having inferior properties in this regard (rapid onset with good tissue penetration, as with lignocaine, being desirable clinical properties). Lipid solubility largely accounts for drug potency, the more lipid-soluble agents (bupivacaine, etidocaine) being capable of clinical blockade at lower concentrations than the relatively less lipid-soluble drugs (lignocaine, mepivacaine) and the even less lipid-soluble agent procaine (high concentration required).

MECHANISMS OF LOCAL ANAESTHETIC DISPOSITION AT THE SITE OF INJECTION

Three mechanisms, which run concurrently, are mainly responsible for the disposition of injected local anaesthetics.

Bulk spread through the tissues

Following injection into an appropriate tissue compartment close to the site of desired action, a bulk spread takes place, which is governed by the macropermeability of local connective tissues.[58,82] This aspect of local anaesthetic disposition is aided by the enzyme hyaluronidase.[52]

Diffusion to the nerve core

Following spread within the extraneural tissue compartments, local anaesthetics diffuse through nerve mantle towards and into the nerve core. This mechanism is affected most by the physicochemical properties described above.

Vascular uptake

Running concurrently with bulk spread and diffusion is vascular uptake of the injected agent into the systemic circulation. The absorption of local anaesthetics from the site of injection is directly related to local blood flow and inversely to tissue binding. Hyperkinetic states as may occur in renal disease, hypertension, hyperthyroidism and certain anxiety states will promote more rapid uptake and therefore shorten duration of action. Inclusion of adrenaline in the injectate by causing vasoconstriction will prolong the action of the shorter-acting agents. Agents with high protein-binding and fat-solubility properties are bound to local tissues; both these factors oppose rapid vascular uptake and prolong duration of action.

Volume, concentration and mass

Volume injected is important in the process of achieving adequate spread of agent around the nerves, and concentration is of primary importance in the development of diffusion gradient for nerve penetrance; mass of injected drug, after the attainment of minimum volumes and concentration, is also a factor in conduction blocks.[9]

ADJUVANT DRUGS TO AUGMENT CLINICAL USE

The three most commonly used adjuvant agents are adrenaline, hyaluronidase and sodium bicarbonate.

Adrenaline

Adrenaline causes blood vessel constriction at, and delays absorption of, local anaes-thetics from the site of injection; peak systemic blood levels of the injected local anaesthesia agent are decreased.[60] The duration of action of all but the long-acting drugs is increased.[10,13] The quality and reliability of blocks are improved,[1,17,65] although the mechanism for this phenomenon is unclear.[51] Adrenaline is more sta-ble in acidic solution and for that reason commercial premixed local anaesthetics containing adrenaline have sodium metabisulphite (allergenic potential also) as an additive; this prevents catecholamine oxidation and an acceptable shelf life is achieved. As a better alternative to prepackaged antioxidant-containing solutions, adrenaline may be freshly added to plain solutions before use to achieve a higher pH and improved tissue penetrance (see above).[24,50] The final concentration of adren-aline in the injectate should not exceed 5 μg/ml (1:200 000), nor should the total amount used exceed 0.2 mg;[39] up to 0.05 mg is commonly all that is required in oph-thalmic regional anaesthesia. This represents 0.1ml of 1:1000 adrenaline (i.e. 100 μg) added (accurately measured in a tuberculin syringe) to 20 ml of local anaes-thetic. Higher concentrations are no more effective and result in systemic side-effects from increased systemic adrenaline levels. The use of adrenaline in orbital regional anaesthesia, although commonly practised, is controversial as it may reduce the blood supply to vital structures of the globe,[20] particularly in the presence of pathological conditions in which vascular compromise is already present.[78] A fall in ocular per-fusion pressure (balance between intraocular pressure and mean local arterial blood pressure) may be associated with the use of adrenaline in intraconal blocks;[35] how-ever, ocular haemodynamics may be more markedly altered following orbital local anaesthetic injection by other factors, even in the absence of adrenaline.[32,33] Local anaesthetics containing adrenaline may be more myotoxic than plain solutions.[85] Adrenaline should be avoided in patients on tricyclic antidepressives, as its cardio-vascular effects may be potentiated. However, in patients taking monoamine oxidase inhibitors, it may be used safely as adrenaline is metabolized by catechol-*o*-methyl tranferase.[77]

Hyaluronidase

The enzyme hyaluronidase is frequently added to local anaesthetics for eye blocks to promote bulk spread of injectate through the tissues. It breaks down collagen bonds and allows anaesthetics to spread across fine connective tissue septal barriers. This action is accomplished by a reversible hydrolysis of extra-cellular hyaluronic acid, which is the intercellular cement substance of connec-tive tissues. To maintain the full activity of the product, commonly supplied in 1-ml glass vials containing 150 turbidity units in solution, refrigeration is impor-tant. Prolonged exposure (in excess of 48 h) to room temperature results in a deterioration of enzyme strength. Autoclaving of solutions results in destruction of enzyme potency. Hyaluronidase is added to local anaesthetic injectate to a concentration of 7.5–15 turbidity units/ml.[20] Sarvela and Nikki compared con-centrations of 7.5 and 15 units hyaluronidase per ml in etidocaine 1.5% and found no advantage to the higher strength.[21] It is a potent enzyme and was used effectively by Hustead in his large practice in the low concentration of 0.5 units/ml.[37] Prior to its introduction into ophthalmic regional anaesthesia, volumes injected into the orbit had to be limited; greatly improved standards of effective anaesthesia and akinesia for ophthalmology (especially cataract extraction), without compromise of intraocular pressure, are made possible by larger volumes of hyaluronidase-containing injectate.[3–5,52,72] Szmyd *et al.* reported a reduction in duration of anaesthesia for ophthalmic surgery;[69] Atkinson's earlier report agreed, but he found that adrenaline in the mixture reversed that tendency.[5] Being of animal origin, hyaluronidase has allergenic potential.[71] A delayed allergic reaction to hyaluronidase of immunoallergic aetiology causing orbital pseudotumour formation has been described.[84] The use of the enzyme is not a substitute for precise anatomic knowledge or poor technique.[8] Because hyaluronidase facilitates spread of injectate along the path of least resistance, the solution must be placed accurately within the appropriate compartment. Hyaluronidase did not enhance brachial plexus block with mepivacaine, nor did it influence plasma levels of local anaesthetics.[56] Most workers find it beneficial for ophthalmic anaesthesia.[52,59] Local anaesthetics containing hyaluronidase may be more myotoxic than enzyme-free solutions.[85]

Sodium bicarbonate

The onset time and penetrance of agents is enhanced by adjusting the pH of the injectate towards the un-ionized basic side by the addition of small amounts of sodium bicarbonate. For each agent there is a pH at which the amount of free base in solution becomes saturated. Increases in pH beyond that point result in precipitation of free base beyond which no further clinical benefit is achievable. In fact, a nuisance factor, blockage of needles by embolization with free base precipitate, presents itself. The literature is equivocal about the effectiveness of pH adjustment in various clinical situations.[6,34,45,67] The author has failed in his practice to see benefit, in orbital blocks, for pH adjustment of local anaesthetics with sodium bicarbonate,[37,40] yet there is considerable support for it in some publications.[80,81] There is lesser pain stimulus during injection when bicarbonate is added.[18,43] Alkalinized solutions should be used within 6 h of their preparation.[51]

DOSAGE OF LOCAL ANAESTHESIA AGENT

The avoidance of toxicity is of paramount importance in the total dose of drug to be administered. The maximum safe dosage for each of the agents, with and without adrenaline, is listed in Table 6.1. In ophthalmologic practice, the required amounts for clinical anaesthesia are always on the safe side of these maximum guidelines, by a wide margin. Possible adverse effects of overdosage are discussed below.

CHOICE OF LOCAL ANAESTHESIA AGENT WITH ADJUVANTS

In choosing a drug or drug combination for orbital regional anaesthesia, the proposed surgical operation will be of paramount importance. For example, surgery for correction of retinal detachment under regional blockade demands the selection of a long-acting agent or drug combination for a surgical time that may exceed 2 h, whereas surgery for a straightforward cataract extraction in the hands of a competent surgeon may only last 15 min and be easily and successfully done with a short-acting local anaesthetic.[42] Further details are discussed in Chapter 7.

ADVERSE REACTIONS TO THE LOCAL ANAESTHETICS

Adverse reactions to the local anaesthetics may arise in three different ways: allergy, tissue toxicity and systemic toxicity.

Allergy

Frequently reported by patients, 'allergy' to local anaesthetics on previous exposure, usually in a dental office, must be evaluated with diligence. It is estimated that 99% of reported adverse reactions do not involve allergic mechanisms.[53] In the author's experience, most have been systemic effects of adrenaline, but other modalities include vasovagal syncope, other drug reactions and surgical oro-facial swelling. True allergy is almost exclusively confined to the ester-linked drugs. Para-aminobenzoic acid (PABA) is a breakdown product of plasma enzymatic cleavage of ester-linked agents and is thought to trigger an allergic reaction in certain individuals. Amide-linked local anaesthetics, on the other hand, are broken down in the liver. However, because methyl-para-aminobenzoic acid (methylparaben) used as preservative in multidose drug vials of some amide-linked preparations is related to PABA, it is best to use preservative-free vials where a history of the problem exists.[38] The author has used only preservative-free amide-linked agents for all orbital blocks and did not have a complication related to allergy in the 10 years of continual practice prior to January 1994, representing 32 500 regional anaesthesia procedures. Nevertheless, two well-documented cases of true allergy to amide drugs have been reported in the literature.[11,55] Sodium metabisulphite, added as an antioxidant to commercially prepared adrenaline-containing solutions and to 1 mg/1 ml adrenaline ampoules, may also be allergenic. The American Regency Company produces 1 mg/1 ml adrenaline ampoules that are antioxidant-free. Where there is a history of a typical histamine-mediated allergic reaction to an ester-linked agent, amide-linked local anaesthetics may be used with safety, as cross-reactivity between these groups does not occur. In the extremely rare event of encountering a true allergic reaction, the appropriate treatment is cessation of further use of the suspected provoking drug, and intramuscular injecton of adrenaline 0.5 mg (for a 70-kg adult) with simultaneous administration of diphenhydramine (0.5–1.0 mg/kg) to block unoccupied histamine receptors. This should be accompanied by general supportive measures such as administration of oxygen, infusion of saline or plasma expander and corticosteroid therapy. Constant monitoring of vital signs is required until recovery is complete.

Tissue toxicity

High concentrations of local anaesthetic agents clearly are cytotoxic, the most vulnerable tissues being nerve and skeletal muscle. In animal research studies, toxic changes are easily produced with supraclinical concentrations of local anaesthetics.[63]

Neurotoxicity

The hallmark of local anaesthesia is that the block is totally reversible. Correctly administered, local anaesthetics of clinical concentration are safe, but animal data indicate that all are potentially neurotoxic.[86] Evidence of neurotoxicity is occasionally seen and depends on type of agent (the ester-linked may be more neurotoxic than the amide-linked anaesthetics), its concentration, the site of injection, osmolarity, pH and whether certain additives, such as vasoconstrictors, antioxidants or preservatives, are present.[26] Electron microscopy studies indicate that the perineurium, Schwann cells and axons themselves may be damaged. Advanced age and disease states enhance susceptibility to neurotoxicity. Toxicity in clinical practice is most commonly seen with spinal anaesthesia.[15] Adrenaline has been investigated as a possible contributor to local anaesthetic neurotoxicity, the suspected mechanism being decreased intraneural blood supply from vasoconstriction.[22] Admixture with the antioxidant sodium bisulphite in the presence of low pH has been shown to be neurotoxic.[28] Commercial adrenaline-containing local anaesthetics include sodium metabisulphite as antioxidant and for this reason should be avoided in orbital regional anaesthesia;[36] as a safer and more effective alternative to these commercial solutions, adrenaline may be added to local anaesthetics freshly before use (pH, toxicity and allergenicity advantages).

In regional anaesthesia techniques in which nerve paraesthesias are sought, damage from direct needle trauma to the nerve, or the associated pressure ischaemia from intraneural injection, may result.[62] Although in ophthalmic regional anaesthesia paraesthesias are not sought, optic nerve damage has been reported (see Chapter 8); in the anterior orbit, the motor nerve to the inferior oblique muscle is vulnerable (see Chapter 1). Needle tips with short bevels, a pin-point tip with side opening, or non-cutting shoulders deflect rather than penetrate nerves;[25,61,74] unfortunately, their use increases patient discomfort in their placement and therefore there is a frequent need to use additional sedation. There are a few reports in the literature of inadvertent needle penetration of the globe followed by injection of clinical concentrations of local anaesthetic intraocularly. The retina, which is specialized nerve tissue, has not undergone toxic change in these circumstances; animal research supports this finding.[41]

Myotoxicity

Much more significant for the ophthalmic anaesthetist, however, is myotoxicity.[79] In young individuals recovery is complete, but in the elderly it may be less successful. Higher local anaesthetic concentrations result in a greater incidence of myotoxicity than lower concentrations; therefore, the strength of agent used in clinical practice should be as low as possible, commensurate with an effective outcome. Whereas myotoxicity of local anaesthesia agents is not a clinical problem in most types of regional anaesthesia, it most certainly is in the field of ophthalmologic practice. Any of the delicate extraocular muscles receiving an intramuscular injection of local anaesthetic may take several weeks to recover and in some the specific paresis may be permanent (author's previously unpublished personal practice experience). The orbicularis oculi muscle is more resistant to toxic damage.[85] Nothing can be more devastating for a cataractous patient and the surgeon involved than to have a perfect optical result, but an associated serious diplopia from globe misalignment. Chapter 8 discusses myotoxicity more extensively.

Systemic toxicity

Toxic effects, when they occur, affect organs with excitable membranes, notably the brain and myocardium. The incidence of systemic toxicity with local anaesthetics is related to total dose given, vascularity of site of injection, drug used, speed of injection, and whether adrenaline has been used as an additive to delay systemic release. The relative toxicity of the agents commonly used in ophthalmologic practice is depicted in Table 6.1. As the milligram amount of local anaesthesia agent (the mass) required for effective clinical results in ophthalmologic practice is relatively small in comparison with regional anaesthesia requirements for most other types of surgery, problems of systemic toxicity are unlikely. Important principles in this and in all uses of local anaesthetics include utilization of a minimum effective dose (well considered choice of drug, its volume and concentration, plus selection of adjuvant drugs), test aspiration before injection, and a slow rate of injection in fractional amounts while maintaining verbal contact with the patient for reporting of possible toxic symptoms (the author injects at a rate of 2 ml/min, which also has the advantage of being more comfortable for the patient than speedier use). Systemic toxicity is most likely to be encountered following unintentional intravascular injection. Slow intravenous injection of the total mass of local anaesthetic, as is usually required for an eye block, would be unlikely to produce other than the mildest of systemic symptoms. However, intra-arterial injection of an orbital arterial vessel has the potential, with retrograde flow to the brain, of producing almost instantaneous and more dramatic sequelae.[2,48]

Central nervous system (CNS) toxicity

Brain tissue is more susceptible to toxic levels of local anaesthetics than myocardium. Progressive central nervous system (CNS) effects, affecting inhibitory and later (with larger dose exposure) facilitatory pathways, produce the following signs and symptoms in approximate order of occurrence: circumoral and tongue numbness and tingling, garrulousness, dizziness, visual and auditory disturbances, drowsiness, confusional state, shivering, muscle twitching and tremors, loss of consciousness, generalized convulsions, coma, respiratory depression and finally apnoea. This serious clinical syndrome can progress very rapidly as respiratory inadequacy and the excessive oxygen demands of convulsing muscles cause acidosis, hyperkalaemia and hypoxia.

Cardiovascular toxicity

Systemic concentrations of local anaesthetics that produce CNS toxicity result in cardiovascular vital sign effects commensurate with the state of convulsive activity. Beta-blockers (e.g. propranolol) or combined alpha- and beta-blockers (e.g. labetalol) may be indicated to control tachycardia, hypertension and dys-rhythmias. Larger local anaesthetic doses exert negative inotropic myocardial and peripheral vasodilator actions, ultimately resulting in cardiac arrest. Bupivacaine is the most cardiotoxic of the local anaesthesia drugs in clinical use.[49] Cardiac dysrhythmias become more severe in the presence of hypoxia, hyperkalaemia and acidosis.

Diazepam given as premedication before regional anaesthesia may increase the seizure threshold.[16] However, the planned dose of local anaesthetic should not be increased based on the prior use of diazepam. The treatment of established systemic toxicity includes appropriate use of ventilatory support using oxygen, with intravenous thiopental, diazepam or suxamethonium to end persistent seizure activity. The primary aim at the onset of seizure activity should be the prevention of the detrimental effects of hypoxia by provision of adequate venti-lation using 100% oxygen.

A form of CNS toxicity, brainstem anaesthesia, may occur with orbital regional anaesthesia.[30] Brainstem anaesthesia is not caused by increasing levels of drug in the systemic circulation (including CNS) but by direct spread of local anaesthetic to the brain from the orbit along submeningeal pathways. The pre-vention and management of brainstem anaesthesia are discussed in Chapter 8.

The above information is provided for safety reasons, as any practitioner using local anaesthetics should know fully of their toxicity potential and how to man-age the established toxicity syndrome. Clinical doses of local anaesthetics as used in eye surgery do not result in high and dangerous systemic levels. The most likely situation that may warrant cardiopulmonary resuscitation is the man-agement of brainstem anaesthesia, which the literature reports as occurring with an incidence of 1 in 350–500 intraconal local anaesthesia injections.[30]

LOCAL ANAESTHETICS COMMONLY USED FOR OPHTHALMIC REGIONAL ANAESTHESIA (Table 6.1)

Lignocaine HCl

Lignocaine (lidocaine in North America; trade name Xylocaine), the first of the amide-linked local anaesthetics, was introduced into clinical practice in the early 1950s. It is commonly used in 1, 1.5 and 2% concentrations, but is also available in North America as a 4% concentration for ophthalmic regional anaesthesia. Its relatively short duration of action in certain circumstances may be a disadvan-tage, but this can be extended by 75% with the addition of adrenaline (see above); in addition, this opposes its inherent vasodilator property. Lignocaine is often regarded as the 'standard' local anaesthetic, because of its fast onset and superb tissue-penetrating properties.

Mepivacaine HCl

Mepivacaine (trade name Carbocaine) is similar to lignocaine in clinical activity and toxicity. Its duration of action is about 50% longer than that of lignocaine because of its lesser inherent vasodilator property. The addition of adrenaline prolongs its action also by about 75%. Unlike lignocaine, mepivacaine is not effective topically.

Bupivacaine HCl

Bupivacaine (trade names Marcaine, Sensorcaine) is an engineered modification of the mepivacaine molecule with increased lipid solubility and protein-binding properties; it therefore has increased potency and a much greater duration of action. Its disadvantages are decreased tissue penetrance with a resultant delayed onset of anaesthesia. Available in 0.25, 0.5 and 0.75% concentrations, the lower concentrations are excellent for sensory anaesthesia; for dependable motor block the higher concentrations are required. The 0.75% concentration is an excellent choice for ophthalmic regional anaesthesia for surgery times in excess of 1.5–2 h. Patients having ophthalmic regional anaesthesia with 0.75% bupivacaine as the sole agent experience a high incidence of diplopia up to, or even beyond, 24 h following blockade. Adrenaline does not prolong the already extended block time of bupivacaine, but is nevertheless used with it for other reasons. Bupivacaine allows for excellent postoperative pain relief compared with the shorter-acting agents.[13] Bupivacaine is more cardiotoxic than lignocaine, but in the doses used in correctly administered ophthalmologic regional anaesthesia this is never seen. In the 0.75% concentration, it is an effective topical corneo-conjunctival anaesthetic.[83]

Etidocaine HCl

Etidocaine (trade name Duranest), available in the Scandinavian countries and the USA, is an engineered modification of the lignocaine molecule with high potency and prolonged duration properties, but, unlike bupivacaine, it has a rapid onset time. It is used clinically in 0.5, 1.0 and 1.5% concentrations. Because of its fast onset and the early availability of motor block compared with bupivacaine it has considerable vogue in ophthalmologic practice.[66,73] As with bupivacaine, patients having ophthalmic regional anaesthesia with etidocaine as the sole agent experience a high incidence of diplopia up to, or even beyond, 24 h following blockade. The drug can be used topically but is rarely used this way.

CLINICAL USE OF MIXTURES OF LOCAL ANAESTHETICS

The compounding of local anaesthesia solutions, despite controversial reports in the literature regarding possible undesirable results,[31] is a common clinical practice.[14] A long-acting but slow-onset agent, typically bupivacaine, is admixed with a fast-onset, shorter-acting agent (such as lignocaine or mepivacaine) in order to produce a mixture incorporating the properties of its constituent parts (i.e. fast onset, long action, excellent postoperative analgesia).[17] In mixtures of local anaesthetics, the final concentrations of each of its constituents is diluted by the presence of the other. Thus 1:1 compounding of lignocaine 2% and bupivacaine 0.5% generates a mixture containing lidocaine 1% and bupivacaine 0.25%. Mulroy states that the toxicity of the drugs contained in a mixture is 'at least additive' and that the mechanisms producing undesirable effects are not fully understood.[51] He advises caution in practising compounding in the light of potential synergistic toxicity. In ophthalmologic regional anaesthesia, in which the total combined mass of drugs required is small, these risks are negligible. The author commonly uses compounding of lignocaine and bupivacaine and is convinced of their safety in combination.[29]

TOPICAL ANAESTHETICS

Topical anaesthesia, essential in the practice of ophthalmology, is used in the testing of intraocular pressure, removal of sutures and small foreign bodies, and in superficial surgery of the conjunctiva and cornea. It is invaluable in preparing the conjunctiva for subsequently painless transconjunctival needle injections. In the early years of the century, much cataract surgery was done with topical cocaine as the sole means of anaesthesia;[36] history is repeating itself, as this practice has again returned (see below and Chapter 7). Table 6.2 displays information about the agents commonly used for topical anaesthesia.

The onset of corneoconjunctival anaesthesia following the instillation of all of the commonly used agents is within 15–20 s and lasts 15–20 min. Stinging is the chief side-effect of topical anaesthetic agents;[78] this may present a problem in paediatric practice. A most useful means of avoiding this stinging is to use proparacaine 0.5% drops (1 ml) diluted in 15 ml sterile balanced salt solution (15 ml plastic bottle readily available in any surgical ophthalmology practice) as a preliminary instillation into the conjunctival sac, prior to the full strength

Table 6.2 Local anaesthetics commonly used for topical corneoconjunctival anaesthesia[a]

Drug	Concentration (%)	Duration (min)	Maximum dose	Corneal toxicity	Miscellaneous
Cocaine	1–4	20	1 mg/kg (20 drops 4%)	++	Vasoconstriction, dilates pupil
Amethocaine	0.5	15	5 mg total (15 drops)	+	Good antibacterial, causes hyperaemia, stings+
Proparacaine	0.5	15	10 mg total (30 drops)	+ −	Poor antibacterial, stings + −
Lignocaine	4	15	3 mg/kg (up to 60 drops)	least	Mild antibacterial, stings + −
Benoxinate	0.4	15	Regular dose up to 12 drops	low	No hyperaemia, stings + −

[a]All are ester-linked agents with the exception of lignocaine.

drops.[36] Ideally, the dilute mixture should be preheated to body temperature before use. Patients should be informed that, during the period of action of the topical anaesthetic, their physiological corneal protective mechanism will be in abeyance; any rubbing of the eye must be discouraged.

Prolonged use of all the commonly used topical agents results in corneal toxicity, cocaine causing the greatest problem, but even proparacaine is not immune.[7] Cell division and migration are inhibited and epithelial defect healing delayed.[57,78] Alteration of lacrimation and tear film instability may also occur; certain preservatives (benzalkonium chloride and chlorobutanol) present in topical corneoconjunctival anaesthetics may be implicated in this effect.[12] If a local tissue reaction to one of these agents occurs, switching to one of the others almost invariably solves the problem. Idiosyncratic reactions are rarely seen, but nevertheless can be dramatic.[47] The rate of drug absorption across mucous membranes is intermediate between intravenous injection and subcutaneous injection and is not influenced by the addition of adrenaline to topical preparations. Therefore, topically administered ophthalmic drugs are capable of attaining clinically significant serum concentrations; side-effects may be experienced, including interaction with patients' other medications.[27] Digital occlusion of the lacrimal puncta at the nasal side of the palpebral fissure is useful in preventing medication from entering the nasolacrimal duct to gain access to further mucosal surfaces from which additional absorption can occur; compression should be maintained for 30 s until the excess medication and tearing have been blinked clear and removed with paper tissue. Particularly with the topical anaesthetics, it is important not to exceed safe clinical doses, as serious and even fatal reactions do occur with overdosing.[24] All drugs are foreign to the human organism and the rationale for their use must be carefully weighed in the risk *vs* benefit balance.[46]

Cocaine HCl

Historically the earliest of the local anaesthetics, cocaine is unique in that, in addition to anaesthesia, the drug promotes vasoconstriction by blocking re-uptake of noradrenaline and adrenaline into sympathetic nerve endings, allowing their accumulation at active receptor sites. Its most common clinical use is as a topical anaesthetic (4–20% concentration) for surface anaesthesia, primarily of the upper respiratory tract. Topical application of cocaine has been considered its only safe clinical use since 1924.[24] Its use for topical corneoconjunctival anaesthesia (limited to 4% maximum) is declining because it produces clouding of the cornea and even ulceration of its surface,[78] and is being replaced by safer alternatives.[76] However, its ability to produce dependable corneal anaesthesia concurrently with conjunctival vasoconstriction and pupil dilatation (sympathomimetic effects) make it a unique and useful clinical tool. No single synthetic topical anaesthetic thus far available can reproduce on its own the unique properties of cocaine.[24] Admixture with adrenaline is controversial and best avoided; although adrenaline delays systemic release of topically applied cocaine, it does so inconsistently. The *Drug Evaluation Handbook* of the American Medical Association suggests a maximum safe dose of 1mg/kg for topical use,[24] whereas twice that amount is recommended as being safe by Watt.[76] Cocaine, released systemically, increases cardiac work simultaneously with reducing oxygen supply from coronary vasoconstriction. Particularly in situations in which there are high levels of endogenous catecholamines, dangerous and even fatal dysrhythmias may occur. Centrally, cocaine causes euphoria and arousal and is biphasic in action, being anticonvulsant at lower doses and convulsant at higher doses. With modern understanding of its addiction potential and toxicity, when these factors are controlled by limitation of access and adherence to appropriate dosage schedules, a restricted place may be found for the drug in contemporary practice. For a comprehensive review article on cocaine, the reader is referred to the publication by Fleming and her colleagues.[24]

Proparacaine HCl

An ester-linked agent, proparacaine 0.5% (trade names Alcaine, Ophthaine), produces a rapid onset of corneoconjunctival anaesthesia with the least amount of stinging (see below). For applanation tonometry, one or two drops given immediately prior to the measurement is all that is required. For deeper anaesthesia, one drop every 5 min for about five doses is required. Facial contact dermatitis is more common with proparacaine than any other topical anaesthetic.[57]

Benoxinate HCl

Ester-linked benoxinate (trade name Dorsacaine) is used in 0.4% solution and is comparable to proparacaine in the amount of stinging that it causes. In combination with 0.25% fluorescein sodium (trade name Fluress), it is commonly used in diagnostic testing, removal of foreign bodies and contact lens fitting.[64]

Amethocaine HCl

Another ester-linked agent, amethocaine 0.5% (tetracaine in North America, trade names Pontocaine, Anethaine), is commonly used for corneoconjunctival anaesthesia and is available in solution and ointment forms; it has a slower onset time and a considerable stinging side-effect when compared with proparacaine. The deeper corneal anaesthesia it produces makes it more suitable for minor surgical procedures. Like cocaine, amethocaine may cause cardiac dysrhythmias or ventricular fibrillation and should be regarded as extremely toxic.[24] A direct action on local blood vessels results in vasodilatation.[76]

Lignocaine HCl

Lignocaine in 4% concentration in water is isotonic and an effective topical anaesthetic with common usage in ophthalmology. Of the available corneoconjunctival anaesthetics, it is the least toxic to the corneal epithelium and produces deep anaesthesia with a relatively long duration of action.[44] For the current vogue of phacoemulsification cataract extraction surgery with small wound clear corneal incision and foldable intraocular lens implantation, carried out under solely topical corneoconjunctival anaesthesia, lignocaine 4% is frequently used.[37]

EUTECTIC MIXTURE OF LOCAL ANAESTHETICS

Topical anaesthesia of mucous membranes is simple to achieve because their penetration barrier to several local anaesthetic agents is weak. Skin is much more resistant, however. The skin barrier can be overcome by mixing solid lignocaine and prilocaine in a way that leaves them liquid at room temperature; this liquid added to a special oil and water emulsion results in a compound, known as eutectic mixture of local anaethetics (EMLA), with the properties necessary to penetrate skin.[19] The ability to penetrate is enhanced by occlusion under a plastic enclosure closely applied to the skin. It has been used to alleviate the pain of percutaneous needle placement for intraconal block.[68]

REFERENCES

1. Aboul-Eish EI. Epinephrine improves the quality of spinal hyperbaric bupivacaine for Cesarean section. *Anesth Analg* 1987; **66**: 395.
2. Aldrete JA, Romo-Salas F, Arora S *et al*. Revese arterial blood flow as a pathway for central nervous system toxic responses following injection of local anesthetics. *Anesth Analg* 1978; **57**: 428.
3. Apel A, Woodward R. Cataract surgery – anaesthesia without hyaluronidase (Letter). *Aust NZ J Ophthalmol* 1991; **19**: 249.
4. Atkinson WS. Local anesthesia in ophthalmology. *Trans Am Ophthmol Soc* 1934; **32**: 399.
5. Atkinson WS. Observations on anesthesia for ocular surgery. *Trans Am Acad Ophthalmol Otolaryngol* 1956; **60**: 376.
6. Benhamou D, Labaille T, Bonhomme L, Perrachon N. Alkalinization of epidural 0.5 per cent bupivacaine for Cesarean section. *Reg Anesth* 1989; **14**: 240.
7. Brent MH, Slomovic AR, Easterbrook M. Keratitis associated with the use of proparacaine hydrochloride. *CMAJ* 1987; **136**: 380.
8. Britton RC, Habif DV. Clinical uses of hyaluronidase: A current review. *Surgery* 1953; **33**: 917.
9. Bromage PR. Mechanism of action of extradural analgesia. *Br J Anaesth* 1975; **47**(suppl.): 199.
10. Bromage PR. *Epidural Analgesia*. W.B. Saunders: Philadelphia, PA, 1978: 358–360.
11. Brown DT, Beamish D, Wildsmith JAW. Allergic reaction to an amide local anaesthetic. *Br J Anaesth* 1981; **53**: 435.
12. Burstein NL. Corneal cytotoxicity of topically applied drugs, vehicles and preservatives. *Surv Ophthalmol* 1980; **25**: 15.
13. Chin GN, Almquist HT. Bupivacaine and lidocaine retrobulbar anesthesia: A double-blind clinical study. *Ophthalmology* 1983; **90**: 369.
14. Cohen SE. The rational use of local anesthetic mixtures. *Reg Anesth* 1979; **4**: 11.
15. Covino BG. Potential neurotoxicity of local anesthetic agents. *Can Anaesth Soc J* 1983; **30**: 111.
16. deJong RH, Heavener JE. Diazepam prevents and aborts lidocaine convulsions in monkeys. *Anesthesiology* 1974; **41**: 226.
17. Donlon JV. Local anesthesia for ophthalmic surgery: Patient preparation and management. *Ann Ophthalmol* 1980; **12**: 1183.
18. Eccarius SG, Gordon ME, Parelman JJ. Bicarbonate-buffered lidocaine–epinephrine–hyaluronidase for eyelid anesthesia. *Ophthalmology* 1990; **97**: 1499.
19. Ehrenstrom GME, Reiz SLA. EMLA – a eutectic mixture of local anesthetics for topical anesthesia. *Acta Anaesth Scand* 1982; **26**: 596.

20. Feitl ME, Krupin T. Neural blockade for ophthalmologic surgery. In *Neural Blockade in Clinical Anesthesia and Management of Pain,* 2nd edn (edited by Cousins MJ, Bridenbaugh PO). JB Lippincott: Philadelphia, PA, 1988: 580.
21. Feitl ME, Krupin T. Retrobulbar anesthesia. *Ophthalmol Clin North Am* 1990; **3:** 83.
22. Fink BR, Aasheim GM, Levy BA. Neural pharmacokinetcs of epinephrine. *Anesthesiology* 1978; **48:** 263.
23. Fink BR. Mechanisms of differential axial blockade in epidural and subarachnoid anesthesia. *Anesthesiology* 1989; **70:** 851.
24. Fleming JA, Byck R, Barash PG. Pharmacolocy and therapeutic applications of cocaine. *Anesthesiology* 1990; **73:** 518.
25. Galindo A, Keilson LR, Mondshine RB, Sawelson HI. Retro-peribulbar anesthesia. *Ophthalmol Clin North Am* 1990; **3:** 71.
26. Gentili F, Hudson AR, Hunter D, Kline DG. Nerve injection injury with local anesthetic agents: A light and electron microscopic, fluorescent microscopic and horseradish peroxidase study. *Neurosurgery* 1980; **6:** 263.
27. Gerber SL, Cantor LB, Brater DC. Systemic drug interactions with topical glaucoma medications. *Surv Ophthalmol* 1990; **35:** 205.
28. Gissen AJ, Datta S, Lambert D. The chloroprocaine controversy. II. Is chloroprocaine neurotoxic? *Reg Anesth* 1984; **9:** 135.
29. Hamilton RC, Gimbel HV, Strunin L. Regional anaesthesia for 12 000 cataract extraction and intraocular lens implantation procedures. *Can J Anaesth* 1988; **35:** 615.
30. Hamilton RC. Brain-stem anesthesia as a complication of regional anesthesia for ophthalmic surgery. *Can J Ophthalmol* 1992; **27:** 323.
31. Hartrick CT, Raj PP, Dirkes WE, Denson DD. Compounding of bupivacaine and mepivacaine for regional anesthesia: A safe practice? *Reg Anesth* 1984; **9:** 94.
32. Hessemer V, Wieth K, Heinrich A, Jacobi KW. Changes in uveal and retinal hemodynamics produced by retrobulbar anesthesia with different injection volumes. *Fortschr Ophthalmol* 1989; **86:** 760.
33. Hessemer V, Heinrich A, Jacobi KW. Ocular circulatory changes induced by retrobulbar anesthesia with and without adrenaline. *Klin Mbl Augenheilk* 1990; **197:** 470.
34. Hilgier M. Alkalinization of bupivacaine for brachial plexus block. *Reg Anesth* 1985; **10:** 59.
35. Hørven I. Ophthalmic artery pressure during retrobulbar anesthesia. *Acta Ophthalmol* 1978; **56:** 574.
36. Hustead RF, Hamilton RC. Pharmacology. In *Ophthalmic Anesthesia* (edited by Gills JP, Hustead RF, Sanders DR). Slack Inc.: Thorofare, NJ, 1993: 69–102.
37. Hustead RF, Hamilton RC. Techniques. In *Ophthalmic Anesthesia* (edited by Gills JP, Hustead RF, Sanders DR). Slack Inc.: Thorofare, NJ, 1993: 103–186.
38. Incaudo G, Schatz M, Patterson R *et al*. Administration of local anesthetics to patients with a history of prior adverse reaction. *J Allergy Clin Immunol* 1978; **61:** 339.
39. Katz RL, Epstein RA. The interaction of anesthetic agents and adrenergic drugs to produce cardiac arrhythmias. *Anesthesiology* 1968; **29:** 763.
40. Lewis P, Hamilton RC, Loken RG *et al*. Comparison of plain with pH-adjusted bupivacaine with hyaluronidase for peribulbar block. *Can J Anaesth* 1992; **39:** 555.
41. Lincoff H, Zweifach P, Brodie S *et al*. Intraocular injection of lidocaine. *Ophthalmology* 1985; **92:** 1587.
42. Livingston MW, Mackool RJ, Schneider H. Anesthetic agents used in cataract surgery (Letter). *J Cataract Refract Surg* 1990; **16:** 272.
43. Manka RL, Gast TJ. Sodium bicarbonate reduces pain associated with ophthalmic nerve blocks. *Refract Corneal Surg* 1991; **7:** 186.
44. Marr WG, Wood R, Senterfit L, Sigelman S. Effect of topical anesthesia on regeneration of corneal epithelium. *Am J Ophthalmol* 1957; **43:** 606.
45. McMorland GH, Douglas MJ, Jeffrey WK *et al*. Effect of pH-adjustment of

bupivacaine on onset and duration of epidural analgesia in parturients. *Can Anaesth Soc J* 1986; **33:** 537.

46. McWhae JA, Chang J, Lipton JH. Drug-induced fatal aplastic anemia following cataract surgery. *Can J Ophthalmol* 1992; **27:** 313.
47. Meyer D, Hamilton RC, Gimbel HV. Myasthenia gravis-like syndrome induced by topical ophthalmic preparations: A case report. *J Clin Neuro-ophthalmol* 1992; **12:** 210.
48. Meyers EF, Ramirez RC, Boniuk I. Grand mal seizures after retrobulbar block. *Arch Ophthalmol* 1978; **96:** 847.
49. Moller RA, Covino BG. Cardiac electrophysiologic effects of lidocaine and bupivacaine. *Anesth Analg* 1988; **67:** 107.
50. Moore DC. The pH of local anesthetic solutions. *Anesth Analg* 1981; **60:** 833.
51. Mulroy MF. Clinical characteristics of local anesthetics. In *Regional Anesthesia: An Illustrated Procedural Guide*. Little, Brown and Company: Boston, MA, 1989: 23–25.
52. Nicoll JMV, Treuren B, Acharya PA *et al*. Retrobulbar anesthesia: The role of hyaluronidase. *Anesth Analg* 1986; **65:** 1324.
53. Philip BK, Covino BG. Local and regional anesthesia. In *Anesthesia for Ambulatory Surgery*, 2nd edn (edited by Wetchler BV). JB Lippincott: Philadelphia, PA, 1991: 357.
54. Raymond SA, Steffensen SC, Gugino LD, Strichartz GR. The role of length of nerve exposed to local anesthetic in impulse blocking action. *Anesth Analg* 1989; **68:** 563.
55. Reynolds F. Allergy reaction to an amide local anaesthetic. *Br J Anaesth* 1981; **53:** 901.
56. Rosenquist RW, Finucane BT, Berman S. Hyaluronidase and axillary brachial block: Effect of latency and plasma levels of mepivacaine (abstract). *Reg Anesth* 1989, **14:** 50.
57. Rossenwasser GOD. Complications of topical ocular anesthetics. *Int Ophthalmol Clin* 1989; **29:** 153.
58. Ropo A, Nikki P, Ruusuvaara P, Kivisaari L. Comparison of retrobulbar and periocular injections of lignocaine by computerised tomography. *Br J Ophthalmol* 1991; **75:** 417.
59. Sarvela J, Nikki P. Hyaluronidase improves regional ophthalmic anaesthesia with etidocaine. *Can J Anaesth* 1992; **39:** 9.
60. Scott DB, Jebson PJR, Braid DP *et al*. Factors affecting plasma levels of lignocaine and prilocaine. *Br J Anaesth* 1972; **44:** 1040.
61. Selander D, Dhunér KG, Lundborg G. Peripheral nerve injury due to injection needles used for regional anesthesia. *Acta Anaesthesiol Scand* 1977; **21:** 182.
62. Selander D, Sjöstrand J. Longitudinal spread of intraneurally injected local anesthetics. *Acta Anaesthesiol Scand* 1978; **22:** 622.
63. Selander D, Brattsand R, Lundborg G *et al*. Local anesthetics: Importance of mode of application, concentration and adrenaline for the appearance of nerve lesions. *Acta Anaesthesiol Scand* 1979; **23:** 127.
64. Schlegel HE, Swan KC. Benoxinate (Dorsacaine) for rapid corneal anesthesia. *Arch Ophthalmol* 1954; **51:** 663.
65. Smith HS, Carpenter RL, Bridenbaugh LD. Failure rate of tetracaine spinal anesthesia with and without epinephrine. *Anesthesiology* 1986; **65:** A193.
66. Smith PH, Smith ER. A comparison of etidocaine and lidocaine for retrobulbar anesthesia. *Ophthalmic Surg* 1983; **14:** 569.
67. Stevens RA, Chester WL, Grueter JA *et al*. The effect of pH adjustment of 0.5 per cent bupivacaine on the latency of epidural anesthesia. *Reg Anesth* 1989; **14:** 236.
68. Sunderraj P, Kirby J, Joyce PW, Watson A. A double-masked evaluation of lignocaine–prilocaine cream (EMLA) used to alleviate the pain of retrobulbar injection. *Br J Ophthalmol* 1991; **75:** 130.
69. Szmyd S, Nelson LB, Calhoun JH, Harley RD. Retrobulbar anesthesia in strabismus surgery. *Arch Ophthalmol* 1984; **102:** 1325.
70. Takman B. The chemistry of local anaesthetic agents. *Br J Anaesth* 1975; **47:** 183.
71. Taylor IS, Pollowitz JA. Allergy to hyaluronidase. *Ophthalmology* 1984; **91:** 1003.
72. Thomson I. Addition of hyaluronidase to lignocaine with adrenaline for retrobulbar anaesthesia in the surgery of senile cataract. *Br J Ophthalmol* 1988; **72:** 700.

73. Thorburn W, Thorn-Alquist AM, Edström H. Etidocaine in retrobulbar anaesthesia: A comparison with mepivacaine. *Acta Ophthalmol* 1976; **54:** 591.

74. Thornton SP. Ocular anesthesia with the Thornton retrobulbar needle. In *Ophthalmic Anesthesia* (edited by Gills JP, Hustead RF, Sanders DR). Slack Inc.: Thorofare, NJ, 1993: 155–159.

75. Tucker GT. Clinically pertinent pharmacology of local anaesthetic drugs. *Curr Opinion Anaesth* 1990; **3:** 727.

76. Watt MJ. The pharmacology of local analgesic agents. In *Practical Regional Analgesia* (edited by Lee JA, Bryce-Smith R). Excerpta Medica: Amsterdam, 1976: 1–32.

77. Watt MJ. The pharmacology of pressor drugs. In *Practical Regional Analgesia* (edited by Lee JA, Bryce-Smith R). Excerpta Medica: Amsterdam, 1976: 33–36.

78. Wilson RP. Complications associated with local and general ophthalmic anesthesia. *Int Ophthalmol Clin* 1992; **32:** 1.

79. Yagiela JA, Benoit PW, Buoncristiani RD *et al*. Comparison of myotoxic effects of lidocaine with epinephrine in rats and humans. *Anesth Analg* 1981; **60:** 471.

80. Zahl K, Jordan A, McGroarty J, Gotta AW. pH-adjusted bupivacaine and hyaluronidase for peribulbar block. *Anesthesiology* 1990; **72:** 230.

81. Zahl K, Jordan A, McGroarty *et al*. Peribulbar anesthesia: Effect of bicarbonate on mixtures of lidocaine, bupivacaine, and hyaluronidase with or without epinephrine. *Ophthalmology* 1991; **98:** 239.

82. Zahl K, Nassif JM, Meltzer MA, Som P. Simulated peribulbar injection of anesthetic. *Ann Ophthalmol* 1991; **23:** 114.

83. Gills JP, Williams DL. Advantage of Marcaine for topical anesthesia. *J Cataract Refract Surg* 1993; **19:** 819.

84. Kempeneers A, Dralands L, Ceuppens J. Hyaluronidase induce orbital pseudotumor as complication of retrobulbar anesthesia. *Bull Soc Belge Ophthalmol* 1992; **243:** 159.

85. McLoon LK, Wirtschafter J. Regional differences in the subacute response of rabbit orbicularis oculi to bupivacaine-induced mytotoxicity as quantified with a neural cell adhesion molecule immunohistochemical marker. *Invest Ophthalmol Vis Sci* 1993; **34:** 3450.

86. Selander D. Neurotoxicity of local anesthetics. *Regional Anesth* 1993; **18:** 461.

CHAPTER 7

Techniques of orbital regional anaesthesia

ROBERT C HAMILTON

HISTORICAL

Pre-1900

A crude alkaloid was extracted from coca leaves in 1855 by Gaedcke, and was purified and named cocaine 5 years later by Neiman, who noted that it 'benumbs the nerves of the tongue, depriving it of feeling and taste'. It was to be another 25 years before Koller, collaborating with Sigmund Freud, reported in August 1884 the use of cocaine as a topical anaesthetic for minor surgery of the conjunctiva.[12] The discovery rapidly spread across the Atlantic where, in New York City, ophthalmologist Dr Herman Knapp published in December of the same year his report of its use in all branches of surgery. This publication included his own report of retrobulbar injection of cocaine for painless enucleation of an eye: 'Cocaine four per cent was instilled, then the globe was rotated toward the nose with forceps and a needle was introduced through the conjunctiva temporally into the muscular cone just posterior to the globe and six minims of a four per cent solution of cocaine were injected. The eye was then enucleated without pain'.[64] Because of serious toxic effects experienced with cocaine injected in larger doses for nerve blocks, particularly in general surgery, this deterred ophthalmologists from injecting local anaesthetics until well into the twentieth century.[12]

Early twentieth century

In 1901 and 1905, respectively, adrenaline and procaine were discovered, and safer blocks became possible but were not introduced into ophthalmology practice for many years. Solely topical corneoconjuctival anaesthesia with cocaine was being employed for cataract extraction procedures, apparently successfully. In 1910, Hirschberg reported thousands of cases and 'encountered only advantages, never a single disadvantage . . .'.[50]

In 1914, van Lint reported his classic facial nerve block technique, removing the problem of forceful contraction of the orbicularis muscle, which had been feared for many years.[12,123] This and other methods of facial muscle akinesia[29] were commonly used as complements to corneoconjunctival topical anaesthesia until the 1930s, by which time retrobulbar blocking using procaine had become widespread.[28] It is salutary to review a few of the classic contributions of earlier generation ophthalmologists in order to appreciate the great insights that they had, despite limitations imposed by the drugs and equipment available at the time, and also because we can learn much that is appropriate to our current practice by studying their methods.

Literature classics in ophthalmic anaesthesia

W S Atkinson published articles on regional anaesthesia for ophthalmologic surgery from 1934 to 1964.[6-14] At the time of his earliest writings procaine was the anaesthetic in use, but hyaluronidase was not available; therefore, the volume of injection had to be limited to around 1.5 ml anaesthetic solution and adrenaline was added to the anaesthetic for its prolongation effect. In 1936, he stressed that for best results the injection should be within the cone and 'just posterior to the globe'. He was well aware from the work of Löwenstein[76] that deep orbital placement of needles could pierce the optic nerve with serious consequences. From the work of Duverger[26] he knew that the optic nerve and apical vessels were in danger when 5-cm needles were used and that the optic nerve was more mobile at a depth of 3.5 cm and could 'always elude' the needle. Atkinson advocated the inferotemporal quadrant as being safe, relatively avascular and having the best angle of approach to the intracone space; the depth range for his needle placement was 2.5–3.5 cm ('depending on the size of the orbit') using a 3.5-cm 25 gauge rounded tip needle with test aspiration before injection.[8] Atkinson designated a retrobular injection at this depth as a 'cone injection' and it included the directive to have the patient turn the eye 'up and away from the site of injection'. Although he taught and promoted this shorter needle method for its safety, he indicated that in 1961 it had not been generally accepted.[12] In the 'up and in' globe position, the intermuscular septum between the inferior and lateral rectus muscles, which he was aware existed only anteriorly, 'moved forward and up out of the way' of the needle entering the cone. In modern practice (see below and Chapter 8) this 'up and in' teaching has been abandoned for safety reasons. With the limitations imposed in the 1930s by non-availability of hyaluronidase, there was often poor akinesia of the globe and inadequate anaesthesia at the superior limbus. To counter this, Atkinson used supplemental subconjunctival local anaesthetic injection at that site to achieve patient comfort. The peribulbar method was described as long ago as 1914 by Allen,[4] but did not come into common practice until 1986.[23]

The 1950s and 1960s

In 1956, Swan emphasized that the term retrobulbar can embrace a variety of depth techniques whose 'effects vary markedly with the site and depth of the injection, with the concentration and quantity of the anaesthetic solution, and with the nature of the added adjuvant'.[117] He singled out three previously described techniques, each employing a different depth of drug placement within the muscle cone: In 1949, Gifford had described a deep apical placement 'most productive of a high percentage of oculomotor blocking' using a 5-cm needle.[35] This block, by removal of extraocular muscle tone, resulted in reduction in intraocular tension. O'Brien's 'retrobulbar' (1934) was immediately behind the globe, could be achieved with a 2.5-cm needle and consequently 'motor effects are absent or minimal'. It produced only sensory and autonomic effects from blockade of the ciliary nerves.[91] Atkinson's 1936 'cone' technique[7] described above was at a depth of about 3 cm and, when administered in sufficient volume and in combination with adrenaline and hyaluronidase (available to Swan in 1956), produced sensory and motor block in addition to hypotony. Swan warned of the risk of serious bleeding from apical vessels with the Gifford technique and of muscle injury from anaesthetic injection directly into an extraocular muscle with any of the techniques. Figure 7.1, taken from Swan's paper, illustrates needles located at the two extremes of retrobulbar placement.

Introduction of lignocaine (lidocaine) and hyaluronidase

Lignocaine was synthesized by Löfgren and Lundqvist in 1943 and first used clinically by Gordh in 1947; this represented a most significant advance.

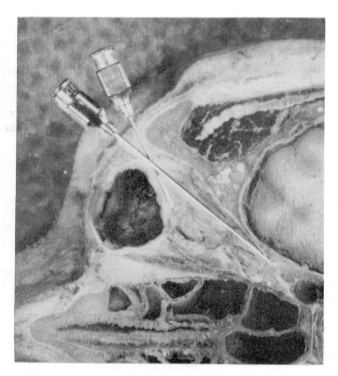

Fig. 7.1. Transverse section through the orbit at the level of the medial and lateral rectus muscles, showing the relative positions of needles in the intracone space, anteriorly (25-mm needle) and apical (50-mm needle). (With permission from ref. 117.)

Atkinson commented on the improved penetrating properties and duration of action of lignocaine over procaine.[11] In the same paper he stated that hyaluronidase, which by then was in widespread use, 'has done more than any other thing in recent years to prevent complications, particularly vitreous loss during intraocular surgery'. Although its use tended to shorten the duration of anaesthesia, this effect was effectively countered by admixture with adrenaline. Larger volumes ('3.0 to 4.0 or more')[12,13] injected within the muscle cone 'until there is a noticeable proptosis' were now possible. With digital pressure following the block the proptosis quickly subsided and greatly improved anaesthesia, akinesia and hypotony resulted, compared with the hitherto low-volume non-hyaluronidase techniques. 'The lowered vitreous pressure was due in a measure to a decrease of blood within the choroid and ciliary body. The decrease of blood was thought to be the result of constriction of the arteries entering the globe caused by epinephrine [adrenaline]. It was also noted that if the concentration of epinephrine in the anaesthetic solution was increased the hypotony increased'.[12] This capacity of adrenaline to produce globe hypotony has since been disputed.[40] If supplemental blocking was required for persistent extraocular movement (most commonly superior rectus), Atkinson preferred to use a superotemporal injection and delayed it until the onset of anaesthesia in the upper lid, about 2 min after the inferotemporal injection, in the interests of patient comfort.[12]

The modern era in ophthalmic regional anaesthesia

With the introduction of mepivacaine in 1957 and its engineered modification, bupivacaine, in 1963, the stage was set for dependable clinical regional anaesthesia to cover a range of surgical times and to provide greatly improved postoperative analgesia. In the USA from the late 1960s onward, cost containment along with the rising population of the elderly became the impetus for the rising popularity of ambulatory surgery facilities. In 1980, those aged 65 years or more represented 11% of the US population; by 2020, this group is expected to constitute 16% of the population.[63] In 1977, Kahn *et al.* reported that 46% of a group of Americans aged over 75 years surveyed had cataracts.[58] Cataract extraction surgery, therefore, accounted for the bulk of this type of anaesthesia. Technical advances in cataract extraction and intraocular lens implantation had made it possible for a surgeon to perform many procedures at one operating session, particularly if an anaesthetist colleague had become competent at orbital regional anaesthesia. Heretofore these blocks had been done by the operating ophthalmologist intermittently between surgeries. A recent survey of those clinics in the USA in which more than 50 cataract surgeries were done weekly found that in 56% the anaesthetist had taken over this traditional role of the ophthalmologist.[68] The number of annual cataract and intraocular lens implantation procedures in USA climbed from 250 000 in 1967 to over 1.3 million in 1992.[53,111]

BASIC ADVICE FOR THE ANAESTHETIST ABOUT TO EMBARK ON OPHTHALMIC REGIONAL ANAESTHESIA

The anaesthetist taking on this type of practice ideally should train well in the basic science disciplines (pharmacology of the ocular and local anaesthetic drugs, physiology of the eye, anatomy of the orbit and its contents) so as not to incur criticism and opposition from ophthalmologists because of a high complication rate.[44,47,71] Would-be practitioners in the art and science of ophthalmic regional anaesthesia, before attempting to assimilate the necessary expertise from books or colleagues who do this type of work occasionally, are encouraged to observe centres operated by personnel with wide experience and knowledge. The goal for each practitioner is to build up an experiential database from which increasingly good judgement can result.

It is essential that the anaesthetist has a good understanding of the operating ophthalmologist's preferred conditions for the surgery. The anaesthesia requirements are dictated by the type and operative technique of the surgery in hand, the surgeon's particular preferences and the wishes of the patient. Many surgeons do not strive for complete akinesia, nor is it necessary in all cases; its achievement by virtue of demanding higher volume orbital injectate may have disadvantages. Again, although most surgeons prefer globe hypotony, there may be some situations where this is undesirable.

Surgeons operating under good regional anaesthesia have to know how to deal with the awake patient on the operating table. O'Brien's (1928) words cannot be improved upon: 'It is unwise to ask repeatedly whether the operation is painful; if it is painful, it is usually not difficult to see that such is the case; while if it is not, it is poor judgement to suggest it to the patient and let him feel that the surgeon does not have confidence in the anesthesia'.[90] The surgeon who knows and trusts a carefully selected staff team should start the operation without fuss and be aware of significant non-verbal responses on the part of the patient.

Patient preparation and practical management

Careful psychological preparation and assessment of the patient are essential. For patients to be relatively accepting of the situation and at ease, they must receive a careful explanation from the physicians and staff of the procedures that lie ahead on the day of surgery.[8] This will include obtaining written informed consent; the word 'informed' implies time spent with patients using some format of explanation. Spaeth suggests that the use of the word 'consent' in the patient–physician relationship is part and parcel of a paternalistic model of medicine; rather, the agreement to proceed with surgery should be seen by patients as their informed choice in response to having trusted their physician.[109] Patients should be given the opportunity to ask questions and receives answers. An excellent British article addresses the issues of informed consent for cataract surgery and includes a suggested form of consent.[45]

Depending on the details of the technique to be used and the intended surgery, preanaesthetic medication may or may not be indicated. It is good routine practice, even where intravenous medications are not part of the planned regime, to set up a fine venous access cannula in the event of unplanned interventions calling for intravenous therapy. Good notekeeping about medical history and health status, type and length of surgical procedure, anaesthetic record and the patient's reaction during the anaesthetic procedure are all important; such data should be systematically recorded. Choice of local anaesthetic drug, its volume of injection, injection sites, decompression pressures, axial length, intraocular pressures, etc., are legitimate items for inclusion in the record. Patients are requested to continue any regular medications right through the operative period, which may include the use of anticoagulants and anti-inflammatory agents (see Chapter 8). The question of whether to maintain patients fasting for some hours prior to short case eye surgery under regional block often will depend on local clinic or hospital regulations. Recent publications are in support of clear fluids being given up to 3 h preoperatively.[77,103] Regular medications are continued up to and on the day of surgery. Hearing aids and dentures are left in place. Patients with dementia and language barriers are discussed in Chapter 5. A foolproof system of drug and solution type and concentration checking in the anaesthetic room and the operating theatre is essential if dangerous errors and damage are to be avoided.[79] Smoothness and safety are ensured by attention to detail. Personal confidence is acquired with repeated use of regional anaesthesia techniques,[91] and, in response to that increased confidence, patients are more stable and reassured, less dependent on premedicant drugs.[83]

It is worthwhile to ask the patient whether there is a history of claustrophobia or, more rarely, panic attacks; it is the author's experience that 25% of people are bothered to some degree with surgical drapes encroaching on their face. Alternative draping techniques can be used[34] or light intravenous sedation administered. Patients should be encouraged to express any concerns in any part of the perioperative period. They must never be left unattended; it is good practice to engage patients in light conversation during both initiation of the anaesthesia and at times during the surgery. In doing so, patients declare their well-being and act as their own monitor. While working with a particular patient, conversations between staff regarding other patients are inappropriate.

Attention to the posture of patients intraoperatively is important. Many undergoing intraocular surgery are elderly; painful arthritis, osteoporosis and kyphosis are common and it is frequently anatomically impossible for them to accommodate themselves with little or no head elevation. The surgeon usually prefers the head in a horizontal plane but this is still achievable with a small pillow under the occiput combined with the necessary extension at the atlanto-occipital joint.[72]

WHAT TYPES OF SURGERY CAN BE UNDERTAKEN UNDER REGIONAL ANAESTHESIA?

Many ophthalmic procedures, such as cataract extraction with introcular lens implantation, corneal transplants, trabeculectomy, lid surgery, strabismus repair and vitrectomy and repair of detached retina (the latter may require postoperative hospital admission; see below), can be performed safely in an outpatient setting using regional anaesthesia with appropriate mild sedation if indicated. Operations extending beyond 1.5–2 h on conscious patients tend to be rather taxing on the elderly; a decision must be made early on as to the preferred method of management (see Chapter 5). A wide range of drugs is now available with which the duration of a safe therapeutic window usually can be predictably planned. For instance, when working with an experienced cataract surgeon doing a series of several uncomplicated cataract extraction and lens implantation procedures, orbital regional anaesthesia adeptly administered using lignocaine 2% with 1:200 000 adrenaline and hyaluronidase 7.5 turbidity units per ml will produce a dependable 90-min therapeutic window of complete akinesia in each case.[73] On the other hand, if regional anaesthesia is the chosen method, for a surgical procedure expected to last 2–2.5 h (e.g. surgery for reattachment of retina), either of the long-acting agents, bupivacaine or etidocaine, should be the agent of choice and it should be used in a high enough concentration to achieve akinesia if this is the wish of the surgeon. Either of these agents will produce a therapeutic window of 3–4 h. Choice of anaesthesia agent, therefore, depends on the surgical requirement; however, the author feels strongly that hyaluronidase as an adjuvant in the injectate is important.[2,9,89]

CURRENT TECHNIQUES

Until recently (see innovative techniques, below) the regional anaesthesia requirements for intraocular surgery, as established in the 1950s and 1960s, were threefold: globe and conjunctival anaesthesia; globe, lid and periorbital akinesia; and intraocular hypotony. An earlier generation of ophthalmologists (as outlined at the start of this chapter) had established that these desirable operating conditions were safely attainable using relatively large volumes of hyaluronidase-containing local anaesthetic injected within the muscle cone. Digital decompression following anaesthetic injection to disperse the agent within the orbit and obtain the benefit of added hypotony was frequently employed. Mechanical orbital decompression devices were introduced in modern times for the more efficient production of hypotony.[18,22,36,80]

Applied anatomy

A matrix of connective tissues, which supports and allows dynamic function of the orbital contents, also controls the mode of anaesthetic injectate spread.[67] Globe and conjunctival anaesthesia (resulting from conduction block of the intraorbital sensory divisions of the ophthalmic branch of the trigeminal nerve) are more easily achieved than globe akinesia (conduction block of intraorbital portions of oculomotor cranial nerves III, IV and VI).

The oculomotor nerves enter the muscle bellies of the four rectus muscles from their conal surface 1.0–1.5 cm from the apex of the orbit (Fig. 7.2). Local anaesthetics in blocking concentration have to reach an exposed 5–10 mm segment of these motor nerves in the posterior intracone space for block of those nerves and akinesia of their supplied muscles to occur. Injectate placed intraconally will achieve motor blocking concentration more easily and with smaller volume than when an extraconal method is used. The motor nerve to the inferior oblique runs a long intraconal course and is therefore relatively easily blocked. However, the motor nerve to the superior oblique muscle (cranial nerve IV; trochlear) runs a short intraorbital, but extraconal, course (Fig. 7.2) before entering the muscle at its superolateral edge; retained activity of this muscle is frequently seen after intraconal local anaesthetic injection because of this anatomical difference.

The sensory and autonomic nerves, as compared with the motor nerves (inferior oblique muscle is an exception), have a longer course from their point of

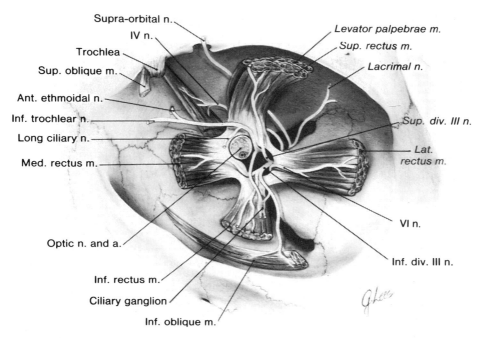

Fig. 7.2. This illustration includes detail of the motor innervation of the extraocular muscles. The four rectus muscles are innervated from their conal surfaces. Note the long course of the nerve to the inferior oblique (branch of Inf. div. III n.). The trochlear nerve (IV n.) remains outside the muscle cone and enters the superior oblique at its superolateral edge. (With permission from ref. 129.)

entry into the orbit at the apex to reach the globe and anterior structures; local anaesthetic injectate therefore has greater potential access to these nerves. Mainly because of these anatomic differences, conduction block of sensory and autonomic nerves precedes that of motor nerves following orbital regional anaesthetic injection. Corneal and perilimbal conjunctival sensation is mediated through the nasociliary nerve, which lies within the cone of muscles; intracone blocks therefore effectively produce anaesthesia of the cornea and the conjunctiva immediately surrounding it. The sensation of the peripheral conjunctiva, however, is supplied through the lacrimal, frontal and infraorbital nerves coursing outside the muscle cone;[8] surgical pain may be experienced in this area following a solely intracone block.[46]

Globe position

For inferotemporal needle placement the globe is best directed in primary gaze or even 'down and out'.[56,93,122] Because the 'down and out' position has the disadvantages of its making an approaching inferotemporal needle come into the field of vision of the patient, which may be frightening, as well as placing the cornea in the way, a recent argument has been made for the 'down and in' globe position (see Chapter 8).[74]

Site and depth of injection

Relatively avascular areas of the orbit must be chosen for injection if the incidence of haematoma formation is to be kept to a minimum. These are confined to the anterior orbit in the inferotemporal and superotemporal quadrants, and the compartment on the nasal side of the medial rectus muscle; needles must never be inserted deeply to the orbital apex (see Chapters 1 and 8).

Intracone (retrobulbar) block

In this chapter, the term 'intracone' will be used, rather than the more vague term 'retrobulbar', to indicate the space behind the globe within the geometric confines of the four rectus muscles. Intraconal block will imply needle tip and injectate placement within that space. A straight needle, mounted on a syringe containing the chosen anaesthesia mixture, is introduced either transconjunctivally or transcutaneously, into the inferotemporal quadrant of the orbit commencing at the junction of the lateral third and medial two-thirds of the inferior orbit rim and running tangentially to the globe. Passing initially close to the orbit floor and medially, the globe equator is passed; at this time the angle of direction is adjusted upward, as illustrated in Fig. 7.3, and the needle advanced to enter

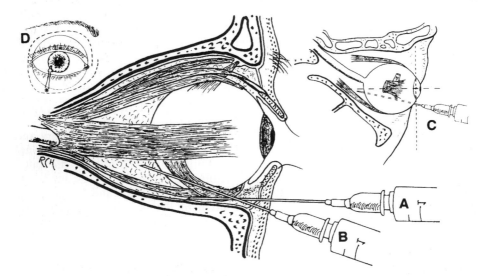

Fig. 7.3. Globe in primary gaze. Transcutaneous approach to the intracone space with a straight needle. The path of the needle is close to the orbit floor until the globe equator is passed (A), after which its angle of direction is adjusted upward and medially and advanced to enter the intracone space posterior to the globe (B). The needle tip approaches but does not pass the mid-sagittal plane of the globe (C). Needle entry point at the junction of the medial two-thirds and lateral third of the inferior orbital rim (D). (With permission from Gimbel Educational Services.)

within the cone of muscles posterior to the globe. It should be aimed at an imaginary point behind the globe on the axis formed by the central pupil and the macula, with care taken not to cross the mid-sagittal plane of the eye.[102] See Fig. 7.13, page 125, for the author's suggested modification of the inferotemporal intracone injection,.

Pericone (peribulbar; periocular) block

With this method of orbital regional anaesthesia, local anaesthetic agents or mixtures are deposited within the orbit but do not enter the geometric confines of the cone of rectus muscles. Introduced as a safer method than intraconal blocking so as to avoid serious complications, such complications nevertheless have been reported (see Chapter 8). The term 'pericone' will be used in this chapter as it is a less ambiguous name for the method than either peribulbar or periocular. Knowledge of orbital anatomy is every bit as important as with the older method and there are disadvantages to using periconal blocking (see below).

In 1986, Davis and Mandel were the first to publish a paper on the pericone block method. Calling the block technique posterior peribulbar, they used two intraorbital needle placements outside the muscle cone, one above and one below the cone each to a depth of 3.5 cm, with a total of up to 10 ml solution injected.[23] Bloomberg has more recently championed the cause of shorter needle pericone regional anaesthesia, and calls his technique periocular block.[16] With Bloomberg's method, a 2.5-cm 25 or 27 gauge needle enters the orbit inferotemporally and is directed 'deliberately toward the orbit floor' to a depth of 2 cm; a single 8–10 ml injection is given. He states that only 5% of patients require supplemental blocking. Other authors report up to 50% failure to achieve akinesia with periconal blocking.[75,124] Onset of akinesia is considerably slower than with intraconal block.[5,61] The volume requirement is greater[116] and more variable,[51,113] the supplementation rate to achieve total akinesia is higher[3,69] and the incidence of chemosis is greater.[5,124,125] There are many variations of the pericone technique, a common one being placement in two locations, one in the superior orbit and one in the inferior orbit. The author's suggested placements of dual pericone needles are illustrated in Figs 7.4 and 7.5. Whichever form of pericone block is used, it is worth noting that there is insufficient space between the lateral rectus and inferior rectus muscles and the lateral and inferior walls of the orbit, respectively (Fig. 7.6), to place injectate there without risking injury to the muscles (see myotoxicity; Chapters 6 and 8).

Differences between young adult patients compared with the elderly

With both intracone and pericone blocks, younger adult patients present more of a challenge in the achievement of total akinesia than the elderly[3,85] because of more dense connective tissues hindering the access of anaesthetics to the oculomotor nerves (see connective tissues; Chapter 1).

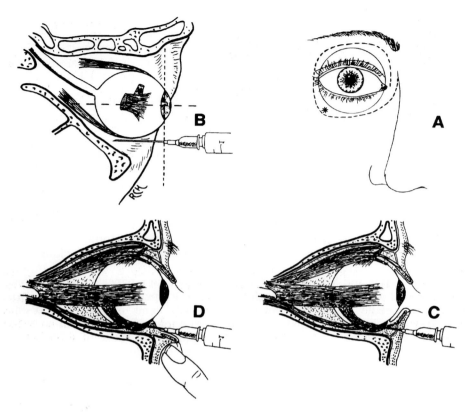

Fig. 7.4.   Author's suggested two-needle pericone technique: Needle 1. A 27 gauge 20–25 mm sharp disposable needle enters the orbit at the lower temporal orbit rim, slightly up from the orbit floor (A) and very close to the bone. The needle passes backwards in a sagittal plane (B) and parallel to the orbit floor (C, D), passing the globe equator to a depth controlled by observing the needle/hub junction reach the plane of the iris (B). The technique is equally applicable to the transcutaneous (C) or transconjunctival (D) route. (With permission from Gimbel Educational Services.)

Transcutaneous seventh nerve blockade

Techniques combining transcutaneous seventh nerve blockade and corneoconjunctival topical anaesthesia held sway in an earlier era (see above). Various methods of seventh nerve block were introduced (in chronological order) by van Lint,[123] Wright,[126] O'Brien,[91] Atkinson,[10] Nadbath and Rehman[87] and Spaeth.[108] Figure 7.7 shows the distribution of the facial nerve from its emergence from the base of the skull at the stylomastoid foramen to its teminal branches with the facial musculature, including the orbicularis oculi. Listing from proximal to distal the techniques are: Nadbath and Rehman, Spaeth, O'Brien, Wright/Atkinson, van Lint. Figure 7.7 illustrates the performance of a van Lint block, for which the originator carefully indicated that the injectate

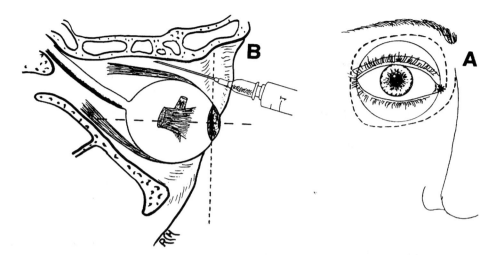

Fig. 7.5. Author's suggested two-needle pericone technique: Needle 2. A 27 gauge 20–25 mm sharp disposable needle enters transconjunctivally on the medial side of the caruncle at the extreme medial side of the palpebral fissure (A). With the bevel facing the orbit wall, it passes backward in the transverse plane, directed at a 5-degree angle away from the sagittal plane and towards the medial orbit wall (B). Depth of insertion is controlled by observing the needle/hub junction reach the plane of the iris (B). (With permission from Gimbel Educational Services.)

must be deposited close to the bone and deep to the orbicularis to be effective. Although the historic and traditional concept of globe anaesthesia/akinesia and orbicularis muscle akinesia being provided by separate interventions is still commonly practised, this need not be so. Given the acceptability, when hyaluronidase is admixed with local anaesthetics, of higher volumes injected into the orbit used in combination with orbital decompression devices, it has been observed that effective spread from the orbit through the orbital septum occurs, thus achieving akinesia of the orbicularis oculi musculature.[37,78,82,92] The medial pericone block (see below) is particularly effective in obtunding tone in the central orbicularis muscle. The injectate spreads out from the orbit, with the help of hyaluronidase, in a plane deep to the orbicularis muscle, to abolish lid closure muscle activity by conduction blockade of terminal divisions of the seventh nerve entering from the muscle's deep surface. In an occasional patient, who exhibits strong recruitment of the more peripheral fibres of orbicularis oculi and/or excessive use of the brow musculature, supplemental transcutaneous blocking of the orbicularis may be necessary (I recommend the van Lint technique). However, in the vast majority of cases, sufficient blockade of the lid closure musculature is achieved from spread outwards from the orbit; painful transcutaneous seventh nerve block through the sensitive facial skin is thus avoided and found to be unnecessary.

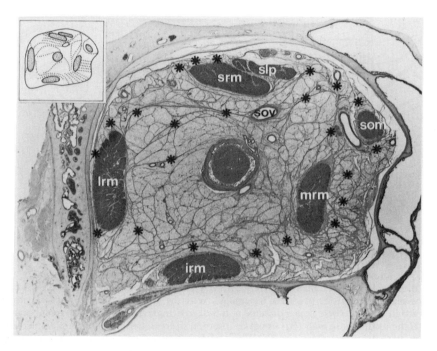

Fig. 7.6.   Cross-section or the orbit 2.6 mm posterior to the hind surface of the globe. Note the proximity of the lateral rectus muscle (lrm) and inferior rectus muscle (irm) to the bony orbit. Note also the connective tissue hammock carrying the superior opthalmic vein (sov) diagonally across the superior orbit from anteronasal to posterotemporal. slp, levator palpebrae superioris muscle; srm, superior rectus muscle; som, superior oblique muscle; mrm, medial rectus muscle; *connective tissue septa. (With permission from ref. 130.)

Needle type and syringe size

Traditional teaching favoured dull-tipped, intermediate-gauge needles with the supposed advantages that blood vessels were pushed aside rather than traumatized and that tissue planes could be more accurately defined. Although a commonly held belief among ophthalmologists,[24,62] it is not true that it is more difficult to penetrate the globe, the optic nerve sheath or blood vessels with a blunt needle.[44] In 1991, Grizzard *et al.* reporting on iatrogenic ocular injuries, found that penetration or perforation of the eye from use of larger dull needles caused more serious damage than when fine disposable ones were implicated, and questioned the arguments in the earlier literature that advocated their use.[44] Because disposable cutting needles produce minimal tissue distortion, little or no pain results. Any needle advanced within the confines of the orbit has the potential of serious complication; therefore, any serious practitioner of ophthalmic regional anaesthesia must understand the anatomy of the orbit and its contents. Grizzard states that tactile discrimination is progressively reduced with increasing needle size; the increased resistance caused by a blunt needle is not appreciated because of the necessarily greater preload (Weber-Fechner law).[43] Special

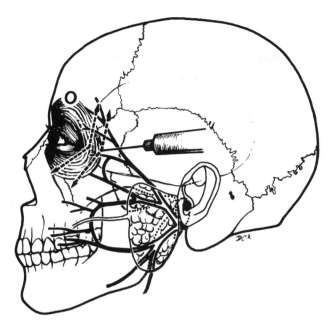

Fig. 7.7. Extracranial path of the facial nerve. Detail of van Lint block technique is shown. O, orbicularis muscle. (With permission from ref. 131.)

attention should be paid to the length of needle entering beyond the orbital rim; a distance of 31 mm as measured from the orbit rim should never be exceeded.[59] The medial directioning of a needle advancing from an inferotemporal entry must be such that the mid-sagittal plane of the eye (Fig. 7.8) is not crossed.[43,102] All needles used for intracone or pericone placement should be orientated tangentially to the globe with the bevel opening facing towards the globe.[37,46] Tangential alignment is most easily achieved in transconjunctival techniques.[37,46]

In modern practice, plastic disposable syringes are most commonly used. The force required to inject fluid at a given rate through a given needle mounted on two syringes, differing only in their total capacity (one having a greater plunger cross-sectional area than the other), is less with the smaller of the two. Because less force has to be exerted, a change in resistance to injectate flow is more easily detected by the injecting hand when using a needle mounted on a smaller syringe as compared with a larger size. The fingers serve as transducers, relaying information to the sensory cortex of the anaesthetist.[17] This ability to detect more easily any change in resistance to injection is important in the avoidance of complications.

Is sedation prior to regional anaesthesia required?

In some practices, various combinations of intravenous tranquillizers, opiate narcotics and even rapid- and short-acting anaesthetics are used just prior to the

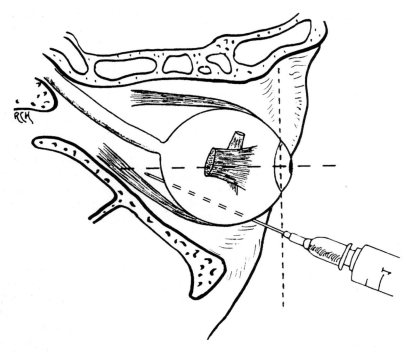

Fig. 7.8.   This 31-mm needle is advanced beyond the equator of the globe, and then directed towards an imaginary point behind the macula, being careful not to cross the mid-sagittal plane of the eye. In a globe with normal axial length as illustrated here, when the needle/hub junction has reached the plane of the iris the tip of the needle lies 5–7 mm beyond the hind surface of the globe. (With permission from Gimbel Educational Services.)

orbital blocks being administered.[16] This usually means that the block method being used is associated with considerable discomfort, which the anaesthetist in charge feels is best covered by some form of significant but short-acting sedation. Opiate narcotics should be avoided in the ambulatory setting because of the associated increased incidence of nausea and vomiting; if they have to be used, antiemetics should be included.

In other practices, pain-free methods of regional anaesthesia induction are used;[32,54] therefore, sedative medications, either parenterally or orally, are not routinely used. Cooperation, especially in the elderly, is usually better in the absence of preoperative sedative medication.[32]

Before any regional anaesthetic is administered, facilities must be present to support a full resuscitation (monitor, defibrillator), including a manual resuscitation bag, masks, and oral, nasal and endotracheal airways along with laryngoscopes. Sources of 100% oxygen and suction, intravenous fluids and the equipment to start an infusion, drugs for cardiopulmonary resuscitation and management of convulsions are all needed and best housed in a well-organized mobile crash cart.[95]

To stress the importance of attention to detail, all aspects of patient care for an outpatient having cataract extraction and intraocular lens implantation under regional anaesthesia at the Gimbel Clinic (where 4500 surgical procedures are performed annually) are discussed in the following paragraphs.

The outpatient cataract experience

Following medical referral an appointment is set up which, for a typical patient at the clinic, lasts 3 days. On each of the 3 days, staff maintain as far as is possible friendly rapport with the patient so as to make the experience non-clinical and minimally stressful. In the weeks between referral and the appointment, in response to a form letter from the anaesthetist detailing the fitness requirements, a preoperative history and physical examination done by the family physician is forwarded to the clinic for appraisal. It is essential that the patient is accompanied on all visits during the 3-day appointment by a responsible adult.

Day prior to surgery

On the first day, tests are done: visual acuity check without correction; a manifest refraction testing; possibly a cycloplegic refraction test; measurement of globe dimension (axial length), from anterior face of cornea to anterior surface of retina using A-scan ultrasound technology ('normal' eye has an axial length of 23.5 mm, but sizes fairly commonly encountered clinically are from 19 to 33 mm); slit lamp and ophthalmoscopic fundus examination; and applanation tonometry (normal intraocular pressures range from 10 to 25 mmHg). Much emphasis is placed on preliminary patient education, verbally by clinic staff and by audiovisual aids; an informed patient is a calm one. After the completion of the tests, the patient takes away written information, drug prescriptions and instructions pertinent to the evening before surgery.

Day of surgery

On the day of surgery, there is no curtailment of regular meals (which incidentally makes the management of the stable diabetic virtually like that of the regular patient), gowning is not part of the routine (street clothes are worn into the operating theatre, footware covered with paper overshoes) and the friendly rapport continued. In the 10 years prior to January 1994, 36 000 cataract extraction surgeries were undertaken with unrestricted preoperative feeding, and no incidents occurred to suggest that this was an unsafe practice. The author's regional block technique is a minimal pain stimulus method on a mainly ageing clientele. Preoperative sedation is used only in patients showing obvious evidence of anxiety (as initially assessed by the receptionist and then by the anaesthetist). In these patients, about 5% of the total, oral diazepam is given in a dose of 2.0–5.0 mg according to age and physical status. The act of taking this in itself often has a calming placebo effect, apart altogether from the desired pharmacological action. The low usage of preoperative sedation is dependent on good preoperative patient education, to a large extent enhanced by word of mouth promotion of former patients.

On arriving at the reception room of the surgical suite, patients sign a consent form outlining potential surgical and anaesthesia complications and walk to the block room. They recline on a motorized contoured dental chair for the block procedure. An adhesive label displaying their name and bilateral axial length measurements is applied to their clothing over the shoulder on the side to be blocked and a small adhesive red tag to the forehead on the side of the proposed surgery. The anaesthetist's nurse assistant institutes checking of vital signs using noninvasive blood pressure monitoring; these data and a note of bilateral eyelid margin preblock distances above the central cornea are entered in the anaesthesia record (for later comparison if postoperative ptosis occurs). Appropriate eyedrops are then instilled prior to the first injection of local anaesthetic.

Prior to and during the induction of regional anaesthesia, a lead 1 electrocardiogram (wrist bracelet electrodes) monitor is attached, the interpretation of which is also entered in the record. Following establishment of full block (details below), patients walk to a holding area, from where they are drawn (remaining ambulatory) to the operating room as required. The operating table is a modified dental chair. Dental chairs, because of the comfort engendered by their contoured shape, are well accepted by patients, particularly the elderly who commonly have painful arthritic joints. Oxygen enrichment of humidified air under the drapes at a flow of up to 10 l/min is adjusted to correct arterial desaturation levels (SaO_2 <92%).[1] During surgery noninvasive blood pressure, lead 1 electrocardiogram (wrist electrodes), pulse wave and pulse oximetric monitoring are routine. For the period of the surgery, the person or persons who have accompanied the patient have the option (most accept) of observing from a room adjacent to the operating theatre separated by a common glass wall; there is two-way electronic voice communication between the relatives and the patient.

Following surgery the patient, remaining ambulatory, returns to the holding area and is joined again by the accompanying responsible adult where they remain for 10–15 min in a routine case; together they receive written and verbal postoperative instructions from a member of staff. These include details of management of the occlusive dressing that is applied to the eye after surgery. The patient's vital signs are recorded in the anaesthesia record, following which the anaesthetist's signature confirms a satisfactory status for discharge. The occlusive eye dressing is usually left in place until the next morning.

First postoperative day

On the first postoperative day, the occlusive eye dressing is removed by the patient or accompanying person prior to returning to the clinic; this allows a period of time for blinking to clear away residual ointment, etc., prior to the routine postoperative checks on day 3, which include intraocular pressure measurement, visual acuity testing and slitlamp examination.

Block details

Combined intraconal / periconal method

For graphic representation of the technique, please refer to the flowchart opposite. The author has personally provided ocular regional anaesthesia for 32 000 cataract extraction and intraocular lens implantation procedures in the 10 years

Regional Ophthalmic Anaesthesia for Cataract Extraction - - Flow Chart

(with permission from Gimbel Educational Services)

ALL ORBITAL BLOCKS ARE WITH EYE IN PRIMARY GAZE POSITION WITH NEEDLES ALIGNED TANGENTIALLY TO THE GLOBE

Routes of Delivery and Monitoring

- The inferotemporal intracone and the medial compartment pericone blocks are given transconjunctival.

- The superotemporal pericone block is given transcutaneous.

- Digital monitoring of orbital pressure during each injection governs the total volume used. Injections should be terminated if orbit shows significant resistance to retropulsation of the globe.

KEY:
INJECT
INSPECT

TOPICAL ANAESTHESIA OF CONJUNCTIVA WITH 0.5% PROPARACAINE

ADDITIONAL DROPS

↓

Q-TIP™ soaked in 0.5% PROPARACAINE TO INFERIOR FORNIX

↓

30 gauge 12 mm "PAINLESS LOCAL" BLOCK 1.0 ml

↓

27 gauge 31 mm INFEROTEMPORAL INTRACONE BLOCK 3.0 - 4.0 ml

↓

Anaesthetic Mixtures

"Painless Local"

| Alcon BSS™ | 10 parts |
| Anaesthetic mixture | 1 part |

Regional Block

Depending on the requirement, a choice from one of the following local anesthetics (or combination) can be used:

LIDOCAINE		2.0%	√
MEPIVACAINE		2.0%	√
LIDOCAINE	4.0%	Ratio	√
BUPIVACAINE	0.75%	1:1	
BUPIVACAINE		0.75%	√

combined with:

HYALURONIDASE 7.5 u/ml

and (unless contraindicated):

EPINEPHRINE 1:200,000

GENTLE MASSAGE OF THE GLOBE APPLIED TO GAUZE WIPES OVERLYING CLOSED LIDS FOR 2 MIN FOLLOWED BY INSPECTION

AKINESIA OF GLOBE BUT NOT ORBICULARIS OCULI MUSCLE	TORQUE ONLY OF SUPERIOR OBLIQUE AND/OR OTHER MINOR EXTRAOCULAR MUSCLE ACTIVITY	RETAINED ACTION MAINLY IN THE SUPERIOR RECTUS AND LEVATOR MUSCLE OF THE UPPER LID	RETAINED ACTIVITY IN RECTUS MUSCLES
30 gauge 12 mm MEDIAL COMPARTMENT PERICONE BLOCK 2.0 - 4.0 ml	30 gauge 25 mm MEDIAL COMPARTMENT PERICONE BLOCK 2.0 - 4.0 ml	27 gauge 31 mm SUPEROTEMPORAL PERICONE BLOCK 2.0 - 4.0 ml	27 gauge 31 mm REPEAT INFEROTEMPORAL INTRACONE BLOCK 2.0 ml

Direct observation until ophthalmic block is complete

15 minutes of continuous decompression time using the Honan Balloon™ at a setting of 30 mm Hg, prior to the commencement of surgery

since the surgical centre opened in January 1984. In 1988, a report on the management of the first 12 000 anaesthesias was published.[46] Five distinct techniques of injection were studied, following which it was determined that a method combining an initial intraconal injection with a secondary periconal supplementation was most suited to the rapid turnover practice. Loots *et al.*, following their extensive experience, also uphold this combined block method.[75] Definitive seventh nerve blocking is not used as sufficient spread to orbicularis oculi muscle follows appropriate intraorbital injection placment.[37,78,82] Because fine sharp disposable needles are used, there is potential for doing much damage to vital structures. A technique with solely periconal placement may be a more prudent alternative for the relatively inexperienced practitioner.

Applied anatomy

The bony anatomy of the orbit and its relationship to the globe is the basis of the method. It consists of a preliminary injection of anaesthetic mixture diluted with balanced salt solution (the type available in ophthalmologists' offices for intraocular instillation),[135] followed by two full-strength local anaesthetic injections, the first an inferotemporal intraconal injection and the second a periconal injection. The rationale for this three-needle technique is to provide effective (low supplementation rate) and safe (low complication rate) anaesthesia and akinesia according to the requirements listed above. The method is virtually painfree; as a result, preoperative and intraoperative sedation are usually not necessary, as outlined above. The no-sedation or minimal-sedation approach gets around the problem of patients falling into deep sleep during surgery, and awakening precipitously with potential detrimental effects to the surgery in hand.[100]

Figure 7.9 illustrates a superimposed outline of the globe and orbit rim. The rim can be seen to have a basic, albeit lop-sided, quadrilateral shape. The space available for needle access to the globe equator and to deeper orbit structures,

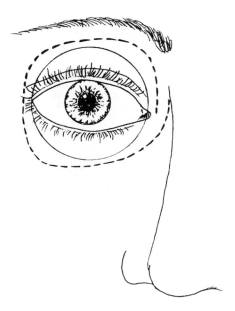

Fig. 7.9.   The outline of the globe is superimposed on a template of the orbital rim. (With permission from Gimbel Educational Services.)

between the globe and the orbit rim, is greatest at the inferotemporal quadrant (Figs 7.9, 7.10); this area is also suitable because it is relatively avascular. For needle access to the intracone compartment, the inferotemporal quadrant is again the route of choice because the lateral orbit rim is set back in line with the globe equator (Fig. 7.11). Figure 7.11 also demonstrates that the orbit, in sagittal section, is C-shaped rather than U-shaped with the greater overhang superiorly. The orbit floor (inferior orbit wall) rises at an angle of 10 degrees from front to back (Fig. 7.12). To avoid trauma to the inferior oblique muscle, or its motor nerve, an inferotemporal needle placement should be lateral to the sagittal plane of the lateral limbus. In the method used by the author, the needle entry point is much further to the temporal side than with the classic Atkinson technique,[7] and in fact is slightly up on the temporal orbit rim (Fig. 7.13A) Figure 7.13 shows the path of a needle appropriately placed (just inferior to the lower border of the lateral rectus muscle and well clear of the belly of the inferior oblique muscle and of the inferotemporal vortex vein; see Chapter 1).[112] Injection into any of the extraocular muscles must be assiduously avoided, otherwise myotoxicity may result in prolonged diplopia, which may be permanent (see Chapters 6 and 8).

Only relatively avascular areas of the anterior orbit should be used for needle placement (vessels increase in size as the apex is approached; also, the end vessels of the ophthalmic artery system are located in the superonasal orbit quadrant, and so this quadrant should therefore not be used for needle placement). In the anterior orbit, the inferotemporal, superotemporal and medial locations have relatively low vascularity (see Chapter 1)

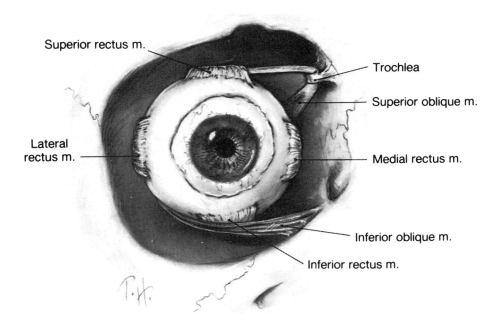

Fig. 7.10. Frontal view showing quadrilateral shape of the orbit rim and its orientation to the extraocular muscles. (With permission from ref. 132.)

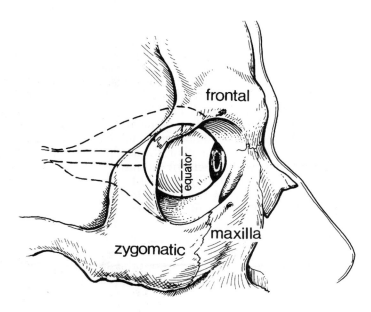

Fig. 7.11.   The lateral orbital rim is set back in line with the globe equator making an infero-temporal approach to the intracone space the route of choice. (With permission from ref. 43.)

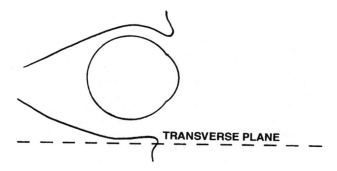

Fig. 7.12.   The orbit floor rises at an angle of 10 degrees to the transverse plane. (With permission from Gimbel Educational Services.)

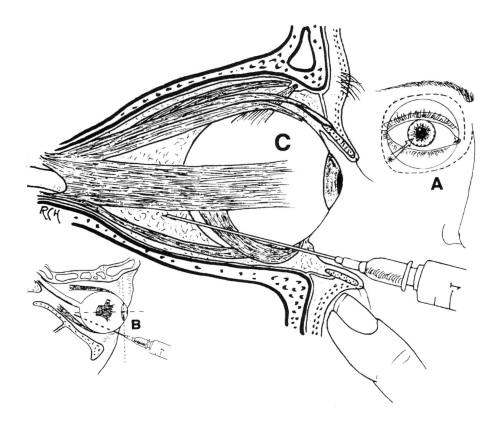

Fig. 7.13. The author's technique of inferotemporal intracone injection. The needle tip is inserted at the lower temporal orbit rim, slightly up from the orbit floor (A) and very close to the bone. In this illustration the conjunctival route is being used with needle tip entry just behind the inferior tarsal plate (if the transcutaneous route were used, the lower lid would not be retracted and needle tip entry would be inferior to the tarsal plate). With either the transconjunctival or the transcutaneous route, the needle track passes initially backwards in the sagittal plane with a 10-degree elevation from the transverse plane until the globe equator is passed. Following this, the needle is directed with medial and slightly upward components aiming for an imaginary point behind the globe on the axis formed by the pupil and the macula, so that the needle tip approaches but does not pass the mid-sagittal plane of the globe as visualized at the start in primary gaze position (A, B). The needle enters the intracone space by passing through the intermuscular septum just inferior to the lower border of the lateral rectus muscle (C). The globe is observed continuously during needle placement to detect globe rotation that would indicate engagement of the sclera by the needle tip. During needle placement, continuing observation of the relationship between the needle/hub junction and the plane of the iris establishes an appropriate depth of orbit insertion (B). (With permission from Gimbel Educational Services.)

Needle selection

Three conventional inexpensive sharp disposable needles (30 gauge 12 mm, 27 gauge 31 mm and 30 gauge 25 mm, in that order) are used. (Some anaesthetists may prefer to substitute a 25 gauge size instead of the 27 gauge, but its length should not exceed 31 mm.[59]) The author routinely modifies the 27 gauge needle with a 10-degree bend at its mid-point (see details below).

Anaesthesia mixture and syringe preparation

Any of the full potency local anaesthetics in common use for ophthalmic regional anaesthesia (Chapter 6) may be used, the eventual choice depending on availability, patient age and desired duration of effect. The author prefers to add adrenaline (final concentration 1:200 000) to the chosen mixture just before use; hyaluronidase is an essential component (see above). Lignocaine/bupivacaine mixtures provide fast-onset anaesthesia with excellent postoperative analgesia and recovery of full eyelid protective reflexes 8 h after the block. For surgical colleagues who prefer more rapid return of eyelid reflexes, lignocaine or mepivacaine with adrenaline and hyaluronidase may be used; however, the postoperative analgesia will be less good and the available akinesia time, especially with the lignocaine, limited to about 2 h following the block. A separate solution ('painless local'[54]) is made up by adding 1.5 ml of any full-strength local anaesthetic to a 15-ml plastic bottle of balanced salt solution (available for intraocular use in ophthalmologists' offices).[135] Sarvela and Nikki suggest a more potent 'painless local' consisting of 10 ml balanced salt solution admixed with 3.3 ml lignocaine 2% and 0.3 ml sodium bicarbonate (1 mEq/ml).[102] Dilute painless anaesthetic solutions are extremely helpful in patient management (if used as the first injection) in three ways: without producing any stinging stimulus, excellent analgesia in the area injected results; patients, having experienced no pain, relax and have confidence in their anaesthetist for the subsequent procedures; and the anaesthetist obtains objective evidence of the patient's psychological status by observing their reactivity to being approached with a needle and receiving a minor stimulus.

In readiness for the author's regional anaesthesia technique, each patient will require one 3-ml disposable plastic syringe containing 1 ml 'painless local' solution and two 5-ml disposable plastic syringes each containing 4 ml full-potency local anaesthetic mixture. A 30 gauge 12-mm needle is firmly mounted on the 3-ml syringe and a 27 gauge 31-mm needle and a 30 gauge 25-mm needle, respectively, on the 5-ml syringes.

Needle modification

When doing the inferotemporal transconjunctival intracone injection, an excellent aid to getting the needle tip behind the eye more easily is to use a needle modified in the following way: the 27 gauge 31-mm needle is bent to an angle of 10 degrees half way along its length following its insertion inside a sterile 18 gauge needle (this is most easily accomplished with both needles mounted on syringes). The bevel of the needle should be in the concavity of the bend (Fig. 7.14). The needle hub is marked with an indelible fibreglass pen to indicate the location of the bevel of the needle and the orientation of its angled distal half; an

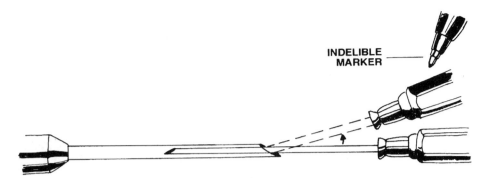

INDELIBLE
MARKER

Fig. 7.14.   A 27 gauge 31-mm needle is bent to an angle of 10 degrees half way along its length by insertion inside a sterile 18 gauge needle. The bevel of the 27 gauge needle should be in the concavity of the bend. The needle hub is marked with an indelible fibreglass pen to indicate the location of the bevel of the needle and the orientation of its angled distal half. (With permission from Gimbel Educational Services.)

alternative method to marking the hub is to mount the needle on a non-luer lock syringe with a predetermined reference point on the syringe aligned with the bent distal half of the needle.

Preblock inspection of the globe and eyelids

Whereas most of the author's inferotemporal blocks are done transconjunctivally, this is not universally so. If on digital retraction of the patient's lower eyelid in a downward and outward direction the eyelid margin is found to be tightly held against the globe, if the globe is deeply recessed within the orbit, if there is a wide lateral canthal fold (see Chapter 1), or if the patient is blinking uncontrollably, the author uses a transcutaneous approach for the intracone injection. In all cases, the axial length measurement of the globe is carefully noted; in the presence of high myopia, an alternative technique may be more prudent (see below).

Three-injection sequence for regional orbital anaesthesia and akinesia

The reader may refer to the flowchart on p. 121 for graphic representation of the following three subsections.

First injection: 'Painless local'

Following topical anaesthesia drops and appropriate ocular medications instilled into the conjunctival sac, a cotton tip applicator soaked with topical anaesthetic (proparacaine 0.5%) is held in the inferotemporal conjunctival fornix for 15–20 s to reinforce sufficiently deep conjunctival anaesthesia for the needle to follow. The patient is informed that the anaesthetist's finger will be felt retracting the

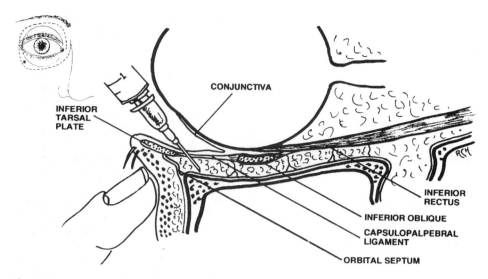

Fig. 7.15.   After gently retracting the lower eyelid with a finger, the tip of the 30 gauge 12-mm needle enters transconjunctivally and inferotemporally just behind the inferior tarsal plate with the shaft of the needle arranged tangentially to the globe. The initial injection is of 1.0 ml 'painless local' at a depth of 1 cm from the conjunctiva. The needle has easily and painlessly (because of preliminary topical anaesthesia drops) penetrated the conjunctiva, and deep to it the capsulopalpebral fascia. The needle entry point is at the lower end of the lateral orbit rim (small insert). Landmarks for transcutaneous injection of 'painless local' are the same, but without lower eyelid retraction. (With permission from Gimbel Educational Services.)

lower eyelid (Fig. 7.15) and that some movement of the lid will be experienced. The injection is of 1.0 ml 'painless local' transconjunctivally and inferotemporally through the 30 gauge 12-mm needle, the tip entering just behind the inferior tarsal plate with the shaft of the needle arranged tangentially to the globe (Fig. 7.15). The needle easily and painlessly (because of preliminary topical anaesthesia drops) penetrates the conjunctiva, and deep to it the capsulo-palpebral fascia; 1.0 ml 'painless local' is deposited at a depth of 1 cm from the conjunctiva (Fig. 7.15) and the needle withdrawn. It is good practice to check routinely for a few seconds after each injection and needle withdrawal for any evidence of bleeding. For established anaesthesia to develop there should be a delay of 1–2 min before proceeding with the second injection. In those patients in whom it has been decided to use a transcutaneous approach for the block, 1 ml 'painless local' is injected through the skin overlying the inferotemporal orbit rim.

Second injection: Inferotemporal intraconal

The safety of this part of the procedure is in its emphasis on the proximity of the needle to the orbit wall at first entry and until the globe equator is passed. In the figures which follow, the intracone needles are shown with the author's custom bend. However, for those anaesthetists who prefer to use a 31-mm straight needle, the identical principles, as described below, apply. Figure 7.15 illustrates the use of this modified needle to achieve the intracone needle tip placement. The anaesthetist at all times is aware of the orientation of the bent distal half by virtue of the ink mark or the syringe alignment. A needle modified as described places less stretch on tissues during its placement than does a straight needle, thus reducing the chances of bleeding into the tissues.[116] Utilizing the above instructions, whether the regular straight needle or its modified version is used, a central intracone location of the needle tip (well above the orbit floor) is achieved and makes for improved evenness of injectate spread within the cone and a greatly reduced incidence of conjunctival chemosis commonly seen in periconal techniques. Furthermore, by maintaining needle direction directed 10 degrees upward from the transverse plane (and parallel to the orbit floor) commencing at the inferotemporal entry point, inferior rectus needle trauma is avoided (see Chapter 8).

The legend of Fig. 7.16 gives detailed step-by-step instruction of the technique. The author most commonly uses a transconjunctival approach, using a 27 gauge 31-mm disposable needle mounted firmly on a 5.0-ml syringe containing 4 ml anaesthesia mixture. The inferotemporal orbit rim is palpated and its relationship to the globe noted, including the orientation of the globe equator to the lateral orbit rim (Fig. 7.11). The mid-sagittal plane of the globe is visualized (dotted line in Fig. 7.8) with the patient's eye in primary gaze.[122] The needle tip is inserted close to the inferotemporal orbit rim. With either the transconjunctival or the transcutaneous route, the needle tip passes inferior to the lower border of the lateral rectus muscle and posterior to the equator of the globe (Fig. 7.16). It is important to observe the globe continuously (on the side being blocked) during needle placement, to advance slowly and always with tangential alignment of the needle to the globe in order to detect globe rotation or other movement that might indicate engagement of the needle tip in sclera. The needle while being inserted should be parallel to the orbit floor (i.e. at a 10-degree rise from the transverse plane).

The needle placement is in two stages, a preliminary short posterior directioning in the sagittal plane until the globe equator has been passed, followed by the assumption of a medial component in the angle of direction of the needle and syringe assembly, aiming for an imaginary point behind the globe on the axis formed by the pupil and the macula,[102] so that the needle tip approaches but does not pass the mid-sagittal plane of the globe as visualized at the start in primary gaze position (Fig. 7.8). As an extra precaution, although the author does not find this necessary, in protecting the optic nerve the patient may redirect the eye being blocked downward and outward[122] (or by a recent suggestion, downward and inward[74]) for this second stage of the needle placement. With the globe depressed and abducted,[105] or depressed and adducted,[74] the optic nerve moves into a position in the intraconal space further from the needle tip than would be the case with the eye in primary gaze.

During needle placement, continuing observation of the relationship between the needle/hub junction and the plane of the iris is used to measure the appropriate depth of needle insertion into the orbit (Fig. 7.16). On attainment of the final needle tip location, the hub of the needle is firmly held between finger and thumb against the zygoma. The angle of the medial component of directioning of the needle and syringe assembly with relation to the skull is not altered. For a globe with normal axial length, the needle tip will now have reached a position

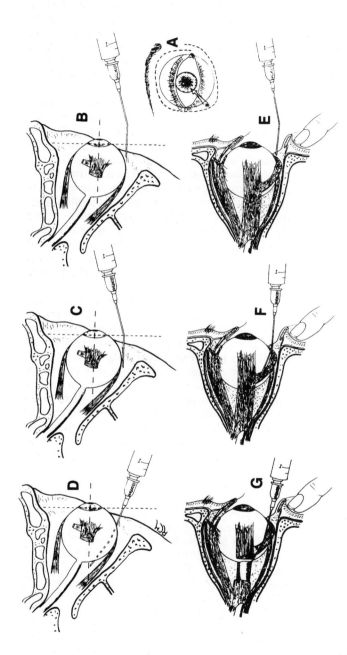

Fig. 7.16. Inferotemporal intracone block with custom-bent 27 gauge 31-mm sharp disposable needle. The figure illustrates the transconjunctival approach with lower eyelid retraction, but is equally applicable to transcutaneous injection. The needle tip enters at the lower temporal orbit rim, slightly up from the orbit floor (A) and very close to the bone. Views B, C and D are from above; views E, F and G are from the temporal side. The leading half of the needle is advanced in the sagittal plane and parallel to the orbit floor (B, E), until the needle bend has reached the plane of the iris (C, F), indicating that the globe equator has been passed. The needle tip is now directed with medial and slightly upward components (A) aiming for an imaginary point behind the globe on the axis formed by the pupil and the macula, so that the needle tip approaches but does not pass the mid-sagittal plane of the globe as visualized at the start in primary gaze position (D, G). The needle enters the intracone space by passing through the intermuscular septum just inferior to the lower border of the lateral rectus muscle (F, G). The globe is continuously observed during needle placement to detect globe rotation that would indicate engagement of the sclera by the needle tip. During needle placement, continuing observation of the relationship between the needle/hub junction and the plane of the iris establishes an appropriate depth of orbit insertion (D, G). (With permission from Gimbel Educational Services.)

within the intracone compartment 5–7 mm behind the hind surface of the globe (Fig. 7.16D). For longer (myopic) globes, identical depth placement according to the iris plane is used and the results are found to be excellent. In high myopes, however, it may be more prudent to use a solely pericone blocking method. Katsev *et al.* stressed the importance of avoiding needle insertion beyond a depth of 31 mm from the inferior orbit rim in the interests of avoiding trauma to the optic nerve.[59] By using the iris plane depth check as described, this rule will automatically be respected.

Following negative test aspiration, injection is commenced to confirm absence of abnormal resistance or presence of atypical discomfort; if any is suspected, the needle tip should be relocated. While monitoring visually and digitally the increasing orbit volume and intraconal pressure (globe between finger and thumb of the non-injecting hand), 3.0–4.0 ml of the anaesthesia mixture is injected very slowly (2 min) until a bulging of the superior orbital sulcus with filling out of the upper eyelid crease and some degree of ptosis and proptosis (the latter of which rapidly subsides) are seen. The needle is withdrawn and a check for bleeding made. In the event that bleeding occurs following this or any of the injections, immediate digital compression should be instituted to minimize any potential pressure build-up. In placing this second needle, no attempt is made to contact the periorbita or bone of the orbit floor as this is inappropriate (infra-orbital canal or fissure may be entered resulting in unpleasant infraorbital nerve paraesthesia).

Following a 2-min period of gentle massage of the globe applied to gauze wipes overlying the closed lids, the effectiveness of the block is assessed in the usual manner by checking globe movements, superior levator activity and orbicularis oculi function. If movement is confined to torque movements of the globe indicating ongoing partial function of the superior oblique muscle (as explained above) or residual activity in the orbicularis oculi muscle, these will be effectively abolished by the complementary pericone injection to follow. Those patients showing strong retention of only superior rectus and levator palpebrae superioris activity are best managed with a superotemporal pericone injection (see below). The author routinely uses a third injection (pericone) to complement the intracone block; a medial pericone injection is used in about 95% of my patients and a superotemporal pericone block in the remaining 5%.

Third injection: Medial pericone injection (95%)

Injection of local anaesthesics into the fat compartment on the nasal side of the medial rectus muscle (see orbital connective tissues; Chapter 1) has distinct advantages because of the arrangement of connective tissues in, and relative avascularity of, the area.[52] Bulk spread of local anaesthetic injected into this discrete medial compartment occurs to the orbital apex posteriorly, but is restricted from direct spread laterally to the intracone compartment (Fig. 7.17) Access of local anaesthetics to the motor nerve supply of the superior oblique muscle and superior rectus/levator complex is facilitated. Concurrently, local anaesthetic injectate spreads through two 'hernial orifices' above and below the medial check ligament in the connective tissue diaphragm that surrounds the globe just anterior to its equator (Fig. 7.18; see connective tissues, Chapter 1), and through the orbital septum, into the upper and lower eyelids in a tissue plane on the deep surface of the orbicularis oculi muscle where the fine terminal motor branches of the seventh nerve are readily blocked.[98] Additionally, the medial compartment block promotes spread of anaesthesia to block sensation of the peripheral conjunctiva, including the lacrimal and frontal nerves, thus effectively abolishing intraoperative discomfort sometimes observed in low-volume solely intracone techniques.[46] This compartment in the area injected is devoid of significant blood vessels. A portion of the superior ophthalmic vein and the end vessels of the ophthalmic artery system – namely, the anterior ethmoidal, supra- and infratrochlear arteries – are present in the medial fat compartment but superior to this

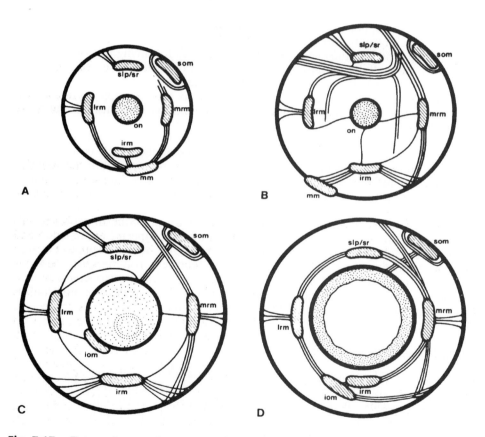

Fig. 7.17. Extraocular muscle connective tissue system. Highly schematic representation of coronal sections: A, near the orbital apex; B, near the posterior pole of the globe; C, mid-way between the posterior pole and equator of the globe; D, at the globe equator. slp/sr, levator palpebrae superioris/superior rectus complex; lrm, lateral rectus muscle; iom, inferior oblique muscle; irm, inferior rectus muscle; mm, Müller's muscle; mrm, medial rectus muscle; som, superior oblique muscle; on, optic nerve. (With permission from ref. 67.)

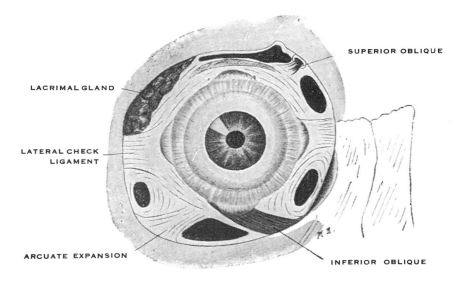

Fig. 7.18. The connective tissue diaphragm situated just anterior to the globe equator demonstrating 'hernial orifices' within it. The eyelids and orbital septum have been removed. (With permission from ref. 133.)

location. These vessels can be traumatized by needles inserted into the superior nasal quadrant of the orbit. The incidence of bleeding seen following 30 gauge needle injections in this area is negligible and always, if it occurs, minor in nature.[52]

Figure 7.19 depicts detailed surface anatomy at the medial canthus. A specialized portion of conjunctiva called the caruncle occupies the extreme medial end of the palpebral fissure; upper and lower lacrimal canaliculi are present within the margins of the upper and lower eyelids, respectively, and merge as the common canaliculus on the nasal side of the medial canthus, and it in turn opens into the lacrimal sac. The needle entry point for the medial orbital pericone block is through a small depression immediately medial to the caruncle. This depression is medial to the sagittal plane of the medial equator of the globe in almost all patients; if in doubt, contact with the periosteum on the medial wall of the orbit, by angling the needle tip in that direction, will confirm clearance from sclera. No complication related to involvement of any part of the tear duct system, nor globe penetration, has been encountered. The medial compartment block is an effective and safe method of complementing the preliminary inferior temporal block and is painless because the conjunctival entry point is innervated by the nasociliary nerve, which lies inside the cone of muscles and is already well blocked by the foregoing intracone injection.

A 30 gauge 25-mm needle is mounted on a 5-ml syringe containing 4 ml of full-strength local anaesthetic mixture. With the bevel opening facing the nasal side of the orbit, the needle tip enters transconjunctivally, through the small depression on the nasal side of the caruncle at the medial end of the palpebral fissure. The needle is advanced in the transverse plane and directed towards the

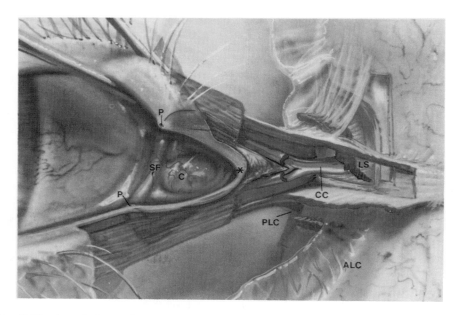

Fig. 7.19.   Detailed superficial anatomy at the medial canthus. C, caruncle; P, punctum; SF, semilunar fold; CC, common canaliculus; LS, lacrimal sac; ALC, anterior lacrimal crest; PLC, posterior lacrimal crest; *medial canthus. (With permission from ref. 134.)

mid-line of the skull at the occiput.[102] Figures 7.20 and 7.21 illustrate the needle direction and placement. The approximately 5-degree angle towards the medial orbit wall directs the needle so as to avoid penetration of the medial rectus muscle or its sheath, since injection into it could result in myotoxicity with resultant prolonged paralysis or paresis. If bony contact is made with the medial orbit wall, the needle is withdrawn slightly and redirected with a lesser medial inclination; this allows the needle tip to be free in fatty tissue once more. Minimal temporary resistance will be felt as the needle traverses the medial check ligament. The medial compartment is 4–10 mm wide anteriorly at the globe equator, 3–8 mm wide at the hind surface of the eye and rapidly becomes narrower as the medial rectus reaches its bony origin posteriorly.

Provided the angle of insertion as described is obeyed entry within the belly or sheath of the medical rectus muscle does not occur. A volume of 2–4ml is injected, the chosen amount depending on the degree of block required, always employing the minimal amount and injecting slowly (and monitoring digitally the changing orbital volume) so as not to impede the desired goal of intraocular hypotony. Part of the injected volume invariably dissects hydraulically into the fascial plane anterior to the orbital septum and posterior to the orbicularis muscle leading to upper and lower lid akinesia and anaesthesia.[98] Residual activity in the extraocular musculature persisting after the initial inferior temporal block is effectively abolished in most cases following the medial compartment block within 5 min.

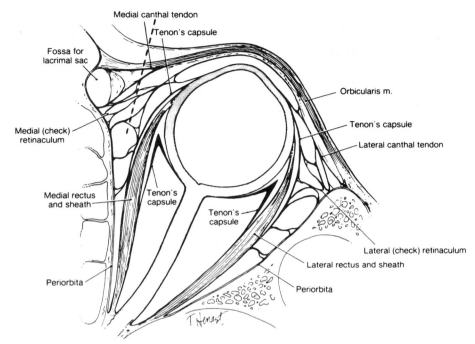

Medial canthal tendon
Tenon's capsule
Fossa for lacrimal sac
Orbicularis m.
Tenon's capsule
Medial (check) retinaculum
Lateral canthal tendon
Tenon's capsule
Medial rectus and sheath
Tenon's capsule
Lateral (check) retinaculum
Lateral rectus and sheath
Periorbita
Periorbita

Fig. 7.20. Schematic transverse section of the orbit. The dotted line represents the path and depth of penetration of a 30 gauge sharp disposable needle traversing the medial check ligament and entering the medial compartment of the nasal side of the medial rectus muscle. (Modified with permission from ref. 132.)

The medial orbital pericone block provides effective abolition of residual activity in the superior oblique muscle, frequently missed in blocks performed through the inferior temporal quadrant. It avoids an unacceptable incidence of lid ecchymoses, frequently seen with blocks performed transcutaneously in the superior nasal quadrant. It achieves excellent periorbital akinesia in the orbicularis oculi musculature, without the pain and other complications that can occur with transcutaneous seventh nerve blockade. By being effective in low volume, it preserves more easily the attainment of the goal of intraocular hypotony. Finally, by promoting spread of anaesthetic solution in the peripheral orbit with additional conduction blockade in the frontal and lacrimal nerve distributions, intraoperative patient comfort is enhanced.

Fourth injection: Superotemporal pericone injection (5%)

In patients in whom there is strong retained activity in the superior rectus and levator palpebrae superioris muscles, a pericone injection of 3–4 ml of anaesthetic mixture is used. The explanation of the phenomenon is the failure of the intracone (second) injection to reach in sufficient concentration the superior

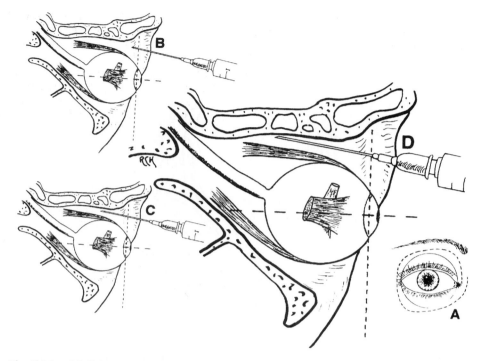

Fig. 7.21. Medial pericone block. Needle entry point is on the medial side of the caruncle at the extreme medial angle of the palpebral fisure (A, B). With the bevel facing the medial orbit wall, the needle advances in the transverse plane, directed towards the mid-line of the skull at the occiput, which is at about 5 degrees toward the medial orbit wall (B, C, D). Continuing observation of the relationship between the needle/hub junction and the plane of the iris controls appropriate depth of insertion (D). In a globe of normal axial length, the 25-mm needle tip will be at the depth of the hind surface of the eye. The eye in the drawing is 23.5 mm in diameter and the needle is 25 mm long. (With permission from Gimbel Educational Services.)

branch of the oculomotor nerve (see Chapter 1); in these individuals, it may be that the connective tissue hammock for the superior ophthalmic vein (Fig. 7.6) is unusually well developed and is only partially permeable to local anaesthetic approaching from within the central cone compartment. This block technique gains access to the nerve from above.

On this occasion, and only for this location of block, it is appropriate to 'walk' the needle tip along the periorbita. The bevel opening of the needle faces the orbit roof. A 27 gauge 31-mm needle is firmly mounted on a 5-ml syringe containing 4 ml anaesthetic mixture. With the eye to be blocked held closed, the needle is held tangential to the upper globe and the needle tip inserted through the skin of the lid at the level of the superior orbit rim and aimed up markedly toward the roof of the orbit (Fig. 7.22) starting 3–4 mm lateral to the sagittal plane of the lateral limbus and with a medial component of about 5 degrees (any more may result in unpleasant paraesthesia from needle tip contact with the frontal nerve or its supraorbital branch). This is also a relatively avascular area lying between the lacrimal vessels on the temporal side and the supraorbital vessels on the nasal side. After making the first bony contact with the orbit roof, the needle is redirected and walked posteriorly with a 5-degree medial component until the needle is at 31 mm depth from the superior orbit rim. Following test aspiration, 3–4 ml solution is injected while monitoring digitally the increasing volume in the orbit and making sure that excessive orbital pressure is not developing. After withdrawing the needle, observe carefully for a few seconds for evidence of haemorrhage.

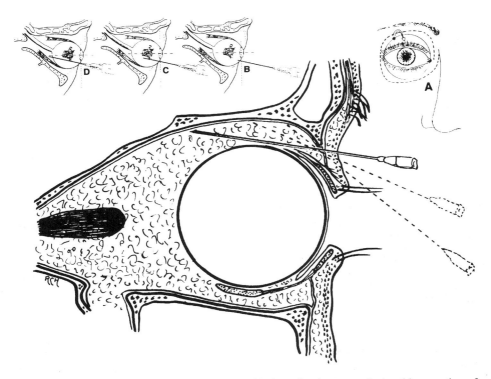

Fig. 7.22. Superotemporal pericone block. Detail of needle placement depicted in a section of the orbit through the lateral limbus at a 5-degree nasal angle from the true sagittal section of the head. The plane is lateral to the cornea and the inferior rectus, superior rectus and levator palpebrae muscles, but the front portion of the levator aponeurosis consisting of anterior (Müller's muscle inserting on the upper edge of the superior tarsal plate) and posterior lamellae is seen. An oblique slice of the lateral rectus muscle appears posteriorly and a cross-section of the inferior oblique muscle below the globe. The needle tip is inserted through the skin of the lid 3 mm lateral to the sagittal plane of the lateral limbus at the level of the superior orbit rim and aimed up markedly towards the roof of the orbit (A), with a medial component of about 5 degrees in a plane lateral to the superior rectus/levator complex (B, C, D). The needle tip 'walks' along the periorbita of the orbit roof (full-size illustration) in curvilinear fashion (A) until the needle tip is at a depth of 25–30 mm, at which point the injection is made with the usual precautions. (With permission from Gimbel Educational Services.)

Final check for globe akinesia

Following the third injection and a brief period of digital massage applied to gauze over the closed eyelids, an assessment of globe movements and orbicularis activity is made. If akinesia has not resulted from the preceding blocks, supplemental injection is indicated, directed to the appropriate quadrant. *Cautionary note:* tactile perception during a repeat intracone injection in the presence of paresis of the extraocular muscles is altered in comparison with that experienced during the preceding primary intracone injection; small rotational movements of the globe are commonly seen. Complaints of discomfort in response to stimuli, as an indicator of erroneous placement (see above), will be markedly obtunded. Having finally achieved akinesia, a 15-min period of continuous decompression follows, with the Honan device at a pressure of 30 mmHg, prior to the patient entering the operating room.

RECENT INNOVATIONS IN REGIONAL ANAESTHESIA FOR OPHTHALMOLOGY

Ongoing reports of the rare but serious complications of intraconal (retrobulbar) anaesthesia stimulated separate editorials in 1988 by Smith in the UK[106] and Lichter in the USA,[70] and introduced the concept of alternative non-akinetic methods of regional anaesthesia for cataract extraction surgery. The techniques published subsequently, which are discussed below, fall into three groups: sub-conjunctival (perilimbal); injection of local anaesthetic by needle or cannula within Tenon's capsule; and solely topical corneoconjunctival anaesthesia. Large-incision intraocular surgery as used in the past required akinesia to avoid loss of globe contents from muscle contraction. The current vogue for non-akinetic methods is made possible by small-incision, closed-system surgical techniques. Furthermore, since small-incision cataract surgery carried out by a gentle surgeon requires anaesthesia solely of the front of the eye, these less invasive methods are gaining favour. History is repeating itself, with topical anaesthesia again being commonly used for cataract extraction (see start of this chapter). However, these newer methods are not universally applicable to all cataract surgery because of patient temperament, lens pathology and surgery type variations.

Sub-conjunctival (perilimbal) injection of local anaesthetics

Several articles published in 1990 and 1991[33,49,94,96,107] advocated (with careful selection of patients) sub-conjunctival injection of local anaesthetics in small volume near the superior limbus, mainly for anterior segment surgery. Open communication between surgeon and patient was important as was minimal use of sedative drugs. Many experienced ophthalmologists would suggest that in its avoidance of intraconal blocks from fear of complications, the subconjunctival method allows exposure to the greater risks associated with performing intraocular surgery in the presence of extraocular muscle activity.[15] Globe perforation associated with the technique has been reported.[127]

Sub-Tenon's block

Anaesthesia for cataract surgery produced by injection beneath Tenon's capsule of small volumes of local anaesthetic were first described by Swan in 1956.[117] He indicated that the sub-Tenon's method produced better iris and anterior segment anaesthesia than did sub-conjunctival injection. Since 1990, the sub-Tenon's injection technique has been used extensively.[121] This injection technique evolved into anaesthesia produced by blunt cannula insertion[115] after surgical dissection into the sub-Tenon's space.[42,81,112] The degree of abolition of extraocular muscle movement is proportional to the volume of injectate. Following placement of local anaesthetic by cannula beneath Tenon's capsule, spread occurs into the anterior intracone space.[114] The disadvantages of the method are an increased incidence of conjunctival chemosis and haemorrhage and the potential of damaging one of the vortex veins.[112] Patients receiving anticoagulant medication should best avoid the technique.[112]

Peripheral orbit anaesthesia may be incomplete; supplemental local anaesthetic injections may be necessary to achieve patient comfort.[104] The various surgical procedures for which it has been advocated include: panretinal photocoagulation;[31,86] strabismus repair;[20,110] trabeculectomy;[97] cataract extraction;[42] and vitreoretinal surgery.[30,81,104] Intravenous sedation was often used during the surgery. General globe mobility is retained, but globe anaesthesia is better than with the sub-conjunctival method described above.

Cataract extraction and intraocular lens implantation under solely topical corneoconjunctival anaesthesia

The most recent step in the evolution of regional anaesthesia for cataract extraction has been the reintroduction by Fichman of solely topical corneoconjunctival anaesthesia.[48] It had been in use, albeit without the advantages of modern technology, in the last century and the first decade of the twentieth century with cocaine, the only available local anaesthesia agent at the time.[50,99] The method is best for lens removal by phacoemulsification with foldable lens implantation though a clear corneal incision of 4 mm width or less. Grabow has listed the advantages and disadvantages of solely topical anaesthesia for cataract extraction.[41] The claimed advantages are: avoidance of the complications of orbital injections; suitability for patients on anticoagulant medication; the appeal of a no-needle procedure; the patient's ability to look in any desired direction at the request of the surgeon; and early visual rehabilitation, especially for the patient with only one sighted eye. Critical non-selection of certain subjects is important, as there must be continuous and open dialogue between the surgeon and the patient throughout the operation. This rules out dementia, deafness and patients with a language barrier; obviously it is not a technique applicable to children. Patients with dense or trauma-induced cataracts, those with small pupils which fail to dilate and those with macular degeneration, are best managed with other forms of anaesthesia.

Surgeons experienced in the technique of intercapsular phacoemulsification, with the appropriate personal psychological traits, with good communication skills and the willingness to talk their patients through the process are most suited to the method. In the clinic in which the author works, the senior surgeon has switched to doing 98% of his cataract extraction procedures with topical corneoconjunctival anaesthesia and scleral tunnel incisions; however, none of the less experienced surgeons has yet requested the method, still preferring akinetic block anaesthesia. The author finds that patients having cataract surgery under topical anaesthesia require more psychological preparation and more frequent anxiolytic premedication for their visit to the operating theatre than do block anaesthesia patients. The amount of sedation, when deemed necessary, is geared to allow retention of intraoperative patient cooperation. Topical agents best suited are lignocaine 4%[41] and bupivacaine 0.75%.[38] The iris and ciliary muscle retain their sensitivity, especially in young and anxious patients.[41] The intraoperative use of intracameral miotic agents is particularly prone to precipitate discomfort from ciliary muscle spasm; to avoid this pain, cataract surgeons using topical anaesthesia are looking for alternatives to miotics. Perhaps the single greatest change involves the surgeon and staff switching to a completely different operating room protocol, including the logistics of operating from the side of the patient and incising the cornea and performing capsulorhexis with full globe motility.[41] Unlike in orbital regional anaesthesia by injection, there is no reduction in optic nerve function and hence an awareness of the brightness of the microscope light which can be disturbing to some patients; by starting off with reduced illumination and bringing it up gradually, this problem can usually be overcome.

TECHNIQUE MODIFICATIONS FOR SPECIFIC SURGICAL PROCEDURES USING REGIONAL ANAESTHESIA

For penetrating keratoplasty (corneal grafting), the regional anaesthesia technique requires a dependable therapeutic window of 2–2.5 h, with strict adherence to full anaesthesia and complete lid and globe akinesia. Specific eyedrops to be instilled in the conjunctival sac will be requested by the surgeon and will usually include a miotic agent. Induction of preoperative osmotic diuresis is commonly used to aid production of ocular hypotony. Likewise, an orbital decompression device is usually utilized. Moderately potent analgesics may be required postoperatively.

For vitreoretinal surgery under regional anaesthesia, a prolonged therapeutic window is necessary. The intraconal, periconal,[5,88] and sub-Tenon's methods[30,81,104] have all been advocated. The duration of planned surgery in itself may mandate in favour of general anaesthesia or a combined regional/intravenous sedation technique in the interests of patient comfort. Patients having vitreoretinal surgery, whether under regional or general anaesthesia, may[55] or may not[19] require hospitalization for optimum care postoperatively. Diabetic patients, particularly those poorly controlled and insulin-dependent, require hospital admission for appropiate metabolic management.[19,55] Patients presenting for vitreoretinal surgery have a relatively high incidence of axial myopia and posterior staphyloma (a bulging of the choroid coat into a thinned and stretched sclera), both of which call for extra caution in needle placement.[5]

For secondary intraocular lens implantation in aphakic patients, the main difference is in the requirement for a different set of conjunctivally instilled agents according to the wishes of the surgeon; the surgery time is usually more protracted than in a standard cataract extraction/intraocular lens implantation procedure, and may warrant the selection of longer-acting anaesthesia agents.

Trabeculectomy is usually performed on an akinetic and anaesthetic globe. In the presence of a previous trabeculectomy bleb, no external pressure should be used. Sub-Tenon's block is an alternative to the full intracone method.[97] Cataract surgery may be combined with trabeculectomy or trabeculotomy designed to reduce intraocular pressure.[39] In the management of glaucoma patients for intraocular surgery, orbital decompression devices are best omitted. Acceptably low orbital pressure in these patients is achieved by using as low an injectate volume as possible, including hyaluronidase in the anaesthesia mixture, and by permitting sufficient time (at least 15 min) to elapse between completion of the block and the commencement of surgery. Intraocular pressure control requires careful preoperative control of higher intraocular pressures (with, for example, oral acetazolamide and/or topical corneoconjunctival agents); induction of osmotic diuresis with mannitol may be required.

For refractive keratoplasty procedures, topical corneoconjunctival anaesthesia alone is most commonly employed. The radial keratotomy method is associated with moderate corneal postoperative discomfort for 24–36 h, whereas with *Excimer* laser keratectomy, in which the corneal epithelium is removed, more severe pain may result. Recently, in both of these methods of refractive surgery, conjunctival instillation of topical non-steroidal anti-inflammatory agents (ketorolac or diclofenac) combined with the use of a bandage contact lens have proved effective in the reduction of postoperative pain.[27,65,66] Optic nerve needle trauma with resultant blindness has been reported following intraconal anaesthesia used prior to astigmatic keratotomy.[57]

Epikeratophakia requires a therapeutic window of 2–2.5 h with full globe and eyelid akinesia. Moderately potent analgesics are required postoperatively for about 48 h.

For keratomileusis, the surgeon will wish to mark the visual axis on the cornea prior to anaesthesia. The anaesthetist should avoid production of conjunctival chemosis if at all possible. Blocking agents appropriate to a therapeutic window of 2–2.5 h with full akinesia of the globe and eyelids should be used and moderate postoperative analgesics will be required for about 48 h.

Panretinal photocoagulation, used in the management of diabetic retinopathy, is done with the argon laser and is painful in the unanaesthetized eye. Akinetic regional orbital anaesthesia allows for patient comfort and at the same time provides the operator with a non-moving retinal field on which to work with assurance that no rapid globe movement will momentarily expose a relatively healthy area to iatrogenic injury. The author uses an intracone injection of 3–4 ml lignocaine 2% with hyaluronidase for this purpose. Some surgeons prefer a sub-Tenon's block technique.[31,86]

Strabismus repair is commonly carried out under full akinetic/anaesthetic orbital regional anaesthesia,[118,119] but many other methods have been described, including non-akinetic periconal,[101] sub-Tenon's,[20,110] and topical.[25,120] Where an adjustable suture technique is used, general anaesthesia or short-acting local anaesthesia should be used.[21]

Oculoplastic surgery is commonly performed under regional anaesthesia. The principles used are identical to those for ophthalmic regional anaethesia in general. For certain procedures, it may be necessary to preserve levator palpebrae function. Higher concentrations of adrenaline in the injectate may be indicated for surgery to the eyelids to reduce operative bleeding. Repair of orbital floor fractures can be done under regional anaesthesia.[60] Dacryocystorhinostomy should be possible with a full medial pericone block but has not been reported. Painless probing of the tear ducts is easily accomplished following a superficial medial pericone block.

INJECTION OF NEUROLYTIC AGENTS FOR THE PAINFUL EYE

Atkinson advocated small-volume intracone alcohol injection (following preliminary local anaesthetic intracone block) in the management of the painful blind eye where enucleation has been refused or is contraindicated.[7] Its use may even apply to painful seeing eyes.[84] A volume of absolute alcohol not exceeding 2 ml is placed in the anterior to middle intracone compartment; the desired effect is interruption of conduction in the sensory nerves and total sparing of the oculomotor nerves. Pain relief lasting from a few months up to 1 year can be achieved. Hyaluronidase should be omitted both from the preliminary local anaesthetic and the subsequent alcohol injections; otherwise, persistent anaesthesia of the periorbital skin may result. Retrobulbar injection of 25 mg chlorpromazine may be more effective than ethanol for relief of chronic pain in sightless eyes.[128]

REFERENCES

1. Ahmad S, Ahmad A, Benzon HT. Clinical experience with the peribulbar block for ophthalmologic surgery. *Reg Anesth* 1993; **18:** 184.
2. Abelson MB, Paradis A, Mandel E, George M. The effect of hyaluronidase on akinesia during cataract surgery. *Ophthalmic Surg* 1989; **20:** 325.
3. Ali-Melkkilä TM, Virkkilä M, Jyrkkiö H. Regional anesthesia for cataract surgery: Comparison of retrobulbar and peribulbar techniques. *Reg Anesth* 1992; **17:** 219.
4. Allen CW. *Local and Regional Anesthesia.* WB Saunders: Philadelphia, PA, 1914: 625.
5. Arora R, Verma L, Kumar A *et al.* Peribulbar anesthesia in retinal reattachment surgery. *Ophthalmic Surg* 1992; **23:** 499.
6. Atkinson WS. Local anesthesia in ophthalmology. *Trans Am Ophthalmol Soc* 1934; **32:** 399.
7. Atkinson WS. Retrobulbar injection of anesthetic within the muscular cone (cone injection). *Arch Ophthalmol* 1936; **16:** 494.
8. Atkinson WS. Local anesthesia in ophthalmology. *Am J Ophthalmol* 1948; **31:** 1607.
9. Atkinson WS. Use of hyaluronidase with local anesthesia in ophthalmology: Preliminary report. *Arch Ophthalmol* 1949; **42:** 628.
10. Atkinson WS. Akinesia of the orbicularis. *Am J Ophthalmol* 1953; **36:** 1255.
11. Atkinson WS. Observations on anesthesia for ocular surgery. *Trans Am Acad Ophthalmol Otolaryngol* 1956; **60:** 376.

12. Atkinson WS. The development of ophthalmic anesthesia: The Sanford R. Gifford Lecture. *Am J Ophthalmol* 1961; **51**: 1.
13. Atkinson WS. Larger retrobulbar injections (Letter). *Am J Ophthalmol* 1964; **57**: 328.
14. Atkinson WS. Facial nerve block. *Am J Ophthalmol* 1964; **57**: 144.
15. Aquavella JV. Limbal anesthesia for cataract surgery (Commentary). *Ophthalmic Surg* 1990; **21**: 26.
16. Bloomberg LB. Anterior periocular anesthesia: Five years experience. *J Cataract Refract Surg* 1991; **17**: 508.
17. Brown DL, Wedel DJ. Introduction to regional anesthesia. In *Anesthesia,* 3rd ed (edited by Miller RD). Churchill Livingstone: New York, 1990: 1370–1371.
18. Buys NS. Mercury balloon reducer for vitreous and orbital volume control. In *Current Concepts in Cataract Surgery* (edited by Emery J). CV Mosby: St Louis, MO, 1980: 258.
19. Cannon SC, Gross JG, Abramson I *et al*. Evaluation of outpatient experience with vitreoretinal surgery. *Br J Ophthalmol* 1992; **76**: 68.
20. Capo H, Munoz M. Sub-Tenon's lidocaine irrigation for strabismus surgery (Letter). *Ophthalmic Surg* 1992; **23**: 145.
21. Cheng KP, Larson CE, Biglan AW, D'Antonio JA. A prospective, randomized, controlled comparison of retrobulbar and general anesthesia for strabismus surgery. *Ophthalmic Surg* 1992; **23**: 585.
22. Davidson B, Kratz R, Mazzoco T. An evaluation of the Honan intraocular pressure reducer. *Am Intra-ocular Implant Soc J* 1979; **5**: 237.
23. Davis DB, Mandel MR. Posterior peribulbar anesthesia: An alternative to retrobulbar anesthesia. *J Cataract Refract Surg* 1986; **12**: 182.
24. Davis DB, Mandel MR. Posterior perimulbar anesthesia: An alternative to retrobulbar anesthesia. *Geriatr Ophthalmol* 1987; **86**: 61.
25. Diamond GR. Topical anesthesia for strabismus surgery. *J Pediatr Ophthalmol Strabismus* 1989; **26**: 86.
26. Duverger C. *L'anesthésie locale en ophthalmologie*. Masson et Cie: Paris, 1920.
27. Eiferman RA, Hoffman RS, Sher NA. Topical diclofenac reduces pain following photorefractive keratectomy (Letter). *Arch Ophthalmol* 1993; **111**: 1022.
28. Feibel RM. Current concepts in retrobulbar anesthesia. *Surv Ophthalmol* 1985; **30**: 102.
29. Feibel RM. Robert E. Wright and the development of facial nerve akinesia. *Surv Ophthalmol* 1989; **33**: 523.
30. Friedberg MA, Spellman FA, Pilkerton R *et al*. An alternative technique of local anesthesia for vitreoretinal surgery. *Arch Ophthalmol* 1991; **109**: 1615.
31. Friedberg MA, Palmer RM. A new technique of local anesthesia for panretinal photocoagulation. *Ophthalmol Surg* 1991; **22**: 619.
32. Fry RA, Henderson J. Local anaesthesia for eye surgery. *Anaesthesia* 1990; **45**: 14.
33. Furuta M, Toriumi T, Kashiwagi K, Satoh S. Limbal anesthesia for cataract surgery. *Ophthalmic Surg* 1990; **21**: 22.
34. Gayton JK, Tessiniar TS, Ledford JK. Alternative draping technique for claustrophobic patients (Letter). *Ophthalmic Surg* 1990; **21**: 672.
35. Gifford H. Motor block of extraocular muscles by deep orbital injection. *Arch Ophthalmol* 1949; **41**: 5.
36. Gills JP. Constant mild compression of the eye to produce hypotension. *Am Intraocular Implant Soc J* 1979; **5**: 52.
37. Gills JP, Loyd TL. A technique of retrobulbar block with paralysis of orbicularis oculi. *Am Intraocular Implant Soc J* 1983; **9**: 339.
38. Gills JP, Williams DL. Advantage of Marcaine for topical anesthesia. *J Cataract Refract Surg* 1993; **19**: 819.
39. Gimbel HV, Meyer D. Small incision trabeculotomy combined with phacoemulsification and intraocular lens implantation. *J Cataract Refract Surg* 1993; **19**: 92.

40. Gjötterberg M, Ingemansson S-O. Effect on intraocular pressure of retrobulbar injection of Xylocaine with and without adrenaline. *Acta Ophthalmol* 1977; **55**: 709.
41. Grabow HB. Topical anesthesia for cataract surgery. *Eur J Implant Ref Surg* 1993; **5**: 20.
42. Greenbaum S. Parabulbar anesthesia. *Am J Ophthalmol* 1992; **114**: 776.
43. Grizzard WS. Ophthalmic anesthesia. In *Ophthalmology Annual* (edited by Reinecke RD). Raven Press: New York, 1989: 265–294.
44. Grizzard WS, Kirk NM, Pavan PR *et al.* Perforating ocular injuries caused by anesthesia personnel. *Ophthalmology* 1991; **98**: 1011.
45. Guarro M, Aggarwal RK, Misson G *et al.* Patient attitude to 'informed consent' in cataract surgery. *Eur J Implant Surg* 1992; **4**: 184.
46. Hamilton RC, Gimbel HV, Strunin L. Regional anaesthesia for 12,000 cataract extraction and intraocular lens implantation procedures. *Can J Anaesth* 1988; **35**: 615.
47. Hamilton RC. Non-ophthalmologists and orbital regional anesthesia (Letter). *Ophthalmology* 1992; **99**: 169.
48. Harr, D. Topical eyedrops replace injection for anesthesia. *Ocular Surgery News* 1992; **10**: 1, 20.
49. Hatt M. Cataract extraction with intraocular lens implantation under subconjuncival local anaesthesia. *Klin Mbl Augenheilk* 1990; **196**: 307.
50. Hirschberg J. *History of Ophthalmology*. JP Wayenborgh Verlag: Bonn, Germany, 1910: 284.
51. Hulquist CR. Perbulbar block injection volume (Letter). *J Cataract Refract Surg* 1993; **19**: 564.
52. Hustead RF, Hamilton RC, Loken RG. Periocular local anesthesia: Medial orbital as an alternative to superior nasal injection. *J Cataract Refract Surg* 1994; **20**: 197.
53. Hustead RF, Hamilton RC. Pharmacology. In *Ophthalmic Anesthesia* (edited by Gills JP, Hustead RF, Sanders DR). Slack Inc.: Thorofare, NJ, 1993: 69–102.
54. Hustead RF, Hamilton RC. Techniques. In *Ophthalmic Anesthesia* (edited by Gills JP, Hustead RF, Sanders DR). Slack Inc.: Thorofare, NJ, 1993: 103–186.
55. Isernhagen RD, Michels RG, Glaser BM *et al.* Hospitalization requirements after vitreoretinal surgery. *Arch Ophthalmol* 1988; **106**: 767.
56. Javitt JC, Addiego R, Friedberg HL *et al.* Brain stem anesthesia after retrobulbar block. *Ophthalmology* 1987; **94**: 718.
57. Jindra LF. Blindness following retrobulbar anestheisa for astigmatic keratotomy. *Ophthalmic Surg* 1989; **20**: 433.
58. Kahn HA, Leibowitz HM, Geneley JP *et al.* The Framingham eye study. 1. Outline and major prevalence findings. *Am J Epidemiol* 1977; **106**: 17.
59. Katsev DA, Drews RC, Rose BT. An anatomic study of retrobulbar needle path length. *Ophthalmology* 1989; **96**: 1221.
60. Kezirian GM, Hill FD, Hill FJ. Peribulbar anesthesia for the repair of orbital floor fractures. *Ophthalmic Surg* 1991; **22**: 601.
61. Khalil SN. Local anaesthesia for eye surgery (Letter). *Anaesthesia* 1991; **46**: 232.
62. Kimble JA, Morris RE, Witherspoon CD, Feist RM. Globe perforation from peribulbar injection. *Arch Ophthalmol* 1987; **105**: 749.
63. Kline D, Sekular R, Dismukes K. Social issues, human needs, and opportunities for research on the effects of age on vision: An overview. In *Aging and Human Visual Function* (edited by Sekuler R, Kline D, Dismukes K). Alan R. Liss: New York, 1982: 3–6.
64. Knapp H. On cocaine and its use in ophthalmic and general surgery. *Arch Ophthalmol* 1884; **13**: 402.
65. Knaub J. Ketorolac use is found to lessen post-PRK pain. *Ocular Surgery News* 1993; **11**: 64.
66. Knaub J. NSAID provides analgesic effect after radial keratotomy. *Ocular Surgery News* 1993; **11**: 46.
67. Koornneef L. Orbital septa: Anatomy and function. *Ophthalmology* 1979; **86**: 876.

68. Leaming DV. Practice styles and preferences of ASCRS members – 1990 survey. *J Cataract Refract Surg* 1991; **17:** 495.

69. Lebuisson DA. Simplified and safer peribulbar anaesthesia. *Eur J Implant Ref Surg* 1990; **2:** 123.

70. Lichter PR. Avoiding complications from local anesthesia. *Ophthalmology* 1988; **95:** 565.

71. Lichter PR. The relative value of quality care (Editorial). *Ophthalmology* 1991; **98:** 1151.

72. Livingston MW. Optimal management of the conscious patient undergoing intraocular surgery. *Am J Ophthalmol* 1965; **60:** 120.

73. Livingston MW, Mackool RJ, Schneider H. Anesthetic agents used in cataract surgery (Letter). *J Cataract Refract Surg* 1990; **16:** 272.

74. Liu C, Youl B, Moseley I. Magnetic resonance imaging of the optic nerve in extremes of gaze: Implications for the positioning of the globe for retrobulbar anaesthesia. *Br J Ophthalmol* 1992; **76:** 728.

75. Loots JH, Koorts AS, Venter JA. Peribulbar anesthesia: A prospective statistical analysis of the efficacy and predictability of bupivacaine and a lignocaine/bupivacaine mixture. *J Cataract Refract Surg* 1993; **19:** 72.

76. Löwenstein A. Ueber regionaire anesthesia in der orbita. *Klin Monatsbl Augenheilkd* 1908; **46:** 592.

77. Maltby JR, Sutherland AD, Sale JP, Shaffer EA. Preoperative oral fluids: is a five hour fast justified prior to elective surgery? *Anesth Analg* 1986; **65:** 1112.

78. Martin SR, Baker SS, Muenzler WS. Retrobulbar anesthesia and orbicularis akinesia. *Ophthalmic Surg* 1986; **17:** 232.

79. McDonald HR, Schatz H, Johnston RN. Aminoglycoside toxicity. *Sem Ophthalmol* 1993; **8:** 136.

80. McDonnell PJ, Quigley HA, Maumenee AE *et al.* The Honan intraocular pressure reducer: An experimental study. *Arch Ophthalmol* 1985; **103:** 422.

81. Mein CE, Woodcock MG. Local anesthesia for vitreoretinal surgery. *Retina* 1990; **10:** 47.

82. Meyer D, Hamilton RC, Loken RG, Gimbel HV. Effect of combined peribulbar and retrobulbar injection of large volumes of anesthetic agents on the intraocular pressure. *Can J Ophthalmol* 1992; **27:** 230.

83. Meyers EF. Anesthesia. In *Complications in Ophthalmic Surgery* (edited by Krupin T, Waltman SR). JB Lippincott: Philadelphia, PA, 1984:1–22.

84. Michels RG, Maumenee AE. Retrobulbar alcohol injection in seeing eyes. *Trans Am Acad Ophthalmol Otolaryngol* 1973; **77:** 164.

85. Morsman CD, Holden R. The effects of adrenaline, hyaluronidase and age on peribulbar anaesthesia. *Eye* 1992; **6:** 290.

86. Moses KC, Norbury JW. Anesthesia for retinal photocoagulation. *Ophthalmic Surg* 1990; **21:** 156.

87. Nadbath RP, Rehman I. Facial nerve block. *Am J Ophthalmol* 1963; **55:** 143.

88. Nicholson AD, Singh P, Badrinath SS *et al.* Peribulbar anesthesia for primary vitreoretinal surgery. *Ophthalmol Surg* 1992; **23:** 657.

89. Nicoll JMV, Treuren B, Acharya PA *et al.* Retrobulbar anesthesia: The role of hyaluronidase. *Anesth Analg* 1986; **65:** 1324.

90. O'Brien CS. Local anesthesia in opthalmic surgery. *JAMA* 1928; **90:** 8.

91. O'Brien CS. Local anesthesia. *Arch Ophthalmol* 1934; **12:** 240.

92. Otto AJ, Spekreijse H. Volume discrepancies in the orbit and the effect on the intraorbital pressure: An experimental study in the monkey. *Orbit* 1989; **8:** 233.

93. Pautler SE, Grizzard WS, Thompson LN, Wing GL. Blindness from retrobulbar injection into the optic nerve. *Ophthalmic Surg* 1986; **17:** 334.

94. Petersen WC, Yanoff M. Subconjunctival anesthesia: An alternative to retrobulbar and peribulbar techniques. *Ophthalmic Surg* 1991; **22:** 199.

95. Philip BK, Covino BG. Local and regional anesthesia. In *Anesthesia for Ambulatory*

Surgery, 2nd edn (edited by Wetchler BV). JB Lippincott: Philadelphia, PA, 1991: 313.

96. Redmond RM, Dallas NL. Extracapsular cataract extraction without retrobulbar anaesthesia. *Br J Ophthalmol* 1990; **74:** 203.

97. Ritch R, Liebmann JM. Sub-Tenon's anesthesia for trabeculectomy. *Ophthalmic Surg* 1992; **23:** 502.

98. Ropo A. Orbicular muscle akinesia: A comparison, using electromyography, of three techniques. *Ophthalmic Surg* 1992; **23:** 414.

99. Rosen. Editorial review: Anaesthesia for cataract surgery. *Eur J Implant Ref Surg* 1993; **5:** 1.

100. Salmon JF, Mets B, James MFM, Murray ADN. Intravenous sedation for ocular surgery under local anaesthesia. *Br J Ophthalmol* 1992; **76:** 598.

101. Sanders RJ, Nelson LB, Deutsch JA. Peribulbar anesthesia for strabismus surgery. *Am J Ophthalmol* 1990; **109:** 705.

102. Sarvela J, Nikki P. Comparison of two needle lengths in regional ophthalmic anesthesia with etidocaine and hyaluronidase. *Ophthalmic Surg* 1992; **23:** 742.

103. Scarr M, Maltby JR, Jani K, Sutherland LR. Volume and acidity of residual gastric fluid after oral fluid ingestion before elective ambulatory surgery. *CMAJ* 1989; **14:** 1114.

104. Simcock PR, Raymond GL, Lavin MJ. Peribulbar injection and direct infiltration for vitreoretinal surgery. *Arch Ophthalmol* 1992; **110:** 1357.

105. Smiddy WE, Michels RG, Kumar AJ. Magnetic resonance imaging of retrobulbar changes in optic nerve position with eye movement. *Am J Ophthalmol* 1989; **107:** 82.

106. Smith RJH. Why retrobulbar anaesthesia? (Editorial). *Br J Ophthalmol* 1988; **72:** 1.

107. Smith RJH. Cataract extraction without retrobulbar anaesthetic injection. *Br J Ophthalmol* 1990; **74:** 205.

108. Spaeth GL. A new method to achieve complete akinesia of the facial nerve muscles of the eyelids. *Ophthalmic Surg* 1976; **7:** 105.

109. Spaeth GL. Informed choice, not informed consent (Editorial). *Ophthalmic Surg* 1992; **23:** 648.

110. Steele MA, Lavrich JB, Nelson LB, Koller HP. Sub-Tenon's infusion of local anesthetic for strabismus surgery. *Ophthalmic Surg* 1992; **23:** 40.

111. Steinberg EP, Javitt JC, Sharkey PD *et al.* Socioeconomics of ophthalmology: The content and cost of cataract surgery. *Arch Ophthalmol* 1993; **111:** 1041.

112. Stevens JD. A new local anaesthesia technique for cataract extraction by one quadrant sub-Tenon's infiltration. *Br J Ophthalmol* 1992; **76:** 670.

113. Stevens J, Giubilei M, Lanigan L, Hykin P. Sub-Tenon, retrobulbar and peribulbar local anaesthesia: The effect upon intraocular pressure. *Eur J Implant Ref Surg* 1993; **5:** 25.

114. Stevens JD, Restori M. Ultrasound imaging of no-needle 1-quadrant sub-Tenon local anaesthesia for cataract surgery. *Eur J Implant Ref Surg* 1993; **5:** 35.

115. Stevens JD. Curved, sub-Tenon cannula for local anesthesia. *Ophthalmic Surg* 1993; **24:** 121.

116. Straus JG. A new retrobulbar needle and injection technique. *Ophthalmic Surg* 1988; **19:** 134.

117. Swan KC. New drugs and techniques for ocular anesthesia. *Tr Am Acad Ophthalmol Otolaryngol* 1956; **60:** 368.

118. Szmyd SM, Nelson LB, Calhoun JH, Harley RD. Retrobulbar anesthesia in strabismus surgery. *Arch Ophthalmol* 1984; **102:** 1325.

119. Szmyd SM, Nelson LB, Calhoun JH *et al.* Retrobulbar anesthesia in strabismus surgery. II. Use of a short acting anesthetic agent. *Arch Ophthalmol* 1985; **103:** 809.

120. Thorson JC, Jampolsky AB. Topical anesthesia for strabismus surgery. *Tr Am Acad Ophthalmol Otolaryngol* 1966; **70:** 968.

121. Tsuneoka H, Ohki K, Taniuchi O, Kitahara K. Tenon's capsule anaesthesia for cataract surgery with IOL implantation. *Eur J Implant Ref Surg* 1993; **5**: 29.
122. Unsöld R, Stanley JA, DeGroot J. The CT-topography of retrobulbar anesthesia. Graefes *Arch Klin Exp Ophthalmol* 1981; **217**: 125.
123. van Lint: Paralysie palpébrale temporaire provoquée dans l'opération de la cataracte. *Ann d'Ocul* 1914; **151**: 420.
124. Wang HS. Peribulbar anesthesia for ophthalmic procedures. *J Cataract Refract Surg* 1988; **14**: 441.
125. Weiss JL, Deichman CB. A comparison of retrobulbar and periocular anesthesia for cataract surgery. *Arch Ophthalmol* 1989; **107**: 96.
126. Wright RE. Blocking of the facial nerve in cataract operations. *Am J Ophthalmol* 1921; **4**: 445.
127. Yanoff M, Redovan EG. Anterior eyewall perforation during subconjunctival cararact block. *Ophthalmic Surg* 1990; **21**: 362.
128. Waltz KL, Williams GA, Goldey SH *et al*. Alternative to retrobulbar ethanol for blind painful eyes. *Ophthalmology* 1992; **99S**: 153.
129. Miller NR. Walsh and Hoyt's *Clinical Neuro-ophthalmology*, 4th edn, Vol. 1. Williams and Wilkins: Baltimore, MD, 1982.
130. Koornneef L, Grizzard WS. Ophthalmic anesthesia. In *Ophthalmology Annual* (edited by Reinecke RD). Raven Press: New York, 1989: 265–294.
131. Zahl K. Blockade of the orbicularis oculi. *Ophthalmol Clin North Am* 1990; **3**: 93–100.
132. Donaxas MT, Anderson RL. *Clinical Orbital Anatomy*. Williams and Wilkins: Baltimore, MD, 1984: 232.
133. Warwick R. The extraocular muscles. In *Eugene Wolff's Anatomy of the Eye and Orbit*, 7th edn. WB Saunders: Philadelphia, PA, 1976: 273.
134. Zide BM, Jelks GW. *Surgical Anatomy of the Orbit*. Raven Press: New York, 1985: 75.
135. Farley JS, Hustead RF, Becker KE. Diluting lidocaine and mepivacaine in balanced salt solution reduces the pain of intradermal injection. *Reg Anesth* 1994; **19**: 48.

CHAPTER 8

The complications of orbital regional anaesthesia

ROBERT C HAMILTON

INTRODUCTION

Sound knowledge of orbital anatomy, ophthalmic physiology and the pharmacology of the anaesthesia and ophthalmic drugs should be prerequisites before embarking on orbital regional anaesthesia; such information should then be augmented by training in technique[89] obtained in clinical settings from practitioners with wide experience and knowledge in the field. All beginner clinicians have to go through an obligatory 'learning curve'; its gradient can be reduced by exposure to expert instruction and supervision.

The complications of regional anaesthesia for ophthalmology may be systemic, or confined to the orbit and its contents, and may be acute in onset or delayed. They range all the way in importance from the death of the patient to the most trivial. This chapter covers the various presentations that may be experienced, their incidence as reported in the literature, discussions regarding their clinical management, and how best to avoid them in the first place. Some are directly related to the local anaesthetic drugs and administration techniques, whereas others are surgical in nature, occurring only after operative intervention. As in other fields of anaesthesia, frequent repetition leads to improvement. The author will indicate errors that he has made and will analyse them in the hope that his unfortunate experience may help others: 'The only true failure is a failure to learn something from the experience'.[37]

In many centres patients routinely receive sedative or narcotic drugs, often intravenously, in order to facilitate anaesthetic techniques. The author advocates that by employing low-stimulus methods, sedative drugs are often unnecessary and intravenous medication only rarely required. Side-effects and complications related to the use and misuse of drugs are thus minimized.[176,215] Excellent surgical outcome is greatly influenced by good anaesthesia; to permit painful surgical stimuli because of incomplete anaesthesia leads to high stress and may provoke serious complications. The most appropriate management of an inadequate block is supplemental injection of further local anaesthetic agent rather than the suppression of reactivity with systemic medication.[48]

PROLOGUE

The eye is naturally well protected within the orbit from injury (Fig. 8.1). However, it is not surprising that medical intervention with needles can result in complications. To achieve the desired goals of globe and adnexal anaesthesia and akinesia, with concurrent hypotony, a two-injection method became the traditionally accepted technique, combining the deposition of a small volume of local anaesthetic at the apex of the orbit with a block of the seventh nerve at some point along its extracranial path. Recent years have seen the advent of new anaesthesia techniques, more effective for the surgeon and more comfortable for the patient. Notable advances include improved anaesthetic agents and the introduction of orbital decompression devices which allow larger volumes of local anaesthetic drug to be injected into the orbit. However, because larger volumes are used, it is all the more important that mechanisms causing complications are fully understood.

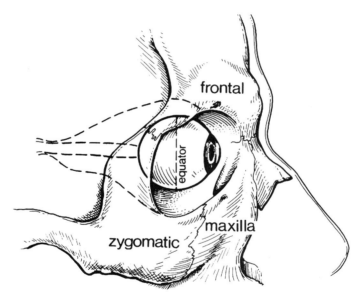

Fig. 8.1. The orbit rim forms a strong bony buttress protecting the vital structures within the orbit. (With permission from ref. 78.)

HISTORY OF INTRACONAL AND PERICONAL TECHNIQUES

Intraconal

Retrobulbar (intraconal) injection of a local anaesthetic was first done in 1884 by Knapp,[118] but failed to become popular until the 1930s when intraconal blocking, first with procaine,[56] and later with lignocaine[177] and bupivacaine,[33,188] became established as an effective method. Intraconal anaesthesia was not without side-effects

Table 8.1   Complications of orbital regional anaesthesia

Complication	Signs and symptoms	Mechanism
Venous haemorrhage	Retrobulbar haematoma	Tearing or puncture of orbital vein
Arterial haemorrhage	Acute massive retrobulbar haematoma with ischaemia	Tearing or puncture of orbital artery
Vascular occlusion	Occlusion of central retinal artery	Retrobular haematoma, intrasheath haematoma
	Transient visual loss and visual field defects	Conduction block by anaesthetic
Optic nerve penetration	Permanent visual loss and visual field defects, optic nerve head swelling, optic atrophy	Ischaemic compression by haematoma, trauma to ciliary arteries, trauma to optic nerve
Penetration or perforation of the globe	Pain, loss of intraocular pressure, intraocular haemorrhage, retinal tear, retinal detachment	Needle penetrates or perforates globe with trauma to the choroid or to the retina
Needle penetration of optic nerve sheath	Increasing or decreasing cardiovascular vital signs, pulmonary oedema, cardiac arrest, shivering, convulsions, hyperreflexia, hemiplegia, paraplegia, quadriplegia, contralateral amaurosis, contralateral oculomotor paralysis, facial palsy, deafness, vertigo, aphasia, loss of neck muscle power, loss of consciousness, vagolysis, respiratory depression, apnoea	Central spread of local anaesthetics along submeningeal pathways
Intravenous injection	Cutaneous numbness, dizziness, confusion, drowsiness, twitching, unconsciousness, convulsions, coma, apnoea, hypoxia, death, hypotension, bradycardia, cardiac standstill, ventricular fibrillation	Central nervous system and cardiovascular toxicity from increasing systemic levels of local anaesthetics
Intra-arterial injection	Acute grand mal convulsive state	Acutely increased cerebral levels of local anaesthetics
Slowing of pulse following strong stimulation	Bradycardia, nausea, increased blood pressure, loss of consciousness, cardiac arrest	Oculocardiac reflex elicited by dull or blunt needle (see text)

and complications.[56] In a 1988 editorial Lichter[133] stated that 'problems still occur from this very basic ophthalmic procedure [retrobulbar injection]. In reviewing the literature on this subject, one realizes that we have not come all that far in standardizing the technique or preventing complications since the first retrobulbar anesthetic was administered over 100 years ago'. The 'up and in' directive of traditional intraconal blocking was exposed as the probable source of many of the complications.[200] A needle advancing from an inferotemporal entry point and aiming for the apex is less prone to contact the optic nerve with the globe in the primary gaze position, whereas the nerve is endangered with the globe elevated and adducted.[7,104,200] Katsev *et al.* recommended that needle length introduced beyond the orbital rim for both intraconal and periconal injections should not exceed 31 mm in order to avoid damage to the optic nerve in all patients.[111]

The most serious complications were brain stem anaesthesia, scleral perforation, retinal vascular occlusion, optic nerve damage, extraocular muscle paresis and retrobulbar haemorrhage; each of these will receive separate attention later in the chapter. Table 8.1 lists the complications, their signs and symptoms and the mechanisms of their causation.

Periconal

Anaesthesia by deliberate local anaesthetic injection outside the muscle cone was first used, in the modern era, in 1971 by Charles Kelman, MD, of New York (personal communication). The method, although clearly described as long ago as 1914 by Allen,[5] was not common practice until after the publication of Davis and Mandel's 1986 article on 'posterior peribulbar anesthesia'.[42] They emphasized the safety features inherent in needle placement in sites more remote from vital orbit structures.

Intraconal vs periconal

Although there are proponents of both intraconal and periconal techniques, safe anaesthesia can be accomplished by both methods; likewise serious complications can arise with both if carried out incorrectly. In a report of 12 000 cataract extraction procedures under regional anaesthesia using one or other of these techniques, or a combination of both, the author found that faster onset was achieved when blocking within the muscle cone;[86] chemosis is more common with periconal blocks.[10,116,206] Much confused thinking has been generated by the fallacious concept of the closed 'cone' consisting of the four rectus muscles and their interconnecting intermuscular septa. Koornneef, in an exhaustive study, failed to find any evidence of a common muscle sheath creating distinct compartments in the posterior orbit. He concluded that the concept of discrete intracone and extracone compartments was erroneous.[121]

NEEDLES AND INJECTION TECHNIQUES

The perception of changes in tissue densities during needle advancement is a vital part of safe regional anaesthesia; it is an acquired skill that requires experience and ongoing practice.[22] Needle advancement within the confines of the orbit is essentially a blind procedure and has the potential of serious complication. Although the complication rate is low, because of the large numbers of eye block procedures carried out annually, even rare complications become significant.[202]

Traditional teaching to ophthalmology and anaesthesia residents tended to follow the Atkinson technique[11] of placing an inferotemporal needle intraconally with the globe elevated and adducted; this was handed down verbally and in texts without detailed instruction in the precision required for safe placement. The Atkinson 'up and in' globe positioning has largely been discredited; nevertheless, despite its dangers, it lingers on in two recent texts.[19,112] During inferotemporal needle insertion with the globe elevated and adducted, the optic nerve is brought closer to the needle tip and the macular area is further exposed to damage.[104,136,200] Optic nerve sheath penetration, optic nerve trauma and ocular penetration or perforation by the needle may result (see various sections below). The posterior pole of the globe is endangered, particularly in the ovoid globes of myopic patients.[78] Many of the serious complications discussed in this chapter will be avoided by having patients direct their eyes in primary gaze position during needle placement and subsequent injection. This has been substantiated by computed tomography scanning and magnetic resonance imaging.[136,186,200]

In the literature there is a considerable lobby for the use of dull needles to reduce the incidence of bleeding.[1,27,43,115] The superiority of blunt- over sharp-tipped needles in reducing the incidence of bleeding has not been demonstrated in a controlled trial. Delicate vessels may be subject to shearing forces created by inserted needles;[20] the author believes that his low incidence of bleeding associated with orbital blocks using fine sharp disposable needles is, among other factors, related to the minimal tissue distortion related to their use. Grizzard states that tactile discrimination is progressively reduced with increasing needle size; the increased resistance caused by a blunt needle is not appreciated because of the necessarily greater preload (Weber-Fechner law).[78] Grizzard *et al.*, reporting on iatrogenic ocular injuries, found that penetration or perforation of the eye from use of larger dull needles caused more serious damage than when fine disposable ones were implicated, and questioned the arguments in the earlier literature that advocated their use.[79] This was the first report in the literature showing an advantage of sharp over blunt needles other than patient comfort.

Traditional teaching favoured dull-tipped, intermediate-gauge needles (23 gauge commonly used), with the supposed advantages that blood vessels were pushed aside rather than traumatized and that tissue planes could be more accurately defined. In the recent literature there are reports of even coarser-diameter, dull-tipped needles (20 and 21 gauge).[18,45] While it is true that scleral penetration is more difficult with blunt-tipped needles, notably those of non-cutting design,[66,202,204] this may not be relevant for a complication so rarely seen. Using blunt-tipped needles does not convey protection against penetration; of the 23 cases reported by Hay *et al.*, 7 were caused by dull needles and of the 11 reported by Grizzard *et al.* 5 implicated this type of needle.[79,90] Because the ratio of resistances of scleral to skin penetration remained the same for the needle tips of both the sharp and dull varieties, Vivian and Canning concluded that it was unlikely that dull needles offered any protection against the complication.[202] Several authors have commented that blunt-tipped needles are painful for the patient.[114,149,202,209] Fine disposable needles are less painful for the patient and with their use oral and intravenous sedative medication often become unnecessary.[161] Intensity of pain increases with the dullness of the needle and the rapidity and volume of the injection.[149] The author has used fine disposable needles in 32 000 cases over the 10 years prior to January 1994 and is convinced of their safety (see Chapter 7).

Special attention should be paid to the length of needle entering beyond the orbital rim and the directioning of the needle.[50,111] Longer needles may reach the orbital apex where the vessels are of larger lumen and the optic nerve and vessels are less mobile (Fig. 8.2); retrobulbar haemorrhage or optic nerve trauma may result. In addition, the rectus muscles converge at the orbital apex into close proximity. Grizzard has described the structures at the apex as being analogous to tightly packed pickles in a jar, rather rigidly held in place and easily pierced.[78] While it is possible to get superb blocks with small volume injection at the apex

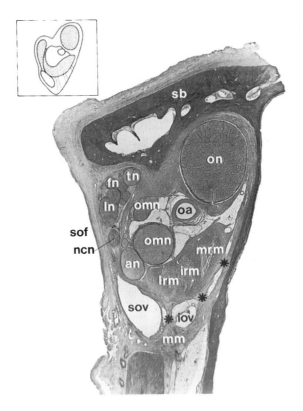

Fig 8.2. Coronal section at the orbital apex 25.4 mm posterior to the hind surface of the globe. Here the vessels are of larger lumen and the optic nerve and vessels more tightly confined. sb, sphenoid bone; on, optic nerve; oa, ophthalmic artery; lrm, irm, mrm, origins of the lateral, inferior and medial rectus muscles at the annulus of Zinn; mm, Müller's muscle (of inferior orbit); sof, superior orbital fissure; ncn, ln, fn, tn, nasociliary, lacrimal, frontal and trochlear nerves; omn, superior and inferior branches of the oculomotor nerve; an, abducens nerve; sov, iov, superior and inferior ophthalmic veins; *connective tissue septa. (With permission from ref. 217.)

of the orbit,[68] the risks are too great. A distance of 31 mm as measured from the orbit rim should never be exceeded,[111] nor should a needle advancing from an inferotemporal entry be allowed to cross the mid-sagittal plane of the eye (Fig. 8.3).[78] All needles used for intraconal and periconal insertion should be orientated tangentially to the globe with the bevel opening faced towards the globe.[70,86] Tangential alignment is most easily achieved in transconjunctival techniques.[70,86] If a tangentially aligned needle contacts the sclera, globe penetration is less likely to occur than with a needle approaching at a greater angle. Having placed the needle at the desired depth, if it is then found that there is an increased resistance above that expected, rather than inject against this resistance it is imperative to reposition the needle tip first.[153,171] All needles in the orbit are potentially hazardous in the wrong hands; careful supervision and training in technique have more relevance in the avoidance of serious complications than the type of needle used.[89] Techniques requiring multiple needle placements are associated with an increased incidence of complications when compared with a single or reduced number of injections.[1,114,193] Commercially produced needles with special tips or of curved design have been developed by ophthalmologists and anaesthetists, each claiming safety advantages.[66,193,199] Siegrist used a curved needle and a transconjunctival approach for orbital blocks in the early 1900s.[5] The author uses a custom-bent needle routinely (see Chapter 7).

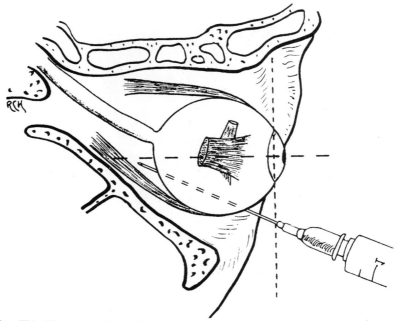

Fig. 8.3. This 31-mm needle is advanced beyond the equator of the globe, and then directed towards an imaginary point behind the macula, being careful not to cross the mid-sagittal plane of the eye. In a globe with normal axial length, as illustrated here, when the needle/hub junction has reached the plane of the iris, the tip of the needle lies 5–7 mm beyond the hind surface of the globe. (With permission from Gimbel Educational Services.)

COMPLICATIONS WITH PERCUTANEOUS SEVENTH NERVE BLOCK

Complications with blocking of the main trunk of the facial nerve after its exit from the stylomastoid foramen have been reported.[120,135] In these there was swallowing difficulty and respiratory obstruction related to unilateral vagus, glossopharyngeal and spinal accessory blockade (Fig. 8.4). For facial blockade at this site it is prudent to inject no deeper than advocated (12 mm) and to avoid hyaluronidase in the injectate.[135,152] Bilateral block must never be done.[164]

There are also five reports of facial nerve paralysis in the literature caused by local anaesthetic blocks, in four patients who had injection of the main trunk[210] and in one blocked by the O'Brien method[156] anterior to the tragus of the ear.[189]

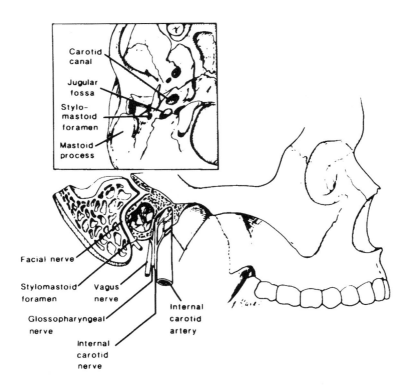

Fig. 8.4.   Anatomical depiction of the proximity of the stylomastoid foramen (facial nerve) to the jugular foramen (vagus, glossopharyngeal and spinal accessory nerves). The latter is not shown. (With permission from ref. 135.)

DIRECT CEREBRAL SPREAD OF LOCAL ANAESTHETICS FROM THE ORBIT

In the late 1960s, some unexpected sequelae of radiologic techniques were reported including the demonstration radiographically of communication from the subdural space of the optic nerve to the chiasm and into the subarachnoid space surrounding the pons and mid-brain.[113,168] Cadaver experiments confirmed these findings.[50,205] Serious central nervous system depression following intra-conal block was reported in several papers commencing in 1980.[15,36,84,145,175,187] The administered dose was insufficient to explain the clinical picture based on systemic drug levels, and the time sequence did not usually support an intra-arterial injection as the explanation[4] (except in one case[148] and possibly a second[171]). An allergic mechanism did not fit, as patients experiencing the problem often had had an uncomplicated operation on the contralateral eye using an identical technique.[104] Although there was knowledge of the meningeal pathway it was not until the mid-1980s that publications came down in favour of that mechanism (Fig. 8.5). Kobet reported a case of brainstem anaesthesia following intra-conal block in which a higher level of lignocaine was found in lumbar cerebrospinal fluid than could be accounted for from systemic distribution.[119] In several large reported series it became clear that the effect of spread of local anaesthetic in the central nervous system during intraconal block depended on the amount of drug entering and the specific area to which it had spread.[2,86,104,153,190,208] An incidence as high as 0.79% is stated in one paper,[208] but

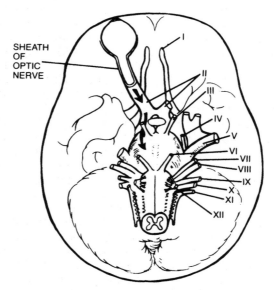

Fig. 8.5.   Illustration of the base of the brain and the pathway for spread of local anaesthetics inadvertently injected into the subarachnoid space surrounding the optic nerve. Note that this pathway includes the cranial nerves, pons and midbrain. (With permission from ref. 104.)

more commonly is reported as one case in 350–500 patients.[2,86,104,153,190] From these sources and others, the author has published a clinical review of the syndrome.[88] Typically, the patient first describes symptoms with onset at about 2 min after the orbital injection. Frequently, the zenith is reached at 10–20 minutes and resolves over 2 to 3 h. As this is a potential complication on each occasion that orbital blocks are performed, patients should not be draped for surgery until 15 min have elapsed after completion of the block, otherwise identification and corrective treatment may be dangerously delayed. Surgery is often possible immediately following recovery from the complication.

An essential prerequisite in all locations where regional ocular anaesthesia is performed is the ability to provide respiratory support and nearby access to cardiopulmonary resuscitation equipment.[56,59,84,104,110,114,119,151] Meyers reported that 5.6% of 1000 patients having cataract extractions under regional anaesthesia generated emergency calls for an anaesthetist.[147] Ophthalmologists most commonly administer orbital blocks; however, with the increasing popularity of fast turnover day-case cataract surgery, anaesthetists have become increasingly involved as the administrators of regional anaesthesia for eye surgery.[85] This frees up the ophthalmologist in a busy practice to use time more efficiently and economically, and the patient has the advantage of undivided and continuing attention. In 1989 and 1990, in more than half of the large volume practices in the USA, the administration of blocks had been delegated to anaesthesia personnel.[126,127]

The clinical picture of brainstem anaesthesia is protean in manifestation[87,154] producing signs which vary[154] from mild confusion,[2] through marked shivering[128] or convulsant behaviour,[2] bilateral brainstem nerve palsies (including motor nerve blocking to the contralateral orbit with amaurosis)[7,60,62,172] or hemi-, para- or quadriplegia,[2] with or without loss of consciousness, to apnoea with marked cardiovascular instability.[36,39,84,178] Two patients given posterior periconal blocks experienced brainstem anaesthesia including apnoea.[44]

Central spread should be suspected if there is onset of any of the following: mental confusion or loss of contact with the patient, signs of extraocular paresis or amaurosis of the contralateral eye, shivering bordering on convulsant behaviour, nausea or vomiting, dysphagia, sudden swings in the cardiovascular vital signs, dyspnoea or respiratory depression.

The above signs may be present in various arrangements; for example, an apnoeic patient may be conscious, or contralateral eye signs may be the only abnormality detected in an otherwise uneventful block. The onset of brainstem anaesthesia should be suspected if there is any indication of loss of patient contact. Ahn and Stanley emphasize the frequent finding of signs of central spread on examination of the contralateral orbit as one of the earliest evidences of the syndrome.[2] If the patient is still conscious, amaurosis may be reported. Usually the contralateral pupil is dilated and areflexic. Oculomotor palsies or frank paralyses may be present in any combination. On confirmation that spread has affected the opposite eye, the physician should immediately be prepared for progression to any degree of development of the syndrome and be ready to provide support including cardiopulmonary resuscitation. Where this is instituted, a favourable outcome is the rule. Should recognition be delayed, then serious sequelae including death could obviously result. Routine provision of pulse oximetric monitoring of oxygen saturation is valuable and desirable in the block room and operating room.[86] Oxygen enrichment of inspired air should be provided to correct arterial desaturation ($SaO_2 < 92\%$).[1] Oxygen enrichment, in either regional or general anaesthesia, used to excess adds to the risk of microscope light phototoxicity and should be avoided.[101]

Treatment of these differing manifestations of central spread includes reassurance, ventilatory support with oxygen, intravenous fluid therapy and pharmacologic circulatory support with vagolytics, vasopressors, vasodilators or adrenergic blocking agents as appropriate and as dictated by close vital sign monitoring.

Cardiac arrest has been reported in three papers,[29,153,175] in one of which cardiopulmonary resuscitation lasting 45 min was required. In animal experiments direct application of local anaesthetics, particularly bupivacaine, to specific areas of the brain had a profound effect on myocardial function.[93,198] Marked increases in arterial blood pressure and heart rate have been reported with brainstem anaesthesia[15,36,39,54,84,104,153,155,175] which in two cases progressed to pulmonary oedema.[36,54] In one of the two cases reported by Cohen *et al.*, new retinal haemorrhages appeared associated with the brainstem anaesthesia.[39] Although death following brainstem anaesthesia has not been reported in the literature, the author has heard of three cases in the years 1991 and 1992, two in different parts of the UK and one in the USA, in each of which an anaesthetist was summoned too late for a successful resuscitation.

The author, using a 38-mm 27 gauge disposable needle observed 20 episodes of central spread in over 16 000 administrations.[87] In subsequent experience with a further 16 000 cataract surgeries under local anaesthesia using a 31-mm needle, brainstem anaesthesia has occurred twice. When using sharp disposable fine needles, the possibility of optic nerve sheath penetration is always there; the dilemma exists that by going a few millimetres deeper, the effectiveness of blocks is greater but the incidence of central spread increases. Any atypical experience of pain in response to injection, or the presence of increased resistance to injection beyond that expected, are indications to re-evaluate the situation and not to proceed without needle tip repositioning; in addition, the anaesthetist should immediately adopt an increased vigilance of the patient's condition.

The dural sheath at the apex of the orbit and along the optic nerve is not impervious to local anaesthetics as evidenced by the incidence of temporary ipsilateral amaurosis following intraconal block.[17,35,131,201] Studies of cortical visual evoked potential also indicate temporary suppression of optic nerve conduction, which is greater with intracone blockade than with pericone.[9,173] The optic nerve has not been examined directly following cases of brainstem anaesthesia and there is no reported incidence of obvious optic nerve trauma, such as optic neuropathy or nerve sheath haemorrhage. In fact, in known cases of optic nerve trauma, a totally different clinical picture is seen (next paragraph) and in this circumstance central spread has not been reported.[117,190,196]

Brainstem anaesthesia has been reported when the injectate did not contain hyaluronidase; therefore, this enzyme does not seem to be a factor in the causation of the complication.[2,153]

Much is known about prevention of this syndrome. Unsöld and her co-workers in 1981 exposed the danger of the elevated, adducted globe, the traditional Atkinson directive, during inferotemporal needle placement.[200] This position places the optic nerve in closer proximity to the advancing needle. They demonstrated in computed tomography studies in fresh cadavers that with the globe in primary gaze (and even more so depressed and abducted), the optic nerve is less vulnerable. Recently, Liu and his colleagues confirmed these findings with *in vivo* studies using magnetic resonance imaging in a single subject.[136] Because the 'down and out' position advocated by Unsöld *et al.* has the disadvantages of its making an approaching inferotemporal needle come into the field of vision of the patient, which may be frightening, as well as placing the cornea in the way, Lui *et al.* suggest a 'down and in' globe position which also places the anterior optic nerve in a safer position in the intracone space. Avoidance of deep penetration of the orbit in any technique is advisable both to prevent this and other serious block complications. Katsev *et al.* advised that maximum penetration from the orbit rim should be 31 mm.[111] In the presence of resistance, injection should be withheld and the needle tip relocated.[153,171] Modern techniques avoid deep orbital placement and instead advocate accurate injection at limited orbital depth and using increased volume of injectate in order to achieve critical blocking concentration at the apex.[87]

SCLERAL PENETRATION AND PERFORATION

To avoid scleral penetration (entrance wound only) or perforation (entrance and exit wounds) the importance of block technique[89] and needle type are stressed (see Needles and injection techniques above). 'The equator of the globe, with the eye in the primary position, is the greatest diameter in the coronal plane. Any needle entering the orbital region anteriorly must be directed in such a manner as to avoid encountering the sclera. Only by accurately judging the position of the equator can a needle be inserted in safety'.[89]

The complication is more likely in patients with elongated myopic eyes. Patients presenting for retinal detachment and radial keratotomy surgery will have a higher propensity of longer globes than patients having cataract surgery. Particularly at risk are myopic patients with staphyloma.[10,166] The author also finds that patients with recessed eyes and those with tight lower eyelids are more challenging and may be at increased risk of ocular penetration. It may be that in these cases a pericone needle placement may be safer than intracone. Ultrasonography of patients with high myopia is effective in the diagnosis of staphyloma;[3] if this condition is found to be present it may be prudent to perform intracone injections with the patient's gaze directed downward and outward,[3] to utilize the pericone method[10], or to opt for general anaesthesia. The reported incidence of globe penetration and perforation in the literature ranges from none in a series of 2000 periconal anaesthesias[42] through 1 in a series of 12 000 comprising both peri- and intraconal,[86] and 1 in a series of 1000,[38] to 3 in a series of 4000 intraconal blocks.[166] Duker *et al.* state that in myopic patients the incidence may be as high as 1 in 140.[52] The true incidence is not known since most cases are not reported.[124] There are many case reports of the complication with both the intraconal[52,79,90,181] and the periconal methods.[44,52,67,79,90,108,115,214] Non-akinetic anaesthesia methods have been developed recently (see Chapter 7), partly to avoid the serious complications related to full akinetic ophthalmic regional anaesthesia, including scleral penetration/perforation.[64] Anterior eyewall penetration has been reported with one of these methods.[212] Many surgeons remain concerned about the risk to the eye when non-akinetic techniques are used for intraocular surgery.[8]

A safe prerequisite to regional anaesthesia of the orbit is to know the axial length measurement of the eye prior to the block to warn of the higher risk in longer-than-average eyes. In cataract surgery, a precise axial length measurement is usually available for the purposes of intraocular lens power calculations. In other than cataract procedures where the axial length is not precisely known, close attention to the dioptre power of patients' spectacles or contact lenses will provide valuable clues to globe dimensions. Fine disposable needles, which are less painful for the patient, have been proven to be relatively safe; however, excellent knowledge of orbital anatomy is essential. Grizzard *et al.*, reporting on iatrogenic ocular injuries, found that penetrations or perforations caused by larger dull needles resulted in more serious permanent damage than when such injuries resulted from the use of fine disposable ones.[79] The diagnosis of penetration may be suspected in the presence of hypotony, poor red reflex, vitreous haemorrhage, and 'poking through sensation';[181] however, more than 50% of iatrogenic needle penetrations of the globe go unrecognized at the time of their occurrence.[72] The patient may report marked pain at the time of the perforation[182] and particularly if anaesthetic is injected intraocularly. Fundoscopy confirms the diagnosis if the media are sufficiently clear. Cases involving retinal tears only and minimal blood can be managed with laser photocoagulation, cryotherapy or, on occasion, observation only. When so much blood is present that the fundus is not visible, early vitrectomy may be indicated. Without surgical intervention, vitreous haemorrhage following penetrating injury frequently leads to proliferative vitreoretinopathy with resultant detachment of the retina. If retinal detachment is present, whether with clear or cloudy media, prompt surgical treatment is indicated. The appropriate management of scleral penetration and perforation is complex and often drawn out over some weeks, involving difficult judgement calls on the part of the ophthalmologist; for details of management, the reader is referred to Rinkoff, Doft and Lobes.[169] The author has twice had experience with this complication:

The first case involved the right eye of a woman in her early 60s scheduled for cataract extraction; it has been reported in the literature[86] and occurred at a time when the author had performed about 2000 orbital regional anaesthesias. The axial length of the eye was 32 mm and, in the performance of an intracone block, perforation (entrance and exit) of the globe occurred, although not recognized at the time. Thin sclera had offered no detectable resistance to the sharp 27 gauge disposable needle, and since the needle tip was within the cone and no unusual subjective sensation was reported, evidence of block onset was normal. Because on inspecting the eye 10 min after routine orbit decompression marked globe hypotony was observed (cornea indented and floppy), the ophthalmologist was immediately alerted. The media were sufficiently clear for entrance and exit wounds to be visualized; the entrance wound was at the globe equator and the exit temporal to the macula. There was intraretinal haemorrhage but no retinal tear and no bleeding into the vitreous. Surgery was postponed and over the subsequent weeks a full resolution of the injury took place without loss of visual acuity or instability of the retina. The patient elected to go elsewhere for removal of her cataract under general anaesthesia. Legal action was settled by payment of a small sum to cover travelling, accommodation and inconvenience expenses.

The second case, involving the right eye of a woman in her mid-70s scheduled for cataract extraction, happened after the author had had experience with 23 000 surgeries under regional anaesthesia and has hitherto not been reported in the literature. The globe had an axial length of 28 mm. The patient had narrow horizontal palpebral apertures, wide lateral canthal folds and tight lower eyelid margins. Unwisely, it was decided to use a transconjunctival inferotemporal approach to the intracone space. During needle placement the patient was experiencing some discomfort but not at a level indicative of a problem. At this stage only about 8 mm of the needle had been advanced and it was decided to inject a little local so as to decrease the discomfort. In doing so there was marked atypical pain and the needle was carefully withdrawn, during which it was obvious that it had been inside the globe (entrance through the sclera had been imperceptible). The ophthalmologist was alerted and confirmed by indirect ophthalmoscopy that there was an entrance wound at 8.30 at the equator. There was blood in the vitreous inferotemporally, a subretinal haemorrhage and inferior retinal elevation, but no retinal detachment. Cataract surgery was cancelled. It was felt that prognosis was good and it was decided to follow the progress of the complication with serial ultrasound scanning and intervene as indicated. Scanning was negative at weekly intervals for 4 weeks but was indicative of retinal detachment at the subsequent examination. A retinal specialist at this time felt that the prognosis was so poor as not to warrant vitreoretinal surgery; a second retinal specialist was consulted who did operate and found the retina completely detached and irreversibly devitalized. Legal action was settled by payment of a sum commensurate with the age of the patient and the visual status of her left eye. This most unfortunate event was, nevertheless, a learning experience for the author. The globe penetration which occurred was brought on by attempting inappropriate transconjunctival access to the intracone space in a myopic patient with narrow horizontal palpebral apertures and wide lateral canthal folds. An inferotemporal transcutaneous approach would have avoided the complication.

RETROBULBAR HAEMORRHAGE, RETINAL VASCULAR OCCLUSION, OPTIC NERVE TRAUMA, AND OPTIC ATROPHY

Retrobulbar haemorrhages vary in severity. Some are of venous origin and spread slowly. Signs of severe arterial haemorrhage are a rapid and taut orbital swelling, marked proptosis with immobility of the globe and massive blood staining of the lids and conjunctiva.[56] Serious impairment of the vascular supply to the globe may result.[76,122] By constant vigilance and keen observation of the signs immediately following needle withdrawal, bleeding may be minimized and confined by rapid application of digital pressure over a gauze pad applied to the closed lids. The incidence of serious retrobulbar bleeding is reported as 1–3% in one paper[150] and as 0.44% in a series of 12 500 cases.[53] No doubt with traditional techniques, using 22 and 23 gauge dull needles directed deeply towards the apex, vessels may not have been easily penentrated, but when this occurs serious bleeding could rapidly ensue. Gentle and smooth needle insertion without pivotal or slicing movement is less likely to cause bleeding.[53,150] A strong argument can be made in favour of fine disposable needles over those of larger gauge,[78,86,161] on the grounds that if a vessel is perforated, then the amount of bleeding that occurs through a small rent is of lesser amount and less precipitous. The author, by using precision depth placement of fine disposable needles in relatively avascular areas of the anterior orbit, has not encountered serious retrobular hemorrhage in the past 8 years and 25 000 cases. The added advantages of fine-needle techniques are the reduced or absent need for sedation and decreased pain during the administration.

To reduce the incidence of bleeding, it is essential to avoid needle insertion in the more vascular areas of the orbit. The apex contains the largest vessels entering and exiting the orbit. When serious bleeding occurs in this area, there is not only the problem of increased general orbital pressure making surgery difficult, but also the potential for obstruction to the blood supply to and from the globe affecting the retina. Investigation of the established retrobulbar haemorrhage includes intraocular pressure measurement, and ophthalmoscopy to check the retinal circulation, if the media are sufficiently clear. Management may include osmotic diuresis, anterior paracentesis to lower intraocular pressure although this is somewhat controversial,[56] and lateral canthotomy to allow drainage of the blood or more extensive surgical decompression of the orbit.[56] Liu has suggested using a small surgical clamp to break through the orbit floor into the maxillary sinus as an effective method of managing severe retrobulbar haemorrhage.[137] Klein *et al.* and Cowley *et al.* reported retinal vascular occlusion in the absence of retrobulbar haemorrhage following intraconal injection of local anaesthetics in patients with severe hematological, or vascular disorders, and postulated either trauma to the central retinal artery or pharmacologic or compressive effects of the injected solution as the cause.[40,117] Frank optic nerve injury after intraconal injection of anaesthetic agents may occur, along with serious compromise of the blood supply to the globe. Computerized scanning or ultrasonography may reveal a dilated optic nerve sheath suggesting intrasheath haemorrhage.[78,94,161,196] The appearance of the retinal fundus following an intrasheath injection may resemble Purtscher's retinopathy, which is a condition thought to be related to rapid elevation of venous pressure.[78,129] Surgical decompression of the nerve sheath may be indicated. In some cases, the increased orbital pressure due to a retrobulbar haemorrhage may tamponade the small nutrient vessels in the optic nerve, explaining those cases of profound visual loss in which the findings of retinal vascular occlusion were not seen and late optic atrophy developed.[30,56] Other factors in cases of this latter type may be postoperative glaucoma[30,91] and pre-existing small vessel disease such as diabetes. However, not all cases of late optic atrophy are easily explainable.[34] Jarrett and Brockhurst reported 11 cases of unexplained optic atrophy following scleral buckling under general anaesthesia.[103]

MINOR BLEEDING PHENOMENA

The anterior orbit has smaller vessels than exist posteriorly. Three anterior orbital locations are relatively avascular: the inferotemporal quadrant, superotemporally in the sagittal plane of the lateral limbus, and directly nasally in the compartment on the nasal side of the medial rectus muscle. By using small needles (27 and 30 gauge) in one or more of these three locations, the author has reduced the incidence of minor bleeding (including retrobulbar and anterior orbital haemorrhages, subconjuctival bleeding and lid ecchymoses) from a published incidence of 2.75%[86] to 1.0%. The superonasal area should be avoided because the end vessels of the ophthalmic artery system are located there, as is the complex trochlear mechanism of the superior oblique muscle (see Chapter 1). Lid ecchymosis is one of the most disconcerting sequelae of intraconal or periconal anaesthesia, making patient and family complaint common. Minor bruising phenomena can largely be eliminated using the relatively avascular areas, as described, for needle placement. Nevertheless, if bruising occurs, the patient and accompanying person(s) should be notified at the time, and reassurance given that the surgical outcome will not be affected and that the bruising will clear spontaneously within a few days.

STEROID AND ANTIBIOTIC INJECTIONS

Orbital injections of depot steroid medications and antibiotics are frequently employed at the time of ophthalmic surgery for their anti-inflammatory and anti-infective properties. Their inadvertent injection into the vitreous has serious implications.[21,28,102,180] On the other hand, the intraocular injection of anaesthetics appears to be better tolerated.[16,56,134,179] In delivering steroids and antibiotics in the planned extraocular location, it is important to avoid intravascular placement of the needle tip. Aspiration prior to injection is advised. There are many reports of retinal, ciliary and choroidal arterial embolism of these medications, often with irreversible vision deterioration.[26,55,143,150,183,195] An inflammatory response to injected antibiotic involving the inferior rectus muscle and causing prolonged diplopia has been reported.[123]

The management of inadvertent intraocular drug injection is lucidly discussed by Schechter,[179] whose article is highly recommended. Intraocular antibiotics are used to treat established endophthalmitis and are being increasingly used prophylactically in its prevention. The preparation of the special concentration required must be done correctly and is probably best delegated to a pharmacist so as to avoid devastating and irreversible retinotoxic iatrogenic damage.[141]

EXTRAOCULAR MUSCLE MALFUNCTION (EXCLUDING PTOSIS)

Strabismus after cataract surgery may result from diverse aetiology,[82] which may be divided into four broad categories:

1. Disorders pre-existing the surgery, but rendered asymptomatic by the dense media (e.g. thyroid eye disease, cranial nerve palsy, myasthenia).
2. Disorders secondary to prolonged vision deprivation by the cataract (e.g. central disruption of binocular vision).
3. Disorders caused by extraocular muscle trauma or damage related to anaesthesia needles or surgical involvement.

4. Disorders resulting from mismatch of optical characteristics of the two eyes after surgery (e.g. aphakia/pseudophakia, anisophoria, colour/brightness disparity).

In the evaluation of ocular motility disorders, traction testing – using corneoconjunctival topical anaesthesia – is indispensible and has two components: force generation, in which the contractile strength of the extraocular muscles is assessed (patient must be awake and cooperative), and passive range of motion, which examines the elastic properties of the muscles and other orbital tissues (patient awake or under anaesthesia).[142]

Prolonged extraocular muscle malfunction may follow regional anaesthesia of the orbit.[31,86,167] Diplopia and ptosis are common for 24–48 h postoperatively when long-acting local anaesthetics have been used in large volume, indicating the protein-binding properties of these agents. However, when this persists for days or weeks, or fails to recover, it may be evidence of toxic change within muscle. In those patients in whom muscle recovery is delayed more than 6 weeks, fully 25% turn out to be permanent.[197] It is indeed a complication of the greatest magnitude for a patient to have a perfect optical result and end up with devastating diplopia because the eyes are misaligned. Animal and human investigation of myotoxicity of local anaesthetics has been published.[32,61,165,211]

Local anaesthetics containing hyaluronidase and/or adrenaline may be more myotoxic than plain solutions.[216] Higher concentrations of local anaesthetic agents are more likely to result in myotoxicity.[211] A common cause of prolonged muscle malfunction, whatever concentration has been used, is intramuscular injection. Several papers emphasize the avoidance of injection into any of the delicate orbital muscles.[61,156,157,165] It is imperative to have a good three dimensional knowledge of the anatomy of the orbit and its contents to place injections accurately. Of particular note are the number of articles indicating damage to the inferior rectus muscle,[24,46,77,82,83,157] which probably indicates that the needle tip has not cleared the inferior rectus muscle to lie free in the intracone compartment. The author emphasizes the importance of setting an adequate angle of elevation (parallel to the orbit floor) for the placement of the inferotemporal intracone injection. Part of the rationale for his use of a custom-bent needle (see Chapter 7) is to avoid damage to the inferior rectus muscle (Fig. 8.6). In his early use of the medial pericone block (see Chapter 7), three patients exhibited medial rectus muscle paresis, almost certainly due to injection into the muscle (one of these failed to recover and required corrective muscle surgery). After modifying the angle of needle insertion during the medial pericone block to assume a 5-degree directioning towards the mid-line (Fig. 8.7), this complication did not recur. The author has observed that 3 and 4% lignocaine may be myotoxic even when intramuscular injection is avoided.

POSTOPERATIVE PTOSIS

Ptosis is common and is as inevitable as cataracts.[191] If defined as a drop of the eyelid margin lower than 2 mm from the superior limbus, then the incidence of ptosis among patients before cataract surgery is reported as being present in 55.5%[109] and 67%.[191] Postoperative ptosis is of multifactorial aetiology, local

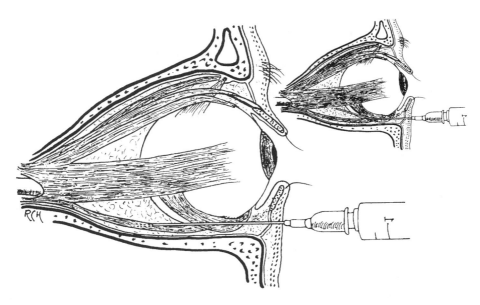

Fig. 8.6.   A straight 31-mm needle being advanced from the inferotemporal quadrant in an attempt to enter the intraconal space has failed to adequately clear the orbit floor. The needle tip has entered the belly of the inferior rectus muscle. Haemorrhage into the muscle with subsequent fibrosis, or intramuscular injection of local anesthetic with subsequent myotoxicity, may result in prolonged or permanent imbalance between the superior and inferior rectus muscles and vertical diplopia. The small insert demonstrates how a custom-bent needle may be helpful in the avoidance of this complication. (With permission from Gimbel Educational Services.)

anaesthesia injections playing only one of these roles. Most postcataract ptosis occurs in patients in whom the levator aponeurosis is already unhealthy (Darrell E. Wolfley MD, Washington, DC, personal communication). Degenerative conditions of the aponeurosis include: disinsertion in the tarsal plate, dehiscence and rarefaction.[47,160,191] Many of these lids would have become ptotic even if cataract surgery had not been performed. The surgery only serves to accelerate a pre-existing condition (Darrell E. Wolfley MD, personal communication). Extension of pre-existing ptosis, or the appearance of a new ptosis, can occur after cataract, anterior or posterior segment, or orbital and oculoplastic surgery.[191] The published incidence of this varies from 0 to 20%.[47,57,109] A lower incidence of postoperative ptosis is seen in surgeries done under general anaesthesia than with local anaesthesia.[6,47] Surgical repair of postoperative ptosis may be necessary if there is interference with vision, but should be delayed for 6 months until a stable state has been reached.[47,109]

Kaplan *et al.* list many factors which may be involved in the production of postoperative ptosis.[109] These include oedema of the eyelid caused by the local anaesthesia or, following on from surgery, effects from pressure applied to the globe and upper lid, pressure exerted by the lid speculum, traction on the superior rectus muscle complex and prolonged postoperative patching. They studied 456 patients and concluded that trauma to the superior rectus muscle complex

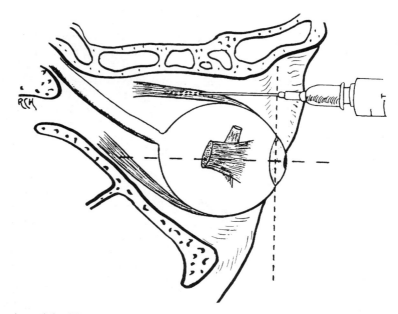

Fig. 8.7. A straight 25-mm 30 gauge needle being advanced in a sagittal plane from the extreme medial end of the palpebral fissure (on the nasal side of the caruncle) has traversed the medial compartment on the nasal side of the medial rectus muscle and entered into the belly of the medial rectus muscle. Haemorrhage into the muscle with subsequent fibrosis, or intramuscular injection of local anesthetic with subsequent myotoxicity, may result in prolonged or permanent malfunction of the medial rectus muscle. (With permission from Gimbel Educational Services.)

was the most critical factor in post operative ptosis. These workers also found that 6 months after surgery, the degree of ptosis had progressed from what it had been immediately after the operation in 12% of patients. Deady *et al.*, however, did not find any evidence of progressive ptosis.[47] Ptosis has even occurred in radial keratomy surgery in which no anaesthetic injections or bridle sutures were used, and was most likely caused by a rigid eyelid speculum.[57] Rainin and Carlson stressed that toxic damage to muscle fibres from direct intramuscular injection of local anaesthetics may account for many cases of transient and permanent ptosis.[165]

The eyelid crease is higher in the presence of ptosis. It is prudent routine practice to chart the positions of the eyelid margins above the central cornea bilaterally before embarking on surgery, possibly including photographic documentation taken close-up. Patients should be informed of the possibility of eyelids drooping temporarily or permanently after surgery; written consent for surgery acknowledging this complication should be obtained. Postoperative entropion, caused by thinning or disinsertion of the capsulopalpebral fascia in the inferior orbit, is directly analogous to upper eyelid ptosis resulting from stretching of the levator aponeurosis.[132]

ORBITAL DECOMPRESSION DEVICES

In intraocular surgery it is considered advantageous if the intraocular pressure is low and pressure fluctuations are kept to a minimum.[140] Phacoemulsification techniques, which require a smaller surgical incision, are associated with smaller swings in intraocular pressure than intracapsular or extracapsular methods. When an eye is opened, the intraocular pressure rapidly approaches that of the atmosphere. If the switch from the pressure prior to opening to atmospheric pressure is a high gradient, stress is inflicted on the choroidal vasculature, thus increasing the risk of haemorrhage (see below), at worst of the expulsive type.[73,207] Atkinson emphasized the attainment of a 'soft eye' in the avoidance of complications, particularly vitreous loss.[12,13]

Following completion of the regional anaesthetic block mechanical orbital decompression devices[25,41,49,69] are commonly used to promote ocular hypotony and a reduction in vitreous volume,[159] especially when larger volumes of orbital injectate have been used. Using an animal model, Otto and Spekreijse studied the effect on intraorbital pressure of volume discrepancies in the orbit.[158] Each time a volume bolus was injected, the intraorbital pressure peaked and rapidly declined in subsequent minutes. Meyer *et al.* confirmed the safety and effectiveness of large-volume intraorbital volumes in a clinical setting.[146]

With decompression devices a drop in pressure occurs in the first 10 min and at a slower rate thereafter; a period of at least 15 min from the initial block should elapse prior to surgery. The customary injection–decompression sequence has proven to be reliable and there are no documented reports of ischaemic insult in the literature.[213] Nevertheless, a concern for the ischaemia-inducing potential exists, as evidenced by the ongoing research on the effects of increased intraocular pressure on ocular perfusion.[23,92,95,96,105,163] Since blood flow to the retina, choroid and optic nerve depend on the balance between the intraocular pressure and the mean local arterial blood pressure, externally applied pressure has the potential to reduce significantly blood flow to these vital areas.[213]

In the presence of significant local arterial disease, orbital haemorrhage or in patients with glaucoma, vascular occlusion may result.[30,195,213] It may be prudent to omit adrenaline from the anaesthesia injectate.[97,100,139]

A compression–injection sequence has been suggested for the safe management for such patients,[213] or the complete avoidance of external decompression in favour of alternative measures. These may include using lower injectate volumes, permitting sufficient time (at least 15 min) to elapse between completion of the block and the commencement of surgery for spontaneous pressure reduction to occur. Non-akinetic anaesthesia techniques which avoid orbital injections may be used if appropriate. Glaucomatous patients may require the preoperative control of higher intraocular pressures using oral acetazolamide and/or topical corneoconjunctival agents, or the induction of osmotic diuresis with mannitol. Cataract surgery may be combined with trabeculectomy or trabeculotomy.[71]

Patients under the age of 40 years have a lower scleral rigidity than older patients and they also may benefit from induced osmotic diuresis (intravenous mannitol or oral glycerol) to achieve optimum operating conditions.[80]

Decompression also promotes akinesia of the periorbital muscles by displacing the anaesthetic mixture from within the orbit into the region of the orbicularis muscle, thus avoiding a separate and painful seventh nerve block. Unlike the extraocular muscles, the orbicularis oculi muscle is relatively safe from local anaesthetic myotoxicity in clinical use.[216]

CORNEAL INJURY

Care must be taken to protect the cornea in the perioperative period. An occlusive dressing should be used after surgery to seal the eyelids shut until such time as their full function has recovered. The amount of time will depend mainly on the duration of action of the chosen anaesthetic. Until a safe protocol of dressing management is established, an occasional incidence of corneal exposure may be seen. Prolonged patching may contribute to the production of ptosis (see above).[109] It is possible that the moist atmosphere beneath a gauze pad provides an ideal culture medium for organism growth.[125] Some experienced surgeons feel it is unnecessary to patch the eye postoperatively[203] but the safety of this decision, from the viewpoint of risk of superficial corneal damage, would depend on the degree of lid akinesia in that surgeon's technique. Regional anaesthesia can suppress lacrimal gland function, making the cornea more susceptible to damage.[27,211] Corneal abrasion pain is a specific eye pain manifesting as the sensation of the presence of a foreign body in the eye, tearing, conjunctivitis and photophobia. Corneal abrasion pain is made worse by blinking. The abraded section of cornea may be seen directly as a dull, nonreflective patch or as a positive area on fluorescein staining. Treatment requries application of antibiotic eye ointment and covering the eye with a patch for at least 48 h. Topical application of anaesthetic drops and steroids to the cornea are contraindicated because they restrict healing.

When using small-wound phacoemulsification cataract extracton with foldable intraocular lens implantation under solely topical anaesthesia (see Chapter 7), care must be taken postoperatively to avoid any corneal exposure while the anaesthesia is still having an effect.[99]

OCULOCARDIAC REFLEX

Meyers states that oculocardiac reflex is the most common complication of intraconal block.[149] The author has not seen this in 32 000 administrations, whether during the blocks, after application of the orbital decompression device or intraoperatively; however, there was an incidence of vasovagal activity of between 0.5 and 0.85% which was twice as common in men as in women and occurred in patients who had a history of fainting.[86] Nicoll *et al.* report similar results based on a series of 6000 patients,[153] and likewise Wong in a series of 8480.[209] It is most likely that dull, larger-gauge needles were the cause in the reported series. Ellis reports that retrobulbar haemorrhage may initiate an oculocardiac reflex.[55] Pearce mentions that, unlike general anaesthesia, the established regional block eliminates any further problem with the oculocardiac reflex.[162] Retrobulbar local anaesthetic injection has been successfully used to abolish the reflex occurring during the course of cataract surgery under general anaesthesia.[106] Incomplete regional anaesthetic block prior to general anaesthesia may fail to abolish the reflex.[14]

INTRAOPERATIVE AND POSTOPERATIVE PAIN

Comparing traditional low-volume with higher-volume techniques, the author reported a twenty-fold reduction in the incidence of pain during surgery, from 2.1% to 0.1%.[86] With the recently described limbal anaesthesia method,[64] which employs a small volume of anaesthetic and does not aim for globe akinesia, it is not surprising that patients may experience iris pain.[130] It is a common practice to administer antibiotic by subconjunctival injection at the end of surgery; this often results in considerable pain and may result in irritation at this site postoperatively. Friedberg *et al.* described a simple technique in which the antibiotic is given at the commencement of surgery, with the avoidance of pain.[63] As a painless alternative, some surgeons prefer intraocular antibiotic therapy at the time of surgery, using appropriately diluted preparations designed for such use.

With modern surgical techniques there is minimal tissue disruption and therefore minimal postoperative discomfort after the local anaesthetic has worn off; Livingston *et al.* have advocated that short-acting agents are sufficient for routine cataract extraction practice.[138] However, the patient is noticeably more comfortable if there is a small concentration of bupivacaine in the anaesthetic mixture. High concentrations of bupivacaine or etidocaine for cataract surgery are probably best avoided because of the incidence of diplopia at 24 h, risk of corneal abrasion and possible promotion of ptosis with prolonged patching. However, for more prolonged surgeries, as required in some retinal operations, the use of long-acting agents may be necessary. Bupivacaine may be administered by the surgeon during operations under general anaesthesia as an effective means of postoperative analgesia.[51]

SUPRACHOROIDAL HAEMORRHAGE

The pathophysiology of suprachoroidal haemorrhage occurring with intraocular surgery has only recently been explained, although the condition has been known for 200 years.[74] The balance between intraocular pressure and vortex vein drainage is paramount; with the eye surgically opened, pooling of fluid in the choroid may result. Probably commencing as a choroidal effusion, it later progresses to the rupture of a ciliary artery from the stress inflicted upon it.[74,207] When the bleeding is of sufficient magnitude to cause extrusion of intraocular contents, it is known as an 'expulsive' haemorrhage.[207] The incidence of the complication is reported as 0.2% in cataract extraction surgery and 0.73% in glaucoma filtering procedures.[207] In the presence of ageing vessels associated with systemic arterial hypertension or prolonged intraocular hypertension, there is increased risk for this surgical complication. High-quality anaesthesia, whether regional or general, is important in providing optimal surgical conditions; however, the complication may occur under either form of anaesthesia even when expertly administered. Preoperative control of the above undesirable characteristics by the judicious use of medications is indicated. The author finds that anxiolytics and oral nifedipine 10 mg (fast-onset by piercing a hole in the capsule and squeezing the contents on to the patient's tongue followed by a low-volume drink to aid rapid passage to the stomach for absorption) are effective in most cases, aiming for a reduction to the 170 mmHg systolic level. For more resistant hypertension, intravenous labetolol or esmalol is suggested, the former drug being easier to administer and one-tenth the cost.[185] Excessive arterial pressure reduction, however, must be avoided because resultant reduced arterial flow may contribute to ischaemic damage to vital ocular structures, especially in the presence of vascular pathology.[30] For ocular hypertension not fully controlled with regular therapy, osmotic diuresis with mannitol is suggested.

Because of the smaller dimension of the surgical wound with phacoemulsification techniques, suprachoroidal bleeding can more easily be brought under control.[207] In patients identified as being at increased risk of the complication and in whom large incision surgery is planned, the prudent ophthalmologist will use preplaced sutures so that the eye can be immediately closed if the complication is suspected. If the intraocular contents can be repositioned without retinal detachment, ultimate visual outcome is often satisfactory.

During surgery, choroidal bleeding may be precipitated by 'bucking', coughing or sneezing, or restlessness from a full urinary bladder. Intravenous lignocaine is the drug of choice in the management of persistent cough in bronchitic patients for whom regional anaesthesia is the chosen method.[58,192] The lung, which has a high affinity for local anaesthetics, is the first major organ exposed to the local anaesthetics following their intravenous administration.[107]

The appearance of suprachoroidal haemorrhage with iris prolapse is a surgical emergency calling for globe closure simultaneously with vigorous pharmacological aqueous suppression. Intravenous acetazolamide may be used; intravenous mannitol is an alternative, 3 min following which vitreous volume will effectively reduce.[98] If vitreous haemorrhage or loss has occurred, it is prudent to obtain a vitreoretinal consultation.

It is preferable not to have to resort to immediate surgical drainage of a suprachoroidal haemorrhage; however, an inability to gain adequate control of intraocular pressure or severe pain may predicate sclerotomy drainage of the ultrasonographically identified quadrant. Although the optimal timing for operative intervention is not known, it is easier to evacuate a massive suprachoroidal clot after a delay of 7–10 days to allow for liquefaction.[207]

USE OF ANTICOAGULANT AND ANTIPLATELET THERAPY

It has been common practice in surgery, including ophthalmic surgery, to reduce or discontinue anticoagulant therapy for some days prior to an operation. The safety of this action for the cataract surgery patient has been questioned.[81,144] Discontinuation of anticoagulant medication may result in thrombotic complications such as cerebral vascular accident, pulmonary embolism and death.[194] In two reports, the minor haemorrhagic complications associated with continuance of anticoagulants had no long-term effects on visual acuity.[65,170] This implies that the risk of stopping anticoagulants for this type of surgery is probably greater than any risk imposed by their continuance. It is suggested that the prothrombin time should not exceed twice normal.[174] It would seem prudent when these cases are done with regional anaesthesia to pay particular attention to the above principles of using fine needles with injections given in avascular areas; cataract surgery on these patients should, if possible, be done using the small incision phacoemulsification method. If appropriate, topical corneoconjunctival anaesthesia combined with clear corneal small-incision surgery with implantation of a foldable intraocular lens is an excellent choice for the anticoagulated patient.[75] The sub-Tenon's method of regional anaesthesia, on the other hand would be ill-advised for patients taking anticoagulant or antiplatelet medications (see Chapter 7).

Patients on antiplatelet therapy may also continue their drugs through cataract surgery if medical reasons dictate.[184]

SUMMARY

Guidelines for successful orbital regional anaesthesia are summarized in Table 8.2 in a 'DOs and DON'Ts' format.

Table 8.2   The DOs and DON'Ts of ophthalmic regional anaesthesia

DON'Ts	DOs
Use the 'up and in' globe position for inferotemporal intraconal blocking	Use primary gaze position, or consider 'down and out' or 'down and in' (see text)
Attempt without anatomical knowledge	Use a precision technique based on sound anatomical knowledge
Fail to check axial length	Measure axial length (thinner sclera with long ovoid myopic eyes)
Fail to check for globe anomalies or previous surgical intervention	Take extra caution in patients known to have staphyloma, coloboma or scleral buckle
Inject with other than tangential alignment to the globe	Align needles tangentially to the globe for all injections
Use the superonasal quadrant	Use avascular injection sites
Inject at the orbital apex using long needles	Inject no longer than 31 mm from the inferior orbital rim
Use dull coarse needles	Use fine sharp needles in combination with good anatomical knowledge for better tactile discrimination, patient comfort and a lower incidence of tissue trauma and haemorrhage
Inject into extraocular muscles	Avoid extraocular muscles
Use unnecessarily high concentrations of anaesthetic agents	Use a well-thought out technique, volume and concentration of chosen anaethestic agent

REFERENCES

1. Ahmad S, Ahmad A, Benzon HT. Clinical experience with the peribulbar block for ophthalmologic surgery. *Reg Anesth* 1993; **18:** 184.
2. Ahn JC, Stanley JA. Subarachnoid injection as a complication of retrobulbar anesthesia. *Am J Ophthalmol* 1987; **103:** 225.
3. Alberth B, Damjanovich J. Complications of retrobulbar injections. *Klin Mbl Augenheilk* 1990; **196:** 92.
4. Aldrete JA, Romo-Salas F, Arora S, Wilson R, Rutherford R. Reverse arterial blood flow as a pathway for central nervous system toxic responses following injection of local anesthetics. *Anesth Analg* 1978; **57:** 428.
5. Allen CW. *Local and Regional Anesthesia.* WB Saunders: Philadelphia, PA, 1914: 625.
6. Alpar JJ. Acquired ptosis following cataract and glaucoma surgery. *Glaucoma* 1982; **4:** 66.
7. Antoszyk AN, Buckley EG. Contralateral decreased visual acuity and extraocular muscle palsies following retrobulbar anesthesia. *Ophthalmology* 1986; **93:** 462.
8. Aquavella JV. Limbal anesthesia for cataract surgery (Commentary). *Ophthalmic Surg* 1990; **21:** 26.
9. Arora R, Verma L, Kumar A Kunte R. Peribulbar anesthesia and optic nerve conduction. *J Cataract Refract Surg* 1991; **17:** 506.
10. Arora R, Verma L, Kumar A *et al.* Peribulbar anesthesia in retinal reattachment surgery. *Ophthalmic Surg* 1992; **23:** 499.
11. Atkinson WS. Retrobulbar injection of anesthetic within the muscular cone (cone injection). *Arch Ophthalmol* 1936; **16:** 494.
12. Atkinson WS. Akinesia of the orbicularis. *Am J Ophthalmol* 1953; 36: 1255.
13. Atkinson WS. Observations on anesthesia for ocular surgery. *Trans Am Acad Ophthalmol Otolaryng* 1956; **60:** 376.
14. Batterbury M, Wong D, Williams R *et al.* Peribulbar anaesthesia: Failure to abolish the oculocardiac reflex. *Eye* 1992; **6:** 293.
15. Beltranena HP, Vega MJ, Kirk N, Blankenship G. Inadvertent intravascular bupivacaine injection following retrobulbar block. *Reg Anesth* 1981; **6:** 149.
16. Berg P, Kroll P, Kuchle HJ. Iatrogenic eye perforations in para- and retrobulbar injections. *Klin Mbl Augenheilk* 1986; **189:** 170.
17. Brent BD, Singh H. The effect of retrobulbar anesthesia on visual acutiy in planned extracapsular cataract extraction. *Ophthalmic Surg* 1991; **22:** 392.
18. Breslin CW, Hershenfeld S. Effect of retrobulbar anesthesia on ocular tension. *Can J Ophthalmol* 1983; **18:** 223.
19. Brown DL. In *Atlas of Regional Anesthesia.* WB Saunders: Philadelphia, PA, 1992: 157–163.
20. Brown GC. Complications of retrobulbar injection. In *Current Therapy in Ophthalmic Surgery* (edited by Spaeth GL, Katz LJ, Parker KW). BC Decker Inc: Toronto, 1989: 11–13.
21. Brown GC, Eagle RC, Shakin EP *et al.* Retinal toxicity of intravitreal gentamicin. *Arch Ophthalmol* 1990; **108:** 1740.
22. Brown DL, Wedel DJ. Introduction to regional anesthesia. In *Anesthesia,* 3rd edn (edited by Miller RD). Churchill Livingstone: New York, 1990: 1370–1371.
23. Bucci MG, Ducoli P, Manni GL *et al.* Recovery time after photostress in induced ocular hypertension. *Glaucoma* 1992; **14:** 17.
24. Burns CL, Seigel LA. Inferior rectus recession for vertical tropia after cataract surgery. *Ophthalmology* 1988; **95:** 1120.
25. Buys NS. Mercury balloon reducer for vitreous and orbital volume control. In *Current Concepts in Cataract Surgery* (edited by Emery J). CV Mosby: St Louis, MO, 1980, 258.

26. Byers B. Blindness secondary to steroid injections into the nasal turbinates. *Arch Ophthalmol* 1979; **97:** 79.
27. Callahan A. Ultrasharp disposable needles (Letter). *Am J Ophthalmol* 1966; **62:** 173.
28. Campochiaro PA, Conway BP. Aminoglycoside toxicity – a survey of retinal specialists: Implications for ocular use. *Arch Ophthalmol* 1991; **109:** 946.
29. Cardan E, Pop R, Negrutiu S. Prolonged haemodynamic disturbance following attempted retrobulbar block. *Anaesthesia* 1987; **42:** 668.
30. Carl JR. Optic neuropathy following cataracat extraction. *Sem Ophthalmol* 1993; **8:** 144.
31. Carlson BM, Emerick S, Komorowski TE *et al*. Extraocular muscle regeneration in primates. *Ophthalmology* 1992; **99:** 582.
32. Carlson BM, Rainin EA. Rat extraocular muscle regeneration. *Arch Ophthalmol* 1985; **103:** 1373.
33. Carolan JA, Cerasoli JR, Houle TV. Bupivacaine in retrobulbar anesthesia. *Ann Ophthalmol* 1974; **6:** 843.
34. Carroll FD. Optic nerve complications of cataract extraction. *Trans Am Acad Ophthalmol Otolaryngol* 1973; **77:** 623.
35. Carroll FD, de Roetth A Jr. The effect of retrobulbar injections of procaine on the optic nerve. *Trans Am Acad Ophthalmol Otolaryngol* 1955; **59:** 356.
36. Chang J-L, Gonzalez-Abola E, Larson CE, Lobes L. Brain stem anesthesia following retrobulbar block. *Anesthesiology* 1984; **61:** 789.
37. Charlton JE. The management of regional anaesthesia. In *Principles and Practice of Regional Anaesthesia* (edited by Wildsmith JAW, Armitage EN). Churchill Livingstone: Edinburgh, 1987: 37–61.
38. Cibis PA. Discussion. In *Controversial Aspects of the Management of Retinal Detactments* (edited by Schepens CL, Regan CDJ). Little, Brown: Boston, MA, 1965: 251.
39. Cohen SM, Sousa FJ, Kelly NE, Wendel RT. Respiratory arrest and new retinal hemorrhages after retrobulbar anesthesia. *Am J Ophthalmol* 1992; **113:** 209.
40. Cowley M, Campochiara PA, Newman SA *et al*. Retinal vascular occlusion without retrobulbar or optic sheath hemorrhage after retrobulbar injection of lidocaine. *Ophthalmic Surg* 1988; **19:** 859.
41. Davidson B, Kratz R, Mazzoco T. An evaluation of the Honan intraocular pressure reducer. *Am Intraocular Implant Soc J* 1979; **5:** 237.
42. Davis DB, Mandel MR. Posterior peribulbar anesthesia: An alternative to retrobulbar anesthesia. *J Cataract Refract Surg* 1986; **12:** 182.
43. Davis DB, Mandel MR. Posterior peribulbar anesthesia: An alternative to retrobulbar anesthesia. *Geriatr Ophthalmol* 1987; **86:** 61.
44. Davis DB, Mandel MR. Peribulbar: Reducing complications. *Ocular Surgery News* 1989; **7:** 21.
45. Davison JA. Acute intraoperative suprachoroidal hemorrhage in capsular bag phacoemulsification. *J Cataract Refract Surg* 1993; **19:** 534.
46. de Faber J-THN, von Noorden GK. Inferior rectus muscle palsy after retrobulbar anesthesia for cataract surgery (Letter). *Am J Ophthalmol* 1991; **112:** 209.
47. Deady JP, Price NJ, Sutton GA. Ptosis following cataract and trabeculotomy surgery. *Br J Ophthalmol* 1989; **73:** 283.
48. Donlon JV. Local anesthesia for ophthalmic surgery: Patient preparation and management. *Ann Ophthalmol* 1980; **12:** 1183.
49. Drews RC. The Nerf ball for preoperative reduction of introcular pressure. *Ophthalmic Surg* 1982; **13:** 761.
50. Drysdale DB. Experimental subdural retrobulbar injection of anesthetic. *Ann Ophthalmol* 1984; **16:** 716.
51. Duker JS, Nielsen J, Vander JF *et al*. Retrobulbar bupivacaine irrigation for postoperative pain after scleral buckling surgery: A prospective study. *Ophthalmology* 1991; **98:** 514.

52. Duker JS, Belmont JB, Benson WE *et al.* Inadvertent globe perforation during retro-bulbar and peribulbar anesthesia. *Ophthalmology* 1991; **98**: 519.
53. Edge KR, Nicoll JMV. Retrobulbar hemorrhage after 12,500 retrobulbar blocks. *Anesth Analg* 1993; **76**: 1019.
54. Elk JR, Wood J, Holladay JT. Pulmonary edema following retrobulbar block. *J Cataract Refract Surg* 1988; **14**: 216.
55. Ellis PP. Occlusion of the central retinal artery after retrobulbar corticosteroid injection. *Am J Ophthalmol* 1978; **85**: 352.
56. Feibel RM. Current concepts in retrobulbar anesthesia. *Surv Ophthalmol* 1985; **30**: 102.
57. Feibel RM, Custer PL, Gordon MO. Postcataract ptosis: A randomized, double-masked comparison of peribulbar and retrobulbar anesthesia. *Ophthalmology* 1993; **100**: 660.
58. Fenton WM. Intravenous lidocaine for control of coughing during standby cataract surgery. *Anesthesiology* 1986; **64**: 847.
59. Fletcher SJ, O'Sullivan G. Grand mal seizure after retrobulbar block. *Anaesthesia* 1990; **45**: 696.
60. Follette JW, LoCascio JA. Bilateral amaurosis following unilateral retrobulbar block. *Anesthesiology* 1985; **63**: 237.
61. Foster AH, Carlson BM. Myotoxicity of local anesthetics and regeneration of the damaged muscle fibers. *Anesth Analg* 1980: **59**: 727.
62. Friedberg HL, Kline OR. Contralateral amaurosis after retrobulbar injection. *Am J Ophthalmol* 1986; **101**: 668.
63. Friedberg HL, Kline OR, Galman BD. Painless cataract surgery (Letter). *J Cataract Refract Surg* 1988; **14**: 100.
64. Furuta M, Toriumi T, Kashiwagi K, Satoh S. Limbal anesthesia for cataract surgery. *Ophthalmic Surg* 1990; **21**: 22.
65. Gainey SP, Robertson DM, Fay W, Ilstrup D. Ocular surgery on patients receiving long-term warfarin therapy. *Am J Ophthalmol* 1989; **108**: 142.
66. Galindo A, Keilson LR, Mondshine RB, Sawelson HI. Retro-peribulbar anesthesia. Special technique and needle design. *Ophthalmol Clin North Am* 1990; **3**: 71.
67. Gentili ME, Brassier J. Is peribulbar block safer than retrobulbar? (Letter) *Reg Anesth* 1992; **17**: 309.
68. Gifford H. Motor block of extraocular muscles by deep orbital injection. *Arch Ophthalmol* 1949; **41**: 5.
69. Gills JP. Constant mild compression of the eye to produce hypotension. *Am Intraocular Implant Soc J* 1979; **5**: 52.
70. Gills JP, Loyd TL. A technique of retrobulbar block with paralysis of orbicularis oculi. *Am Intraocular Implant Soc J* 1983; **9**: 339.
71. Gimbel HV, Meyer D. Small incision trabeculotomy combined with phacoemulsification and intraocular lens implantation. *J Cataract Refract Surg* 1993; **19**: 92.
72. Ginsburg RN, Duker JS. Globe perforation associated with retrobulbar and peribulbar anesthesia. *Sem Ophthalmol* 1993; **8**: 87.
73. Gjötterberg M, Ingemansson S-O. Effect on intraocular pressure of retrobulbar injection of Xylocaine with and without adrenaline. *Acta Ophthalmol* 1977; **55**: 709.
74. Glazer LC, Williams GA. Management of expulsive choroidal hemorrhage. *Sem Ophthalmol* 1993; **8**: 109.
75. Grabow HB. Topical anesthesia for cataract surgery. *Eur J Implant Ref Surg* 1993; **5**: 20.
76. Goldsmith MO. Occlusion of the central retinal artery following retrobulbar anesthesia. *Ophthalmologica* 1967; **153**: 191.
77. Grimmett MR, Lambert SR. Superior rectus muscle overaction after cataract extraction. *Am J Ophthalmol* 1992; **114**: 72.
78. Grizzard WS. Ophthalmic anesthesia. In: *Ophthalmology Annual* (edited by Reinecke RD). Raven Press: NY, 1989: 265–294.

79. Grizzard WS, Kirk NM, Pavan PR *et al.* Perforating ocular injuries caused by anesthesia personnel. *Ophthalmology* 1991; **98**: 1011.
80. Guindon B, Harvey J, Peacocke A *et al.* Factors modifying vitreous pressure in cataract surgery. *Can J Ophthalmol* 1981; **16**: 73.
81. Hall DL, Steen WH, Drummond JW, Byrd WA. Anticoagulants and cataract surgery. *Ophthalmic Surg* 1988; **19**: 221.
82. Hamed LM. Strabismus presenting after cataract surgery. *Ophthalmology* 1991; **98**: 247.
83. Hamed LM, Mancuso A. Inferior rectus muscle contracture syndrome after retrobulbar anesthesia. *Ophthalmology* 1991; **98**: 1506.
84. Hamilton RC. Brain stem anesthesia following retrobulbar blockade. *Anesthesiology* 1985; **63**: 688.
85. Hamilton RC. Non-ophthalmologists and orbital regional anesthesia (Letter). *Ophthalmology* 1992; **99**: 169.
86. Hamilton RC, Gimbel HV, Strunin L. Regional anaesthesia for 12,000 cataract extraction and intraocular lens implantation procedures. *Can J Anaesth* 1988; **35**: 615.
87. Hamilton RC, Gimbel HV, Javitt JC. The prevention of complications of regional anesthesia for ophthalmology. *Ophthalmol Clin North Am* 1990; **3**: 111.
88. Hamilton RC. Brain-stem anesthesia as a complication of regional anesthesia for ophthalmic surgery. *Can J Ophthalmol* 1992; **27**: 323.
89. Hawkesworth NR. Peribulbar anaesthesia (Letter). *Br J Ophthalmol* 1992; **76**: 254.
90. Hay A, Flynn HW Jr, Hoffman JI, Rivera AH. Needle penetration of the globe during retrobulbar and peribulbar injections. *Ophthalmology* 1991; **98**: 1017.
91. Hayreh SS. Anterior ischemic optic neuropathy IV. Occurrence after cataract extraction. *Arch Ophthalmol* 1980; **98**: 1410.
92. Hayreh SS, Kolder HE. Central retinal artery occlusion and retinal tolerance time. *Ophthalmology* 1980; **87**: 75.
93. Heavner JE. Cardiac dysrhythmias induced by infusion of local anesthetics into the lateral cerebral ventral of cats. *Anesth Analg* 1986; **65**: 133.
94. Hersch M, Baer G, Dieckert JP *et al.* Optic nerve enlargement and central retinal artery occlusion secondary to retrobulbar anesthesia. *Ann Ophthalmol* 1989; **21**: 195.
95. Hessemer V, Wieth K, Heinrich A, Jacobi KW. Changes in uveal and retinal hemodynamics produced by retrobulbar anesthesia with different injection volumes. *Fortschr Ophthalmol* 1989; **86**: 760.
96. Hessemer V, Heinrich A, Jacobi KW. Ocular circulatory changes induced by retrobulbar anesthesia with and without adrenaline. *Klin Mbl Augenheilk* 1990; **197**: 470.
97. Heyworth PLO, Seward HC. Local anaesthesia: The ophthalmologist's view. *Eur J Implant Ref Surg* 1993; **5**: 12.
98. Hustead RF, Hamilton RC. Pharmacology. In *Ophthalmic Anesthesia* (edited by Gills JP, Hustead RF, Sanders DR). Slack Inc.: Thorofare, NJ, 1993: 69–102.
99. Hustead RF, Hamilton RC. Techniques. In *Ophthalmic Anesthesia* (edited by Gills JP, Hustead RF, Sanders DR). Slack Inc.: Thorofare, NJ, 1993: 103–186.
100. Hørven I. Ophthalmic artery pressure during retrobublar anesthesia. *Acta Ophthalmol* 1978; **56**: 574.
101. Jaffe GJ, Irvine AR, Wood IS *et al.* Retinal phototoxicity from the operating microscope: The role of inspired oxygen. *Ophthalmology* 1988; **95**: 1130.
102. Jain VK, Mames RN, McGorray S, Giles CL. Inadvertent penetrating injury to the globe with periocular corticosteroid injection. *Ophthalmic Surg* 1991; **22**: 508.
103. Jarrett WH, Brockhurst RJ. Unexplained blindness and optic atrophy following retinal detachment surgery. *Arch Ophthalmol* 1965; **73**: 782–791.
104. Javitt JC, Addiego R, Friedberg HL, Libonati MM, Leahy JJ. Brain stem anesthesia after retrobulbar block. *Ophthalmology* 1987; **94**: 718.
105. Jay WM, Aziz MZ, Green K. Effect of Honan intraocular pressure reducer on ocular and optic nerve blood flow in phakic rabbit eyes. *Acta Ophthalmol* 1986; **64**: 52.

106. Jedeikin RJ, Hoffman S. The oculocardiac reflex in eye-surgery anesthesia. *Anesth Analg* 1977; **56:** 333.
107. Jorfeldt L, Lewis DH, Lofstrom B, Post C. Lung uptake of lidocaine in healthy volunteers. *Acta Anaesthesiol Scand* 1979; **23:** 567.
108. Joseph JP, McHugh JDA, Franks WA, Chignell AH. Perforation of the globe: a complication of peribulbar anaesthesia. *Br J Ophthalmol* 1991; **75:** 504.
109. Kaplan LJ, Jaffe NS, Clayman HM. Ptosis and cataract surgery. *Ophthalmology* 1985; **92:** 237.
110. Kaplan SL. Peribulbar anesthesia. *Ophthalmic Surg* 1988; **19:** 374.
111. Katsev DA, Drews RC, Rose BT. An anatomic study of retrobulbar needle path length. *Ophthalmology* 1989; **96:** 1221.
112. Katz J. In *Atlas of Regional Anesthesia*. Appleton and Lange: Norwalk, CT, 1985: 30–31.
113. Kaufer G, Augustin G. Orbitography: Report of a complication with use of water-soluble contrast material. *Am J Ophthalmol* 1966; **61:** 795.
114. Khalil SN. Local anaesthesia for eye surgery (Letter). *Anaesthesia* 1991; **46:** 232.
115. Kimble JA, Morris RE, Witherspoon CD, Feist RM. Globe perforation from peribulbar injection. *Arch Ophthalmol* 1987; **105:** 749.
116. Kishore K, Agarwal HC, Sood NN *et al.* Evaluation of peribulbar anesthesia in eye camps. *Ophthalmic Surg* 1990; **21:** 566.
117. Klein ML, Jampol LM, Condon PI *et al.* Central retinal artery occlusion without retrobulbar hemorrhage after retrobulbar anesthesia. *Am J Ophthalmol* 1982; **93:** 573.
118. Knapp H. On cocaine and its use in ophthalmic and general surgery. *Arch Ophthalmol* 1884; **13:** 402.
119. Kobet KA. Cerebral spinal fluid recovery of lidocaine and bupivicaine following respiratory arrest subsequent to retrobulbar block. *Ophthalmic Surg* 1987; **18:** 11.
120. Koenig SB, Snyder RW, Kay J. Respiratory distress after a Nadbath block. *Ophthalmology* 1988; **95:** 1285.
121. Koornneef L. New insights in the human orbital connective tissue: Result of a new anatomical approach. *Arch Ophthalmol* 1977; **95:** 1269.
122. Kraushar MF, Seelenfreund MH, Freilich DB. Central retinal artery closure during orbital hemorrhage from retrobulbar injection. *Trans Am Acad Ophthalmol Otolaryngol* 1974; **78:** 65.
123. Kushner BJ. Ocular muscle fibrosis following cataract extraction (Letter). *Arch Ophthalmol* 1988; **106:** 18.
124. Lakhanpal V, Dogra MR. Ocular perforation can occur during peribulbar anesthesia. *Ocular Surgery News* 1991; **9:** 28.
125. Laws DE, Watts MT, Kirkby GR, Lawson J. Is padding necessary cataract extraction? *Br J Ophthalmol* 1989; **73:** 699.
126. Leaming DV. Practice styles and preferences of ASCRS members – 1989 survey. *J Cataract Refract Surg* 1990; **16:** 624.
127. Leaming DV. Practice styles and preferences of ASCRS members – 1990 survey. *J Cataract Refract Surg* 1991; **17:** 495.
128. Lee DS, Kwon NJ. Shivering following retrobulbar block. *Can J Anaesth* 1988; **35:** 294.
129. Lemagne J-M, Michiels X, Van Causenbroech S, Snyers B. Purtscher-like retinopathy after retrobulbar anesthesia. *Ophthalmology* 1990; **97:** 859.
130. Levin ML, in Masket S (ed.). Consultation section. *J Cataract Refract Surg* 1990; **16:** 766.
131. Levin ML, O'Connor PS. Visual acuity after retrobulbar anesthesia. *Ann Ophthalmol* 1989; **11:** 337.
132. Levine MR, Enlow MK, Terman S. Spastic entropion after cataract surgery. *Ann Ophthalmol* 1992; **24:** 195.
133. Lichter PR: Avoiding complications from local anesthesia (Editorial). *Ophthalmology* 1988; **95:** 565.

134. Lincoff H, Zweifach P, Brodie S *et al.* Intraocular injection of lidocaine. *Ophthalmology* 1985; **92:** 1587.
135. Lindquist TD, Kopietz LA, Spigelman AV *et al.* Complications of Nadbath facial nerve block and review of the literature. *Ophthalmic Surg* 1988; **19:** 271.
136. Liu C, Youl B, Moseley I. Magnetic resonance imaging of the optic nerve in extremes of gaze: Implications for the positioning of the globe for retrobulbar anaesthesia. *Br J Ophthalmol* 1992; **76:** 728.
137. Liu D. A simplified technique of orbital decompression for severe retrobulbar hemorrhage. *Am J Ophthalmol* 1993; **116:** 34.
138. Livingston MW, Mackool RJ, Schneider H. Anesthetic agents used in cataract surgery (Letter). *J Cataract Refract Surg* 1990; **16:** 272.
139. Loots JH, Koorts AS, Venter JA. Peribulbar anesthesia: A prospective statistical analysis of the efficacy and predictability of bupivacaine and a lignocaine/bupivacaine mixture. *J Cataract Refract Surg* 1993; **19:** 72.
140. Mackool RJ. Intraocular pressure fluctuations (Letter). *J Cataract Refract Surg* 1993; **19:** 563.
141. McDonald HR, Schatz H, Johnson RN. Aminoglycoside toxicity. *Sem Ophthalmol* 1993; **8:** 136.
142. McKeown CA. Ocular motility disorders and orbital trauma. *Int Ophthalmol Clin* 1992; **32:** 123.
143. McLean EB. Inadvertent injection of corticosteroid into the choroidal vasculature. *Am J Ophthalmol* 1975; **80:** 835.
144. McMahan LB. Anticoagulants and cataract surgery. *J Cataract Refract Surg* 1988; **14:** 569.
145. Mercereau DA. Brain-stem anesthesia complicating retrobulbar block. *Can J Ophthalmol* 1989; **24:** 159.
146. Meyer D, Hamilton RC, Loken RG, Gimbel HV. Effect of combined peribulbar and retrobulbar injection of large volumes of anesthetic agents on the intraocular pressure. *Can J Ophthalmol* 1992; **27:** 230.
147. Meyers EF. Problems during eye surgery under local anesthesia. *Anesthesiol Rev* 1979; **6:** 23.
148. Meyers EF, Ramirez RC, Boniuk I. Grand mal seizures after retrobulbar block. *Arch Ophthalmol* 1978; **96:** 847.
149. Meyers EF. Anesthesia. In *Complications in Ophthalmic Surgery* (edited by Krupin T, Waltman SR). JB Lippincott: Philadelphia, PA, 1984: 1–22.
150. Morgan CM, Schatz H, Vine AK *et al.* Ocular complications associated with retrobulbar injections. *Ophthalmology* 1988; **95:** 660.
151. Morgan GE. Retrobulbar apnea syndrome: A case for the routine presence of an anesthesiologist (Letter). *Reg Anesth* 1990; **15:** 107.
152. Nadbath RP, Rehman I. Facial nerve block. *Am J Ophthalmol* 1963; **55:** 143.
153. Nicoll JMV, Acharya PA, Ahlen K *et al.* Central nervous system complications after 6000 retrobulbar blocks. *Anesth Analg* 1987: **66:** 1298.
154. Nicoll JMV, Acharya PA, Edge KR *et al.* Shivering following retrobulbar block. *Can J Anaesth* 1988; **35:** 671.
155. Nique TA, Bennett CA. Inadvertent brain stem anesthesia following extra-oral trigeminal V2–V3 blocks. *Oral Surg* 1981; **51:** 468.
156. O'Brien CS. Local anesthesia. *Archiv Ophthalmol* 1934; **12:** 240.
157. Ong-Tone L, Pearce WG. Inferior rectus muscle restriction after retrobulbar anesthesia for cataract extraction. *Can J Ophthalmol* 1989; **24:** 162.
158. Otto AJ, Spekreijse H. Volume discrepancies in the orbit and the effect on the intraorbital pressure: An experimental study in the monkey. *Orbit* 1989; **8:** 233.
159. Palay DA, Stulting RD. The effect of external ocular compression on intraocular pressure following retrobulbar anesthesia. *Ophthalmic Surg* 1990; **21:** 503.

160. Paris GL, Quickert MH. Disinsertion of the aponeurosis of the levator palpebrae superioris muscle after cataract extraction. *Am J Ophthalmol* 1976; **81**: 337.
161. Pautler SE, Grizzard WS, Thompson LN, Wing GL. Blindness from retrobulbar injection into the optic nerve. *Ophthalmic Surg* 1986; **17**: 334.
162. Pearce JL. General and local anaesthesia in eye surgery. *Trans Ophthalmol Soc UK* 1982; **102**: 31.
163. Priddy R, Loken RG, Hamilton RC. Ocular pressures and regional anaesthesia. Paper presented at the Xth Congress of the European Society of Cataract and Refractive Surgeons, Paris, September, 1992.
164. Rabinowitz L, Livingston M, Schneider H, Hall A. Respiratory obstruction following the Nadbath facial nerve block (Letter). *Arch Ophthalmol* 1986; **104**: 1115.
165. Rainin EA, Carlson BM. Postoperative diplopia and ptosis: A clinical hypothesis on the myotoxicity of local anesthetics. *Arch Ophthalmol* 1985; **103**: 1337.
166. Ramsay RC, Knobloch WH. Ocular perforation following retrobulbar anesthesia for retinal detachment surgery. *Am J Ophthalmol* 1978; **86**: 61.
167. Rao VA, Kawatra VK. Ocular myotoxic effects of local anesthetics. *Can J Ophthalmol* 1988; **23**: 171.
168. Reed JW, MacMillan AS Jr, Lazenby GW. Transient neurologic complication of positive contrast orbitography. *Arch Ophthalmol* 1969; **81**: 508.
169. Rinkoff JS, Doft BH, Lobes LA. Management of ocular penetration from injection of local anesthesia preceding cataract surgery. *Arch Ophthalmol* 1991; **109**: 1421.
170. Robinson GA, Nylander A. Warfarin and caratact extraction. *Br J Ophthalmol* 1989; **73**: 702.
171. Rodman DJ, Notaro S, Peer GL. Respiratory depression following retrobulbar bupivacaine: Three case reports and literature review. *Ophthalmic Surg* 1987; **18**: 768.
172. Rogers R, Orellana J. Cranial nerve palsy following retrobulbar anesthesia. *Br J Ophthalmol* 1988; **72**: 78.
173. Ropo A, Ruusuvaara P, Setälä K. Visual evoked potentials after retrobulbar or periocular anaesthesia. *Br J Ophthalmol* 1992; **76**: 541.
174. Rosen E. Editorial review: Anaesthesia for cataract surgery. *Eur J Implant Ref Surg* 1993; **5**: 1.
175. Rosenblatt RM, May DR, Barsoumian K. Cardiopulmonary arrest after retrobulbar block. *Am J Ophthalmol* 1980; **90**: 425.
176. Rubin AP. Anaesthesia for cataract surgery – time for change? (Editorial). *Anaesthesia* 1990; **45**: 717.
177. Russell DA Jr, Guyton JS. Retrobulbar injection of lidocaine (Xylocaine) for anesthesia and akinesia. *Am J Ophthalmol* 1954; **38**: 78.
178. Ruusuvaara P, Setälä K, Tarkkanen A. Respiratory arrest after retrobulbar block. *Acta Ophthalmol* 1988; **66**: 223.
179. Schechter RJ. Management of inadvertent intraocular injections. *Ann Ophthalmol* 1985; **17**: 771.
180. Schlaegal TF, Wilson FM. Accidental intraocular injection of depot corticosteroids. *Trans Am Acad Ophthalmol Otolaryngol* 1974; **78**: 847.
181. Schneider ME, Milstein DE, Oyakawa RT *et al*. Ocular perforation from a retrobulbar injection. *Am J Ophthalmol* 1988; **106**: 35.
182. Seelenfreund MH, Freilich DB. Retinal injuries associated with cataract surgery. *Am J Ophthalmol* 1980; **89**: 654.
183. Shorr N, Seiff SR. Central retinal artery occlusion associated with periocular corticosteroid injection for juvenile hemangioma. *Ophthalmic Surg* 1986; **17**: 229.
184. Shuler JD, Paschal JF, Holland GN. Antiplatelet therapy and cataract surgery. *J Cataract Refract Surg* 1992; **18**: 567.
185. Singh PP, Dimich I, Sampson I, Sonnenklar N. A comparison of esmolol and labetolol for the treatment of perioperative hypertension in geriatric ambulatory surgical patients. *Can J Anaesth* 1992; **39**: 559.

186. Smiddy WE, Michels RG, Kumar AJ. Magnetic resonance imaging of retrobulbar changes in optic nerve position with eye movement. *Am J Ophthalmol* 1989; **107**: 82.
187. Smith JL. Retrobulbar Marcaine can cause respiratory arrest. *J Clin Neuro-Ophthalmol* 1981; **1**: 171.
188. Smith RB, Lynn JG Jr. Retrobulbar injection of bupivacaine (Marcaine) for anesthesia and akinesia. *Invest Ophthalmol* 1974; **13**: 157.
189. Spaeth GL. Total facial nerve palsy following modified O'Brien facial nerve block. *Ophthalmic Surg* 1987; **18**: 518.
190. Stanley JA. Subarachnoid injection of retrobulbar anesthetic as a complication of retrobulbar block. *Saudi Bull Ophthalmol* 1987; **2**: 13.
191. Stasior OG. Postoperative ptosis: Etiology, diagnosis, treatment, informed consent. Paper presented at the 4th Annual Scientific Meeting of the Ophthalmic Anesthesia Society, San Antonio, Texas, October 1990.
192. Stewart RH, Kimbrough RL, Engstrom PF *et al.* Lidocaine: An anti-tussive for ophthalmic surgery. *Ophthalmic Surg* 1988; **19**: 130.
193. Straus JG. A new retrobulbar needle and injection technique. *Ophthalmic Surg* 1988; **19**: 134.
194. Stone LS, Kline OR Jr, Sklar C. Intraocular lenses and anticoagulation and antiplatelet therapy. *Am Intraocul Implant Soc J* 1985; **11**: 165.
195. Sugin SL, Yannuzzi LA. Choroidal ischemia following intraocular surgery. *Sem Ophthalmol* 1993; **8**: 149.
196. Sullivan KL, Brown GC, Forman AR *et al.* Retrobulbar anesthesia and retinal vascular obstruction. *Ophthalmology* 1983; **90**: 373.
197. Tennant JL. Diplopia. Paper presented at the 4th Annual Scientific Meeting of the Ophthalmic Anesthesia Society, San Antonio, Texas, October 1990.
198. Thomas RD, Behbehani MM, Coyle DE, Denson DD. Cardiovascular toxicity of local anesthetics: An alternative hypothesis. *Anesth Analg* 1986; **65**: 444.
199. Thornton SP. Ocular anesthesia with the Thornton retrobulbar needle. In *Ophthalmic Anesthesia* (edited by Gills JP, Hustead RF, Sanders DR). Slack Inc.: Thorofare, NJ, 1993: 155–159.
200. Unsöld R, Stanley JA, DeGroot J. The CT-topography of retrobulbar anesthesia. *Graefes Arch Klin Exp Ophthalmol* 1981; **217**: 125.
201. Verma L, Arora R, Kumar A. Temporary conduction block of optic nerve after retrobulbar anesthesia. *Ophthalmic Surg* 1990; **21**: 109.
202. Vivian AJ, Canning CR. Scleral perforation with retrobulbar needles. *Eur J Implant Ref Surg* 1993; **5**: 39.
203. Wallace RB, in Masket S (ed.). Consultation section. *J Cataract Refract Surg* 1990; **16**: 766.
204. Waller SG, Taboada J, O'Connor P. Retrobulbar anesthesia risk: Do sharp needles really perforate the eye more easily than blunt needles? *Ophthalmology* 1993; **100**: 506.
205. Wang BC, Bogart B, Hillman DE, Turndorf H. Subarachnoid injection – a potential complication of retrobulbar block. *Anesthesiology* 1989; **71**: 845.
206. Weiss JL, Deichman CB. A comparison of retrobulbar and periocular anesthesia for cataract surgery. *Arch Ophthalmol* 1989; **107**: 96.
207. Welch JC, Spaeth GL, Benson WE. Massive suprachoroidal hemorrhage. *Ophthalmology* 1988; **95**: 1202.
208. Wittpenn JR, Rapoza P, Sternberg P, Kuwashima L, Saklad J, Patz A. Respiratory arrest following retrobulbar anesthesia. *Ophthalmology* 1986; **93**: 867.
209. Wong DHW. Review article: Regional anaesthesia for intraocular surgery. *Can J Anaesth* 1993; **40**: 635.
210. Wright RE. Blocking of the main trunk of the facial nerve in cataract operations. *Arch Ophthalmol* 1926; **55**: 555.
211. Yagiela JA, Benoit PW, Buoncristiani RD *et al.* Comparison of myotoxic effects of lidocaine with epinephrine in rats and humans. *Anesth Analg* 1981; **60**: 471.

212. Yanoff M, Redovan EG. Anterior eyewall perforation during subconjunctival cararact block. *Ophthalmic Surg* 1990; **21:** 362.
213. Zabel RW, Clarke WN, Shirley SY, Rock W. Intraocular pressure reduction prior to retrobulbar injection of anesthetic. *Ophthalmic Surg* 1988; **19:** 868.
214. Zaturansky B, Hyams S. Perforation of the globe during the injection of local anesthesia. *Ophthalmic Surg* 1987; **18:** 585.
215. Zeitlin GL, Hobin K, Platt J, Woitkoski N. Accummulation of carbon dioxide during eye surgery. *J Clin Anesth* 1989; **1:** 262.
216. McLoon LK, Wirtschafter J. Regional differences in the subacute response of rabbit orbicularis oculi to bupivacaine-induced mytotoxicity as quantified with a neural cell adhesion molecule immunohistochemical marker. *Invest Ophthalmol Vis Sci* 1993; **34:** 345.
217. Koornneef L, Grizzard WS. Ophthalmic anesthesia. In *Ophthalmology Annual* (edited by Reinecke RD). Raven Press: New York, 1989: 265–294.

CHAPTER 9

General anaesthesia and monitoring

G BARRY SMITH

INTRODUCTION

Many anaesthetists consider that eye anaesthesia on the open globe is difficult and demanding, however, surgeons are tending to operate more and more on closed eyes in which intraocular pressure (IOP) is controlled by the height of an intraocular infusion. Keratoplasty (corneal graft), large perforating injuries and cataract sections which are made deliberately large to facilitate the expression of the lens nucleus, are all exceptions in which there is a risk of vitreous loss or expulsive choroidal haemorrhage. In these operations and also in glaucoma when the IOP is already raised, the anaesthetist must contrive to produce a 'soft' eye in a relaxed and still patient.[14] Modern anaesthetics and surgery have combined to make general anaesthesia in this speciality a safe alternative to local anaesthesia for both patient and surgeon.[10] Good anaesthesia relies on basic fundamentals. The preoperative assessment and a few basic investigations will point out the dangers to be avoided in a group of patients, many of whom have multiple pathology including ischaemic heart disease, airway obstruction or diabetes. Fortunately, the operations for cataract and glaucoma are extremely short, the metabolic disturbance to the patient is minimal and ambulation within a few hours is the rule. Postoperative respiratory complications and thrombotic episodes are no more common with general anaesthesia than they are with local anaesthesia. This is a complete change to figures published only 20 years ago, when prolonged recumbency led to a much greater morbidity. Postoperative complications are now extremely rare.

Attention to the airway, to ventilation, to monitoring and to recovery are vital for success and are dealt with in detail in the following sections.

THE AIRWAY

A clear airway is absolutely mandatory because any resistance to expiration is reflected in raised venous pressure, which is instantly translated into raised intraocular pressure. Access to the head is restricted by drapes, surgical equipment and the surgeon; therefore, until recently, a clear airway could only be guaranteed by the insertion of an endotracheal tube of sufficient diameter to allow easy passive expiration. Many elderly patients have an incompetent oesophagogastric junction which may permit reflux of gastric contents, and to protect the lungs against aspiration the tube must be cuffed. The anaesthetic tubing lies podally over the patient's chest and this increases the curvature required from the traditional Magill pattern endotracheal tube which may, as a result, kink in the back of the mouth or over the lower incisor teeth. For a period anaesthetists overcame this difficulty by using tubes reinforced with a metal or nylon spiral, but during the last few years preformed tubes which have more anatomical shapes such as the RAE and the Oxford tube have become standard. The main problem with preformed tubes is that they are designed for the average patient. In some patients, particularly the endentulous, the right main bronchus may be accidentally intubated, while in a few patients the tube is too short and slips out of the larynx. Inflation of the left lung should be checked by inspection or auscultation of the chest in the fourth costal space in the mid-axillary line. In situations where this is not obvious, the patient should be ventilated for a period with 30% oxygen and the oxygen saturation on the pulse oximeter noted. A saturation of 90% or less suggests a malposition of the tube which may need to be partially or totally withdrawn.

As many eye patients are elderly and have stiff necks, brittle, mobile or reconstructed teeth, laryngoscopy may be difficult or impossible. A well-prepared failed intubation drill and equipment such as gum elastic bougies, a fibre-optic laryngoscope, a variety of tubes and a laryngeal mask are essential.

The anaesthetic tubing must be securely anchored so that it cannot move during the operation and it should be checked for torsional strains which might occlude the tube by twisting. Finally, all connections must be double-checked as movement of the head by the surgeon or pressure of the surgeon's elbow may dislodge a poorly made connection.

LARYNGEAL MASKS

It was providential that laryngeal masks[5-7] and propofol became available at the same time, as they are complementary and mark progress in anaesthesia for surgery of the anterior segment of the eye. Laryngeal masks have the advantage of being easy to position without laryngoscopy, they do not activate the vasopressor and oculotensive reflexes initiated by laryngeal intubation,[8,16] and they have a reduced incidence of sore throat and dental trauma. There are important restrictions on their use, they do not provide a perfect seal to protect the airway from aspiration and should *never* be used in a patient who is suspected of having a full stomach. Similarly, it is *dangerous* to use them in patients in whom it is expected to use inflation pressures of 20 cm of water or more as there is grave risk of gastric inflation.

Insertion of the tube needs a patient with reduced pharyngeal reflexes, usually produced by a suitable dose of propofol, but which may also be obtained by thiopentone and muscle relaxant or by careful local anaesthesia of the pharynx. The originally described position is similar to that for laryngoscopy (i.e. a flexed neck and extended head); however, many anaesthetists find the mask can be passed in a neutral position. The mask is traditionally completely deflated by pressing on a flat surface, well-lubricated and held like a pen with the index finger extended along the tube to the base of the mask. It is then passed up into the palate and, in one continuous movement, on into the pharynx until it meets the resistance of the superior oesophageal sphincter. The tube is held while the cuff is inflated with 20 ml or more of air (which pushes the tube out a little). Patency is then checked by observing the respiration of the spontaneously breathing patient or by gentle inflation with the bag. The tube is then firmly anchored. Obstruction usually means that the epiglottis has been hooked down and the mask can be deflated and reinserted. Various modified methods of insertion have been suggested, such as partial inflation of the cuff, different head positions and lateral rotation of the cuff during insertion to guide it through the fauces. Anaesthesia is then continued with spontaneous respiration or positive pressure respiration. In the latter case, only low inflation pressures should be used and a watch should be kept for accidental inflation of the stomach.

PREMEDICATION

With the advent of day-case surgery, it seems that fewer patients receive a premedicant drug. The majority of elderly patients accept this with equanimity. However, younger patients often seem to need some sedation and in these patients a benzodiazepine orally 1–2 h preoperation usually relieves anxiety and reduces the dose of anaesthetic agent required.

A new departure is the administration of a non-steroidal anti-inflammatory drug, such as indomethacin or diclofenac, orally or rectally before, during or immediately after surgery, to reduce the inflammatory response and as a basis for postoperative analgesia. There are some unresolved problems related to the use of these drugs in relation to wound healing, gastric irritation, anaphylaxis and decreased clot formation. The situation will only become clear when large series are published.

INDUCTION

Thiopentone

Induction with thiopentone 2–7 mg/kg is the benchmark by which other methods can be judged. It produces unconsciousness predictably, side-effects and true allergy are rare, intraocular pressure is reduced and recovery is rapid. It does sensitize the airways to stimuli which may provoke some bronchospasm. Laryngoscopy after thiopentone is marked by a rise in blood pressure and a sharp but temporary rise in IOP. To block this response, some anaesthetists use a small dose of short-acting narcotic such as alfentanil, others use intravenous lignocaine[19,20] and there have been reports of the beneficial results of nifedipine.[4,12,15,24,30,35] Local anaesthesia of the larynx is usually insufficient to block this response.

Etomidate

This drug initially showed great promise as it reduces IOP more than thiopentone.[9,13] Since it was discovered that it depresses the adrenal cortex for 8 h, it has been less favoured. Given in a dose of 0.3 mg/kg, it produces less of a histamine response than thiopentone and allergy is very rare. It is now considered to be more porphyrinogenic than propofol, though it has been given safely to several known porphyrics without any apparent clinical harm.[25] It is not now considered to be safe for use by infusion.

Propofol

The emulsion contains 10 mg/ml and a suitable dose is 3 mg/kg, which may be reduced in extreme old age or when the drug is preceded by a narcotic analgesic such as alfentanil 250 μg.[22,23] It sometimes produces pain or discomfort when injected into small veins. This can be prevented by the admixture of lignocaine 1% 1 ml. It induces sleep rapidly; this is accompanied by a relaxation of the jaw and depression of the pharyngeal and laryngeal reflexes which lasts for a few minutes. This is often associated with a short period of respiratory depression, which is of no consequence if the patient has been preoxygenated. There is also a small depression of the blood pressure and a marked fall in IOP. Recovery is rapid and is associated with a feeling of well-being.[34] It seems at present to be an extremely safe agent and particularly suitable for use with the laryngeal mask and for day surgery. It may be used with muscle relaxants for longer procedures but the advantages are less clear-cut. It reduces the pressor responses to induction and tends to lower IOP during surgery.[22,23,31,32,37]

Ketamine

This induction agent is inappropriate for most eye operations as it tends to raise IOP when given intravenously. It has found an important niche in the management of congenital glaucoma and in the examination of small children.[2,3] The patient retains muscle tone but the airway is not protected against aspiration.

Muscle relaxants

Suxamethonium remains the fastest, shortest acting and most effective muscle relaxant, making it the ideal agent for 'crash inductions' in the presence of a full stomach or when intubation is expected to present problems. It is not used as often as it used to be for routine intubation because of the common side-effect of severe myalgia (the incidence of which may be reduced by a small dose of non-depolarizing relaxant). The other problems are those of prolonged neuromuscular block and the rare but sometimes fatal occurence of hyperthermia. In ophthalmic surgery, there has always been a question over its use in patients with a perforation of the globe because of its known tendency to elevate the IOP by 8–15 cm of water for 10 min.[17,26,28,33,35] This rise is small compared with pressures associated with the squeezing of the eyelids or the rise in pressure caused by coughing, vomiting or laryngoscopy. Although any rise is undesirable, suxamethonium may still be the best option when there is a full stomach, a difficult intubation or an inexperienced anaesthetist.

The anaesthetist is spoilt for choice with an excellent range of curare-like muscle relaxants with different lengths of action. Although gallamine was once prized for its vagal blocking activity, it has been superseded by agents without vagal effects.[11,21,31,39] Modern relaxants have sharper endpoints and it is necessary to identify this with a train-of-four nerve stimulator.

BALANCED ANAESTHESIA

The triad of unconsciousness, muscle relaxation and blockade of painful afferent stimuli provides anaesthesia for every situation. Nitrous oxide in a concentration of 70% is still the most common and convenient means of producing loss of consciousness and 'analgesia' supplemented with the vapour of halothane, enflurane or isoflurane. Halothane is falling from favour because of the fear of the medicolegal consequences of the rare occurrence of hepatic necrosis, particularly after repeated administration. In some countries, it is the only available volatile agent except for ether. It is not always necessary to use a narcotic supplement in ophthalmic anaesthesia when the surgical stimuli are minimal. Narcotics often increase postoperative nausea, but they tend to reduce the rise in ocular tension produced by noxious stimuli in the airway or at the operative site.[12,35]

Nitrous oxide is not suitable for vitrectomies in which the surgeon intends to use air or gas as a means of internal tamponade because nitrous oxide will rapidly diffuse into and out of the bubble.[29,36] In these circumstances, it is either necessary to use a total intravenous technique from the start or to turn off the nitrous oxide before the gas is introduced and substitute it with a more volatile agent and intravenous narcotic.[39]

RECOVERY

Proper staffing of the recovery unit is essential and patients should stay not only until their vital signs are stable, but until they have control of their airway and sufficient self-control not to interfere with their eye.[38] It must be remembered that many of the patients will be somewhat confused as they will be temporarily blinded by their dressings and many older patients may be handicapped by deafness.

Ideally, the monitoring started in theatre should be continued in the recovery unit until stability is achieved. It is a safe routine to administer oxygen-enriched air to all patients until they have cleared their bodies of dissolved nitrous oxide and until it is certain that muscle relaxants have been completely and totally reversed. All patients require continuous pulse oximetry in the recovery area.

It is in the recovery unit that pain and nausea can be assessed and treatment started.[1,18,27] The majority of eye patients complain of soreness and only leading questions suggest to patients that this may be pain needing narcotics. There is a high incidence of nausea and vomiting among patients having surgery to the extraocular muscles; some of these have had droperidol or trifluoperarazine during the operation and may need further antiemetics later. Children who have had squint surgery are a problem, as there is no reliable antiemetic which will not in some instances cause frightening extrapyramidal side-effects such as opisthotonos or oculogyric crisis.

MONITORING

The anaesthetist has less direct access to the patient in ophthalmology than in any other form of surgery. The lighting may be dimmed to reduce corneal reflections or it may be completely extinguished to allow the surgeon to work on the retina. The anaesthetist must have sufficient shielded light to check the identity of drug ampoules, to keep records, to observe flow meters and to perform other essential tasks. All the monitors must be self-illuminated. There is usually a patient's hand available, a radial pulse to palpate and a cannula for access. It is often difficult to observe the respiratory movements directly as the equivalent of a Mayo table covers the thorax. Fortunately, as vitrectomists became more adventurous and demanding, so electronic monitoring became more available.

The safety of the patient depends on the vigilance of the anaesthetist, the meticulous manner in which the equipment is checked before use, the way in which all drugs and infusions are examined, the recording of trends and immediate, appropriate response to any alarm or change in the patient's state.

Finally, I not only recommend the standards for monitoring the anaesthetized patient listed in Table 9.1, but suggest they are mandatory for any patient undergoing this form of surgery.

Table 9.1   Standards of monitoring during anaesthesia and recovery

---

1. Continuous presence of an adequately trained anaesthetist
2. Regular blood pressure and heart rate measurements (recorded)
3. Continuous monitoring of the ECG throughout anaesthesia
4. Continuous analysis of the gas mixture oxygen content
5. Oxygen supply failure alarm (UK)/Ventilator disconnection alarm (USA)
6. Ventilator diconnection alarm (UK)
7. Pulse oximeter
8. Capnography
9. Temperature measurement available
10. Neuromuscular monitoring available
11. Spirometry (tidal volume measurement) (USA)

This list is compiled from the Recommendations of the Association of Anaesthetists of Great Britain and Ireland (1988) and the Standards for patient monitoring during anaesthesia at Harvard Medical School (*JAMA*) 1986; **256:** 1017

REFERENCES

1. Abramowitz MD, Oh TH, Epstein BS, Ruttiman UE, Friendly DA. The antiemetic effects of droperidol following outpatient strabismus surgery in children. *Anesthesiology* 1983; **59:** 579.
2. Apivor D. Ketamine in paediatric ophthalmological surgery. *Anaesthesia* 1973; **28:** 501.
3. Ausinsch B, Rayburn RL, Munson ES, Levy NS. Ketamine and intraocular pressure in children. *Anesth Analg* 1976; **55:** 773.

4. Black TE, Kay B, Healey TEJ: Reducing the haemodynamic responses to laryngoscopy and intubation. *Anaesthesia* 1984; **39:** 883.

5. Brain AIG. The laryngeal mask: A new concept in airway management. *Br J Anaesth* 1983; **55:** 801.

6. Brain AIG, McGhee TD, McAteer EJ, Thomas A, Abu–Saad MAW, Bushman JA. The laryngeal mask airway. *Anaesthesia* 1985; **40:** 356.

7. Brain AIG. Further developments of the laryngeal mask *Anaesthesia* 1989; **44:** 530.

8. Braudie N, Clements EAF, Hodges UM, Andrews BP. The pressor response and laryngeal mask insertion: A comparison with tracheal intubation. *Anaesthesia* 1989; **44:** 551.

9. Calla S, Gupta A, Sen N, Garg IP. Comparison of the effects of etomidate and thiopentone on intraocular pressure. *Br J Anaesth* 1987; **59:** 437.

10. Campbell DNC, Lim N, Kerr Muir M, O'Sullivan G, Falcon M *et al*. A prospective randomised study of local versus general anaesthesia for cataract surgery. *Anaesthesia* 1993; **48:** 422.

11. Craig JF, Cook JH. A comparison of isoflurane and halothane in anaesthesia for intraocular surgery. *Anaesthesia* 1988; **43:** 454.

12. Crawford DC, Fell D, Achola KJ, Smith G. Effects of alfentanil on the pressor and catecholamine responses to tracheal intubation. *Br J Anaesth* 1987; **59:** 707.

13. Criado A, Maseda J, Navarro E, Escarpa A, Avello F. Induction of anaesthesia with etomidate: Haemodynamic study of 36 patients. *Br J Anaesth* 1980; **52:** 803.

14. Cunningham AJ, Barry P. Intraocular pressure – physiology and implications for anaesthetic management. *Can Anaesth Soc J* 1986; **33:** 195.

15. Derbyshire DR, Smith G, Achola KJ. Effect of topical lignocaine on the sympathoadrenal responses to tracheal intubation. *Br J Anaesth* 1987; **59:** 300.

16. Denny NM, Gadelrab R, Complications following general anaesthesia for cataract surgery: A comparison of the laryngeal mask airway with tracheal intubation. *J Roy Soc Med* 1993; **86:** 521.

17. Donlon JV. Succinylcholine and open eye injury. *Anesthesiology* 1986; **64:** 524.

18. Doze VA, Shafer A, White PF. Nausea and vomiting after outpatient anaesthesia – effectiveness of droperidol alone and in conjunction with metoclopramide. *Anesth Analg* 1987; **66:** 541.

19. Drenger B, Pe'er J, Ben Ezra D, Katenelson R, Davidson JT. The effect of intravenous lidocaine on the increase of intraocular pressure induced by tracheal intubation. *Anesth Analg* 1985; **64:** 1211.

20. Drenger B, Gertel M, Pe'er J. Ocular responses after intravenous lidocaine. *Can Anaesth Soc J* 1986; **33:** 219.

21. Earnshaw G. Enflurane, isoflurane and the eye. *Acta Anesthesiol Scand* 1984; **28:** 419.

22. Gillies GWA, Lees NW. The effects of speed of injection on induction with propofol: A comparison with etomidate. *Anaesthesia* 1989; **44:** 386.

23. Guedes Y, Rakotoseheno JC, Leveque M, Mimouni F, Egreteau JP. Changes in the intraocular pressure in the elderly during anaesthesia with propofol. *Anaesthesia* 1988; **43:** 58.

24. Indu B, Batra YK, Puri GD, Singh H. Nifedipine attenuates the intraocular pressure response to intubation following succinylcholine. *Can J Anaesth* 1989; **36:** 269.

25. Harrison GG, Meissner PN, Hift RJ. Anaesthesia for the porphyric patient. *Anaesthesia* 1993; **48:** 417.

26. Jantzen JP, Hackett GH, Earnshaw G. Succinylcholine and open eye injury. *Anesthesiology* 1986; **64:** 524.

27. Korttilla K, Kauste A, Auvinen J. Comparison of domperidone, droperidol and metoclopramide in the prevention and treatment of nausea and vomiting after balanced general anaesthesia. *Anesth Analg* 1979; **58:** 396.

28. Libonati MM, Leahy JJ, Ellison N. Use of succinylcholine in open eye injury. *Anesthesiology* 1985; **62:** 637.

29. Merhige K, Lincoff H, Van Poznak A. Effect of nitrous oxide on gas bubble volume.

Arch Ophthalmol 1985; **103:** 1272.
30. Miller CD, Warren SJ. IV lignocaine fails to attenuate the cardiovascular response to laryngoscopy and tracheal intubation. *Br J Anaesth* 1990; **65:** 216.
31. Mirakhur RK, Elliott P, Shepherd WFI, Archer DB. Intraocular pressure changes during induction of anaesthesia and tracheal intubation: A comparison of thiopentone and propofol followed by vecuronium. *Anaesthesia* 1988; **43:** 54.
32. Oji EO, Holcroft A. The ocular effects of etomidate. *Anaesthesia* 1979; **34:** 245.
33. Paudey K, Badola RP, Kumar S. Time course of intraocular hypertension produced by suxamethonium. *Br J Anaesth* 1972; **44:** 191.
34. Sanders LD, Isaac PA, Yeomans WA, Clyburn PA, Rosen M, Robinson JO. Propofol induced anaesthesia: Double blind comparison of recovery after anaesthesia induced by propofol or thiopentone. *Anaesthesia* 1989; **44:** 200.
35. Sweeny J, Underhill S, Dowd T, Mostafa SM. Modification by fentanyl and alfentanil of the intraocular pressure response to suxamethonium and tracheal intubation. *Br J Anaesth* 1989; **65:** 216.
36. Thaller VT. Effect of nitrous oxide on gas bubble volume. *Arch Ophthalmol* 1985; **103:** 1272.
37. Vanacker B, Dekegel D, Dionys J *et al.* Changes in intraocular pressure associated with the administration of propofol. *Br J Anaesth* 1987; **59:** 1514.
38. Yee DA, Rose DK, Cohen MM, Rogers KH. Recovery room events in eye patients: Should it influence your technique? *Can J Anaesth* 1990; **37:** S80.
39. Zindel G, Meistelman C, Gaudy JH. Effects of increasing enflurane concentrations on intraocular pressure. *Br J Anaesth* 1987; **59:** 440.

CHAPTER 10

Paediatric anaesthesia

CAROLINE A CARR ——————————————————————

INTRODUCTION

Children differ from adults in their anatomy, physiology, drug metabolism and psychological response to hospital admission. This means that anaesthesia for children demands specifically trained staff and special facilities.[1] Neonates should ideally be treated in specialist centres and children under 5 years of age anaesthetized by an experienced consultant anaesthetist. Care of children before and after surgery should be carried out by appropriately trained nursing staff.[2]

GENERAL PRINCIPLES

An understanding of how children differ from adults is necessary before embarking on paediatric anaesthesia. Full details can be found in standard texts of paediatric anaesthesia, but a few points will be dealt with here briefly before proceeding to the particular setting of ophthalmic anaesthesia.[3]

Anatomy

Apart from the obvious difference of overall size, the most important anatomical differences are to be found in the airway. Small children have relatively large heads, short necks, large tongues and narrow nasal passages. The larynx is anteriorly placed with a U-shaped epiglottis angled at 45 degrees; the narrowest part is at the cricoid ring. The trachea is short and the main bronchi are given off at equal angles; the airways are relatively narrow. These make management of a small child's airway quite different from that of an adult and easily obstructed by the inexperienced.

Physiology

Under normal conditions the small child has a high oxygen consumption with a limited capacity to increase the supply (Table 10.1). The neonate has twice the metabolic rate of an adult to provide energy for thermoregulation and growth. The immature myocardium and respiratory system limit the capacity to increase oxygen supply. The proportion of contractile tissue in the heart is much less than in an adult and stroke volume is relatively fixed. Cardiac output therefore varies

Table 10.1 Some physiological variables in children

	Age				
	1 day	*1 week*	*1 month*	*1 year*	*5 years*
Systolic/diastolic BP (mmHg)	65/45	75/50	80/55	85/60	100/65
Haemaglobin (g/dl)	17–22	10–12	11–12	11.5–12.5	11.5–12.5
Heart rate (beats/min)	120	135	160	140	100
Blood volume (ml/kg)	85	80	80	75	70
PaO$_2$ (kPa)	10–10.7	10–10.7	10–10.7	12–13	12–13

with heart rate. In a young child the lungs collapse easily, making gas exchange less efficient, and respiratory muscles fatigue easily. Immature central control of respiration in the infant may result in periodic breathing and sleep apnoea.

Many anaesthetic agents are myocardial depressants and interfere with respiratory function, so anaesthesia may further impair the small child's ability to increase oxygen supply.

Pharmacology

Responses to drugs in children are determined by a large number of factors that change during development.[4] The pharmacokinetics (absorption, distribution, elimination) of administered drugs will be affected by changes in cardiac output, protein binding, membrane permeability, fluid volumes, tissue volumes, hepatic and renal function. The pharmacodynamics (drug–receptor interaction) of administered drugs will be affected by alterations in receptor sensitivity and the availability of normal transmitter substances. These factors change independently of each other during development, which makes it difficult to predict drug effects in a given paediatric age group.

Psychology

A child's response to hospital admission will depend on age and previous experiences in hospital (Table 10.2).[5]

Table 10.2 Phychological responses of children to hospital admission

Infant	Little affected/ may compromise maternal bonding
Toddler/pre-schooler	Upset by change in environment and separation from parent
Schoolchild	Greater ability to communicate, may have a morbid fear of mutilation
Adolescent	May fear loss of self-control, may present a rebellious attitude

SPECIAL CONSIDERATIONS

Quite apart from the implications of paediatric anaesthesia, ophthalmic anaesthesia for children demands several other considerations. Although most children will be ASA categories I or II, associated congenital abnormalities or acquired medical problems will be encountered in a significant number of cases (Table 10.3).[6]

Table 10.3 Paediatric disorders with anaesthetic implications for ophthalmic surgery

Syndrome or disease	Eye problem	Anaesthetic problems
Apert's	Glaucoma, cataracts, strabismus, hypertelorism, proptosis, ectopia lentis	Difficult intubation, cardiac anomalies
Crouzon's	As for Apert's	Upper airway obstruction, difficult intubation
Down's	Cataracts, strabismus, keratoconus	Mental retardation, congenital heart disease
Goldenhar's	Glaucoma, cataracts, strabismus	Difficult intubation, congenital heart disease
Homocystinuria	Strabismus, retinal detachment, glaucoma, optic atrophy	Skeletal and cardiac anomalies, coagulation defects, hypoglycaemia
Lowe's	Cataracts, glaucoma	Severe mental retardation, hypotonia, renal tubular dysfunction
Marfan's	Glaucoma, cataracts, strabismus, retinal detachment, lens subluxation	Skeletal anomalies, cardiac anomalies
Myopathies and muscle disorders	Strabismus, cataracts, ptosis	Respiratory problems, malignant hyperthermia, cardiac conduction defects
Riley Day	Corneal damage secondary to absence of lacrimation	Unstable circulatory system
Rubella	Cataracts	Mental retardation, deafness, cardiac anomalies
Stevens-Johnson	Ocular erosions	Bullous lesions in the airway
Stickler's	Retinal detachment, strabismus	Micrognathia, cleft palate
Sturge-Weber	Glaucoma, vascular malformations	Mental retardation, fits, airway angiomata

The association of ocular problems, particularly squints, with myopathies and myotonias means that although rare, the possibility of malignant hyperthermia occurring during anaesthesia must be kept in mind by the anaesthetist.

The anaesthetist must have an understanding of the eye condition and the operating conditions required. General anaesthesia will be necessary for virtually all ophthalmic procedures in children (even fundoscopy), as cooperation is limited by fear and lack of understanding. During ophthalmic procedures access to the airway is difficult, so most children will have to be intubated or the airway secured in some other way. Most ophthalmic surgery in children is elective and surgical trauma, blood and fluid and electrolyte loss are limited.

Minimal monitoring guidelines have been laid down for monitoring during anaesthesia, but the high incidence of cardiac dysrhythmias associated with ophthalmic surgery makes continuous monitoring of the ECG essential.[7] Many of the simple procedures are considered suitable for day-case surgery.[8]

PREOPERATIVE PREPARATION

Psychological preparation

Before admission to hospital, the child and parents should become familiar with the children's ward. A play therapist can prepare children for anaesthesia and operation by allowing them to see intravenous cannulae, face masks and other items of equipment that will be used at induction of anaesthesia. The use of the eutectic mixture of local anaesthetic – lignocaine–prilocaine (EMLA) – cream can be explained and the fear of intravenous induction reduced.[9] Eye drops that may be used preoperatively can be demonstrated and eye pads and shields that will be applied following surgery explained. Booklets, posters and videos can be used to supplement these explanations. It is particularly important to prepare children and their parents for disfiguring surgery such as enucleation.

The psychological stress of hospital admission can be greatly reduced for children if the planned procedures are carried out on a day-case basis and they know they will be going home with parents afterwards.[10,11]

The preoperative visit by the anaesthetist is important in this psychological preparation, as well as providing an opportunity for assessment of the child's fitness for anaesthesia. If a child is to have repeated visits to theatre, it is ideal for the same anaesthetist to be available on each occasion, as an established rapport will make the induction of anaesthesia less stressful for both child and parents as well as the anaesthetist. The rapport established and the information given to a child will obviously depend on age and ability to understand, but it is important not to give misleading information and to answer questions truthfully. In the same way, parents must be given accurate information as to what is happening and be fully involved in the care of their child while in hospital. In most circumstances, a parent would come to the operating theatre with their child and remain until induction of anaesthesia is complete. Studies show that parents are usually effective at reducing anxiety in their children at induction of anaesthesia and major problems with excessively anxious parents are rare.[12,13]

Anticipation of postoperative pain and its effective relief should be discussed with the parents and the child as appropriate.

Preoperative assessment

The aims of preoperative assessment are to establish that the child is fit for anaesthesia and surgery, to be able to anticipate perioperative problems and to plan the postoperative care. Procedures in children should be carried out as day-cases where ever possible.

The fit normal child (older than 1 month, not premature, and with no associated medical condition) requires minimal investigation. A full history and examination with sickle-cell testing and haemoglobin estimation in the appropriate ethnic groups are sufficient. If there is a history of recent upper respiratory tract infection, it is important to determine if a runny nose is due to allergy or infection. Allergy usually produces chronic symptoms which may have some seasonal variation. Elective procedures should be postponed in the face of recent infection, as there is evidence of increased perioperative complications in these children.[14,15]

The other important points to elicit in the history are a history of asthma or croup, problems with anaesthesia in other family members, the presence of loose teeth and when the child last ate or drank.

Premedication

The aims of premedication are to provide a calm child at induction of anaesthesia and to avoid adverse cardiovascular or respiratory events. Historically, heavy intramuscular sedation was used to overcome the problems of inhalational induction with chloroform and ether. Although less unpleasant, halothane may cause bradycardias or laryngospasm and atropine is necessary prior to inhalation induction. Another important reason for heavy preoperative sedation was the exclusion of parents from the anaesthetic room. It is now universally accepted for parents to be present at the induction of anaesthesia and studies show that this is usually effective in reducing a child's anxiety.[13]

The choice of premedication depends on careful assessment of the individual child and parents and consideration of the proposed procedure. Rigid premedication regimens are best avoided, but guidelines may be proposed (Table 10.4). For most simple ophthalmic procedures in children, opiate premedication is inappropriate and light sedation only is usually more than adequate. The shorter-acting benzodiazepines are effective in producing a calm child who is not too heavily sedated and they are well absorbed orally. Recent studies on the use of midazolam as a premedication in children[16-18] have shown that it has a short elimination half-life of 1.5–2 h, a reliable dose-dependent anxiolytic effect with minimal cardiovascular or respiratory effects, and an anterograde amnesic effect. It is painful on intramuscular injection, rectal instillation may be distressing to the child and, although intranasal administration is rapid, it produces a burning sensation that is unpleasant. Sublingual administration is reliable and produces effects in about 10 min, the oral route produces effects within about 20 min in a dose of 0.5 mg/kg.

The use of EMLA cream, which contains a eutectic mixture of lignocaine and prilocaine, to produce dermal analgesia after topical application prior to venepuncture is widely used in children.[19] Its use has a profound psychological effect on children and their parents preoperatively to reduce the fear of

Table 10.4   Paediatric premedication guidelines

Less than 6 months	No sedation Atropine 0.02 mg/kg (intramuscular in neonates) 30 min pre-induction EMLA
All other children	Atropine 0.02 mg/kg orally for inhalational inductions EMLA
Distressed or anxious children	Temazepam 0.5 mg/kg orally 30 min pre-induction *or* midazolam 0.5 mg/kg orally 20 min pre-induction EMLA
Very distressed children	Morphine 0.25 mg/kg and atropine 0.02 mg/kg intramuscularly 90 min pre-induction *or* papaveretum 0.4 mg/kg and Hyoscine 0.008 mg/kg intramuscularly 60 min pre-induction *or* midazolam 0.2 mg/kg sublingually or intranasally 10–15 min pre-induction EMLA

intravenous induction and if used carefully provides pain-free conditions for venepuncture. The main drawback is that EMLA requires a minimum application time of 1 h under an occlusive dressing and that vasoconstriction occurs at the site. A preparation of amethocaine in the form of a self-adhesive patch has been introduced and initial studies indicate that it has a shorter onset time than EMLA and possibly produces slight vasodilatation at the site of application.[20]

Preoperative fasting

The two factors to be considered when setting a time for preoperative fasting are the dangers of hypoglycaemia and the dangers of regurgitation of gastric contents. The fasting period that can be tolerated without hypoglycaemia will depend on the child's age and medical condition. A healthy child is unlikely to become hypoglycaemic during routine preoperative fasting.[21] Whether it is necessary to withhold fluids for as long as food has been investigated and there is clear evidence that gastric volumes and pH are unchanged if sugar-containing fluids are given for up to 2 h before surgery.[22–24]

A preoperative fasting regimen for children might be suggested as follows: no solid food or milk for 6 h, clear fluids including nonparticulate fruit juices or squashes for up to 2 h preoperatively. Infants and young children should be encouraged to drink sugar-containing fluids at least 4 h preoperatively to ensure hypoglycaemia does not occur perioperatively.

INTRAOPERATIVE MANAGEMENT

Before starting, make sure all the necessary equipment and drugs are ready.

Facemasks

These should be lightweight, easy to use and be available in a range of sizes. The importance of reduced dead-space is negated by the streaming effects of the fresh gas flow within the mask. The black rubber Rendell-Baker-Soucek face-mask is still in common usage, but the clear plastic facemasks are easier to use, especially for mask ventilation, and are cheaper and more pleasant for an inhalation induction (Fig.10.1).

Oropharyngeal airways

A range of sizes of plastic disposable Guedel airways should be available.

Laryngoscopes

A straight blade is needed for infants under 1 year, as the large floppy epiglottis tends to obscure the inlet to the anterior highly placed larynx (Fig. 10.2).

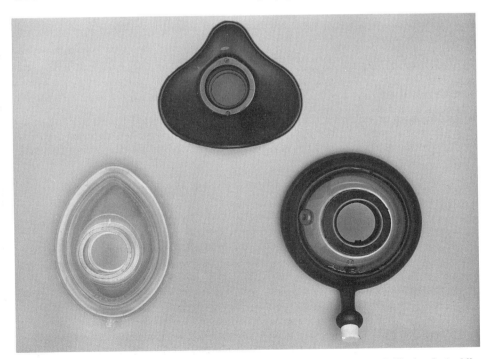

Fig. 10.1. Commonly used paediatric face masks. From left to right: Mallinckrodt (toddler size), MIE Rendell-Baker-Soucek (size 2), Ambu (size 0).

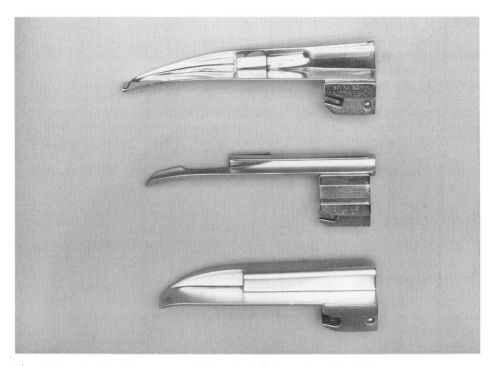

Fig. 10.2. Straight laryngoscope blades for infants and small children. From top down: Robertshaw 1 infant blade (Penlon), Miller 1 infant blade (Penlon), Heine 1 blade (Blease).

Tracheal tubes

For ophthalmic procedures, preformed RAE tubes are best (Fig. 10.3). The connector is well away from the operating field and can be reached without disturbing the operating area. Tube size is usually determined by the following formula (Table 10.5):[25]

$$\text{Internal diameter (mm)} = 4 + \text{age (years)} / 4$$

Table 10.5   Age and tracheal tube size (preformed uncuffed RAE tubes)

Age	Internal diameter (mm)
1–6 months	3.5
6–12 months	4.0
1–2 years	4.5
2–4 years	5.0
4–5.5 years	5.5
5.5–7.5 years	6.0
7.5–9 years	6.5
9+ years	7.0

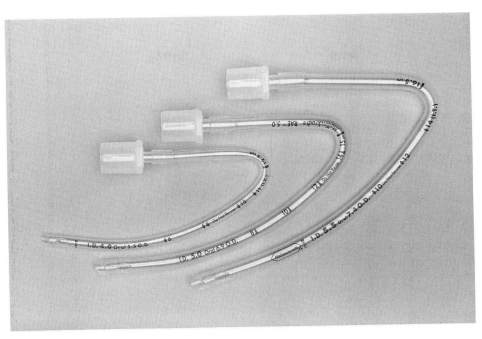

Fig. 10.3. Preformed RAE endotracheal tubes for paediatric ophthalmic surgery.

Although these are the manufacturers' recommended sizes, a size smaller than calculated is often the best fit to allow an air leak around the tube.

Laryngeal masks (Fig. 10.4)

The Brain laryngeal mask airway has become well established in adult anaesthesia as a more secure airway than a conventional airway, with many of the advantages of endotracheal intubation without many of the disadvantages.[26] In paediatric anaesthetic practice, experience is increasing in its use and a reinforced version has been developed particularly for head and neck surgery.[27] Its main advantages are: it can be inserted without the use of muscle relaxants; irritation of the airway due to endotracheal intubation is avoided, which means emergence from anaesthesia without coughing can be achieved; and resistance to breathing with the conventional version is less than through an endotracheal tube.[28] Its main disadvantages are: the airway is not protected from regurgitation; the paediatric sizes are scaled-down adult versions and do not allow for the anatomical differences, thus making a less good fit; it may be more easily displaced during surgery than an endotracheal tube, which would be a problem during intraocular surgery; and possible trauma to the pharyngeal wall with repeated use has been reported.[29–31] The laryngeal mask for paediatric use comes in sizes 1, 2, 2.5 and 3 in the conventional version and sizes 2, 2.5 and 3 in the reinforced

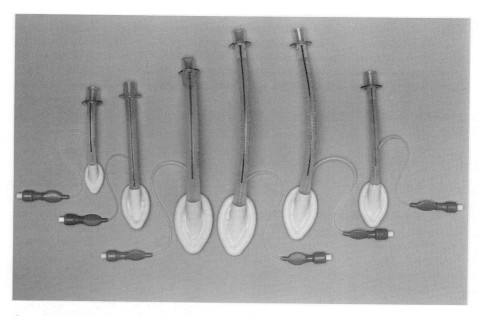

Fig. 10.4.   Standard and reinforced laryngeal mask airways for paediatric ophthalmic surgery.

version. The use of controlled ventilation with the laryngeal mask is another controversial area and is not recommended for lengthy procedures or with the size 1 mask.[32]

Breathing systems

For children up to 5 years of age or 10 kg body mass, the Jackson Rees modification of Ayres T-piece provides a lightweight circuit with few connections and minimal resistance to breathing. A Bain coaxial circuit is most suitable for older children and allows for scavenging. The T-piece is difficult to scavenge and various devices have been developed to avoid the risk of exposing the airway to high pressures. A scavenging dish with no direct contact with the circuit has proved useful.[33]

Ventilators

A T-piece occluding ventilator, such as the Nuffield series 200 ventilator, with a Newton valve is suitable for neonates and children up to 10 kg and will deliver low flows at high rates with control over time intervals. A high-pressure alarm must be used. Most children over 10 kg can be ventilated with adult ventilators set to appropriate volumes and rates. During any lengthy procedure, humidification should be used.

Heat conservation

During ophthalmic surgery, most heat loss will take place from a child's body surface and will occur more rapidly in infants and neonates due to their high surface area to body mass ratio. The head is a particularly important site for heat loss but is usually well covered during these procedures. Warming pads should be used for active warming in all children under 10 kg and for older children during prolonged surgery. The ambient temperature in the operating theatre should be raised as much as allows comfortable working conditions for the theatre staff.

Intravenous access

With the use of EMLA cream it is possible to obtain venous access in most children prior to induction which can then be intravenous. This is often easiest with sharp, fine needles using veins on the back of the hand. Other sites in infants or neonates are the scalp veins or the front of the wrist. Although these needles may have wings by which they can be strapped down, they cannot be relied on and may cut out. There is a wide range of intravenous cannulae available which may be used for induction of anaesthesia or inserted afterwards to provide venous access (Fig. 10.5). All children undergoing ophthalmic procedures should have

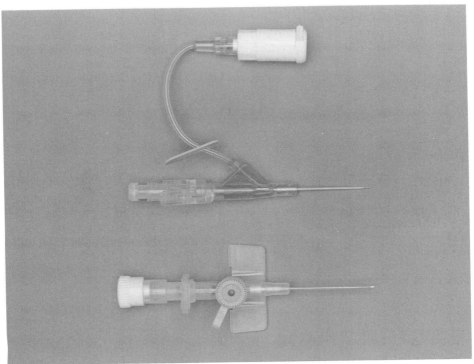

Fig. 10.5. Intravenous cannulae suitable for induction of anaesthesia in children. Above: Wallace Y can 23 g × 22 mm with syringe valve, below: Venflon 2 22 g × 25 mm (BOC Ohmeda).

intravenous access. Gaining access to the cannula site might prove a problem in a very small child due to the operating equipment, and extension tubing may be added or intravenous access established on the dorsum of the foot. In either case, administered drugs will have to be flushed in to ensure rapid entrance to the circulation.

Positioning on the operating table

The operating surgeon will require access to a motionless surgical field for anything from a few minutes to a few hours and may need to move the head at times. Obviously the airway, intravenous access and monitoring must be well secured, the nonoperated eye protected and the head secured on a ring or headrest. In small children, a small pad under the shoulders helps to prevent neck flexion and provides better surgical access as well as avoiding airway obstruction.

Monitoring

This must start at induction of anaesthesia. Even very young children will accept ECG electrodes and a pulse oximeter probe if they are explained and a game made of them. Bradycardias and hypoxia may occur during inhalation induction, or at intubation. During surgery itself, the oculocardiac reflex may be stimulated and ECG monitoring is mandatory.[34] Indirect blood pressure measurement, end-tidal carbon dioxide and temperature monitoring should be routine in all ophthalmic surgery in children. Additionally a precordial stethoscope is useful in small children, and a peripheral nerve stimulator should be used if muscle relaxation is required.

INDUCTION OF ANAESTHESIA

This may be by inhalation or intravenous routes depending on the preference of the anaesthetist and the child. The main aim is to avoid crying and coughing which will raise the intraocular pressure. The avoidance of hospital admission, careful preoperative preparation, the use of premedication in appropriate cases and the presence of a parent in the anaesthetic room will all help to provide a calm cooperative child. Use of EMLA cream makes a smooth intravenous induction a realistic possibility. The importance of skilled help and the cooperation of an informed parent cannot be underestimated. Apart from the consideration of intraocular pressure, a calm induction will make repeated anaesthetics much easier to manage.

Inhalational induction

Halothane is the anaesthetic of choice for an inhalation induction, as coughing and laryngospasm are rare compared with enflurane and isoflurane despite their theoretical advantages. Two new volatile anaesthetics, sevoflurane and desflurane, are undergoing evaluation in children. Sevoflurane on initial tests appears to be suitable for induction of anaesthesia in children. It is non-irritant and due to a lower blood-gas solubility provides a more rapid induction than halothane. The main problems associated with the use of halothane are the possibility of halothane hepatitis following repeated use, and its implication in masseter spasm and malignant hyperthermia.

Masseter spasm and malignant hyperthermia

Masseter spasm is the sustained contracture of the jaw muscles after induction of anaethesia that prevents opening of the mouth for laryngoscopy, although relaxation of the extremities is adequate. The incidence may be as high as 1:100 in children when a halothane induction is followed by intravenous suxamethonium.[35] If this anaesthetic combination is used in children with strabismus this incidence rises to 2.8:100.[36] The coincidence of MH and masseter spasm is about 50%.[37] The incidence of MH in children is usually quoted as 1:10 000–20 000.[66] Obviously a large number of children who develop masseter spasm do not develop MH or the incidence would be much higher.

A child who develops masseter spasm is treated as at risk of developing MH. Elective surgery is cancelled and the anaesthetic stopped. The child is mask ventilated with 100% oxygen and no further anaesthetic given. Temperature, creatine phosphokinase, myoglobin and potassium are monitored for up to 24 hours. If masseter spasm resolves rapidly and other signs of MH are absent, dantrolene is not indicated. Emergency surgery can proceed by discontinuation of all MH triggers, using a nontriggering technique and careful monitoring. Dantrolene should be given prophylactically. The patient and family should be counselled on the implications for future anaesthetics and treated as MH susceptible until further testing. The management of a fulminant episode of MH is outlined in Appendix II.

Halothane hepatitis

Although it is commonly believed that halothane hepatitis does not occur in children, it is now established that it does and can be fatal.[38] The incidence appears to be lower than in adults, 1:82 000 compared with 1:6000–1:22 000, but it is recommended that repeated exposure to halothane is avoided where possible and other techniques may be used.[39] However, many experienced paediatric anaesthetists repeat its use if they believe the benefits outweigh the harm.[40]

Intravenous agents (Table 10.6)

The most commonly used drugs for intravenous induction are thiopentone and propofol. Thiopentone provides a smooth painless induction in doses of 5 mg/kg in premedicated children and up to 7 mg/kg in unpremedicated children. Propofol is particularly useful in day-case anaesthesia because it is associated with a rapid recovery and anti-emesis, but is not licensed for use in children under 3 years of age in the UK.[41] It is used in a dose of 2 mg/kg in premedicated children and 3 mg/kg in unpremedicated children. Following a report of metabolic acidosis and death after the use of propofol for sedation in five paediatric intensive care patients, it is recommended that propofol is no longer used for sedation in children in intensive care.[42]

Table 10.6   Anaesthetic drug doses in children

Intravenous induction agents
Thiopentone   5–7 mg/kg
Propofol   2–4 mg/kg

Ketamine   1–2 mg/kg i.v.
                              up to 10 mg/kg i.m.

Anticholinergic agents
Atropine   0.01–0.02 mg/kg
Glycopyrrolate   0.01 mg/kg

Neuromuscular blocking agents
Suxamethonium   2–3 mg/kg
Atracurium   0.5 mg/kg
Vecuronium   0.1 mg/kg
Mivacurium   0.2 mg/kg
Rocuronium   0.8 mg/kg

Reversal of neuromuscular blockade
Neostigmine   0.05 mg/kg

Intraoperative opiates and other analgesics
Alfentanil   0.02 mg/kg
Fentanyl   0.01 mg/kg
Morphine   0.1–0.2 mg/kg
Ketorolac   0.75 mg/kg
Pethidine   1.0 mg/kg i.m.
Codeine phosphate   1.0 mg/kg i.m. (never i.v.)
Diclofenac   1–2 mg/kg by suppository
Paracetamol   15 mg/kg orally

Anti-emetic agents
Droperidol (i.v.)   up to 0.075 mg/kg
Metoclopramide (i.m.)   under 3 years: 1 mg
                              3–5 years: 2 mg
                              5–9 years: 2.5 mg
                              9–14 years: 5 mg

Ketamine

Ketamine has a useful role in ophthalmic anaesthesia for children. It can be given intravenously in a dose of 1–2 mg/kg or intramuscularly in a dose of 7–10 mg/kg for procedures of short duration without the need for securing the airway. It is often used for measuring the intraocular pressure in congenital glaucoma as it does not spuriously lower the pressure as do all other anaesthetic agents.[43] Premedication with an antisialogogue is necessary to overcome the increased saliva production ketamine produces. Although much less frequent in children than in adults, hallucinations on emergence from ketamine anaesthesia do occur and will make repeated usage difficult.[44]

Anticholinergic agents

Atropine and glycopyrrolate are the anticholinergics of choice as they do not produce sedation as hyoscine can. Their use is to block vagally mediated reflexes as might occur at laryngoscopy, or during eye surgery, and to prevent bradycardia secondary to the administration of suxamethonium, halothane, opioids and propofol.

Preoperative administration of atropine is useful to reduce airway secretions but should be avoided in states of tachycardia or pyrexia. Intravenous administration of atropine 0.02 mg/kg at induction is effective and should be considered in infants of 1 year or less, prior to suxamethonium and before eye surgery. Glycopyrrolate 0.01 mg/kg has some advantages, in that it does not produce central excitatory effects, produces less tachycardia and has a longer duration of action.[45]

Muscle relaxants

To facilitate intubation or intermittent positive pressure ventilation (IPPV), neuromuscular blocking drugs may be used.

Suxamethonium. Despite its many known side-effects, suxamethonium is useful for endotracheal intubation because of its rapid onset and short duration. The recommended dose for infants has been raised to 3 mg/kg and for children to 2 mg/kg to give an equivalent block to 1 mg/kg in adults.[46] The important side-effect in children is bradyarrhythmias, which can occur after a single dose and may be prevented by atropine 0.01 mg/kg intravenously just prior to administration. Hyperkalaemia is not significant in healthy children but may be a problem in the presence of burns, tetanus and paraplegia. Masseter spasm and malignant hyperthermia are associated with the use of suxamethonium. Intraocular pressure rises after the administration of suxamethonium within 1 min, reaches a peak in 3 min and subsides in 7 min. Although it has been used in the presence of an open eye injury, most anaesthetists would avoid suxamethonium if possible.[47,48] Intubation conditions after thiopentone/suxamethonium have been compared to those after propofol/alfentanil in children. Thiopentone 5 mg/kg with suxamethonium 2 mg/kg gave significantly better conditions than propofol 3.5 mg/kg and alfentanil 0.02 mg/kg.[49] In healthy children, however, propofol/alfentanil would provide adequate intubating conditions when suxamethonium should be avoided.[50]

Non-depolarizing muscle relaxants. The short-acting muscle relaxants atracurium and vecuronium are popular in paediatric practice and are particularly satisfactory for ophthalmic procedures and can be easily reversed. Two new drugs, mivacurium and rocuronium, have only been evaluated in older children so far. Mivacurium is partially hydrolysed by plasma cholinesterase, 95% recovery after a dose of 0.2 mg/kg takes 18 min and this is not affected by prolonged infusion, so antagonism of blockade is rarely necessary.[51] Rocuronium is an analogue of vecuronium with an onset of action three times as rapid. With a dose of 0.8 mg/kg in children, block develops in 28 s and lasts 32 min.[52] Muscle relaxants can be avoided altogether in children, as they can be intubated under deep halothane anaesthesia or with an alfentanil/propofol combination, and spontaneous ventilation can be taken over manually or mechanically if necessary.[53]

MAINTENANCE OF ANAESTHESIA

The aims during anaesthesia for ophthalmic surgery in children are to avoid reflex responses to surgery, to control intraocular pressure, to minimize respiratory depression and to avoid postoperative nausea and vomiting. The techniques chosen should reflect these aims. Infants and small children will need to be ventilated for all but the shortest procedures. Inhalational anaesthetics depress ventilation in a dose-dependent fashion and may cause respiratory embarrassment and a rise in intraocular pressure.[54] Older children for extraocular surgery may well be managed with spontaneous ventilation. A balanced technique with small doses of short-acting opiates, such as fentanyl or alfentanil, and low concentrations of inhalational agent in the ventilated child will provide good operating conditions and little postoperative sedation or respiratory depression. Propofol infusions have been used in strabismus surgery to reduce postoperative nausea and vomiting.[41]

Fluid balance

This is not a problem in the healthy child undergoing routine ophthalmic procedures. However, during tumour surgery or dacryocystorrhinostomy, blood loss in very small children may require replacement with colloid or even blood depending on the starting haemoglobin. During prolonged surgery in small children maintenance crystalloid fluids may be necessary, especially if there was lengthy preoperative fasting (Table 10.7).

Table 10.7   Formulae to calculate fluid requirements and acceptable fluid loss in the anaesthetized child

Fluid requirements:	first 10 kg	4 ml/kg/h
	second 10 kg	2 ml/kg/h
	each kg over 20 kg	1 ml/kg/h

$$\text{Allowable blood loss} = \frac{\text{blood volume}}{\text{starting haemoglobin} \times (\text{starting} - \text{target haemoglobin})}$$

EXTUBATION

If an endotracheal tube has been used, coughing and straining on it at the end of surgery will cause a rise in arterial, venous and intraocular pressures and should be avoided. This is best accomplished by extubating while the child is still anaesthetized enough not to respond to the tube but is fully reversed from muscle relaxation if used. Modern operative and suturing techniques will prevent leaks following intraocular surgery if the intraocular pressure is raised moderately. Laryngeal mask airways can be left *in situ* until the child is in command of his airway without stimulation of laryngeal reflexes. Oropharyngeal secretions are retained above the laryngeal mask and coughing can be avoided by suctioning as the mask is removed.

Post-intubation croup

The two main causative factors are traumatic intubation and chemical irritation. These can be avoided by gentle laryngoscopy and the use of the correct size of a plastic, non-reactive, non-cuffed tube. A small air leak should be demonstrable if a positive pressure of 20–30 cm water is applied; if not, the tube should be changed for a size smaller. Stridor usually develops rapidly following extubation, although most day-case units will observe children post-extubation for up to 4 h.[55] If persistent stridor should occur, the child will need hospital admission and treatment with humidification, steroids and if necessary nebulized adrenaline.

POSTOPERATIVE PAIN AND VOMITING

It is important to minimize pain and vomiting postoperatively for humanitarian reasons, but more particularly after eye surgery when crying and retching may damage the eye by raising intraocular pressure. Opiates are not usually required postoperatively but may be administered intramuscularly during the operation to provide smooth emergence from anaesthesia. Of the nonsteroidal anti-inflammatory drugs (NSAIDs) diclofenac is particularly useful, as it can be given by suppository after induction of anaesthesia and provides good postoperative analgesia.[56] The NSAIDs act by inhibiting prostaglandin synthesis, which minimizes the activation and sensitization of peripheral nociception. Ideally, they should be given prior to the painful stimulus (pre-emptive analgesia).[57] Although NSAIDs prolong bleeding time by inhibiting platelet aggregation, increased perioperative bleeding has not been demonstrated. The newer ketorolac is not recommended in children under 16 years but has been used successfully intravenously during surgery.[58] Anti-emetics should be given prophylactically during high-risk operations such as strabismus surgery. Droperidol 0.075 mg/kg intravenously at induction or 30 min before the end of surgery is very effective in reducing the frequency and severity of vomiting.[59,60] Ondansetron and other 5HT3 antagonists are proving successful in the management of nausea and vomiting in paediatric oncology.[61]

POSTOPERATIVE RECOVERY

Experienced trained staff should be responsible for the postoperative recovery of children and this should ideally be in a separate area than that for adults so that parents can be with their child as soon as possible to prevent unnecessary distress and crying. Minimal monitoring of ECG, pulse oximetry and noninvasive blood pressure should continue until recovery of airway reflexes, and added oxygen should be given to avoid hypoxia.[62] If not already given, analgesia and anti-emetics may be needed. It is important to distinguish the distress of thirst, hunger or parental absence from that of pain. This may be difficult in the very young child. When the child is awake, paracetamol suspensions may be given orally. It is only after extensive surgery that parenteral analgesia may be required, which will usually be intramuscularly unless a high-dependency area is available to supervise continuous intravenous infusions of opioids.

If there is no nausea or vomiting, oral fluids may be started as soon as the child requests a drink and, if that is retained, light food can be provided when the child feels hungry. Mobilization will depend on postoperative management of the eye procedure and visual ability (both eyes may be covered). It is expected that most minor procedures will be managed on a day-case basis and the child discharged into the care of parents with appropriate instructions concerning continuing postoperative care.

SPECIFIC SURGICAL PROCEDURES

Examination under anaesthesia (EUA)

Babies and young children will require general anaesthesia for direct fundoscopy, refraction, evaluation of intraocular or intraorbital tumours, for intraocular pressure measurements and the measurement of visual evoked responses (VER) and electroretinography (ERG). It is important to discuss with the surgeon the exact requirements before starting. Some procedures may be short and do not require complete immobility of the head and a technique based on intramuscular ketamine would be suitable. Other procedures may be fairly lengthy or require fixation of the head and use of the operating microscope and a more appropriate technique would involve securing the airway with an endotracheal tube or laryngeal mask airway. If the procedure is likely to proceed to further surgery, the anaesthesia technique may need to be converted half-way through. Such examinations may need to be repeated at regular intervals and it is important to form a rapport with both child and parents and to select a technique of induction of anaesthesia to ensure that the next occasion is not made more difficult. These children will usually be treated on a day-case basis and the parents must have full instructions regarding preoperative fasting. Premedication may be EMLA cream and oral atropine 0.02 mg/kg. Sedation with temazepam 0.5 mg/kg orally or midazolam 0.5 mg/kg orally or 0.2 mg/kg sublingually or intranasally may be necessary in children over 1 year who are distressed. Induction of anaesthesia is intravenous if possible with propofol 3 mg/kg, or alfentanil 0.02 mg/kg and propofol 2–3 mg/kg, and insertion of the appropriate-sized laryngeal mask. If intravenous access is not possible, then an inhalation induction with oxygen, nitrous oxide and halothane and insertion of the laryngeal mask at a suitable level of anaesthesia is performed and intravenous access then obtained. Glycopyrrolate 0.01 mg/kg might be given intravenously at induction to block the oculocardiac reflex. Anaesthesia is maintained with spontaneous respiration and isoflurane. Full monitoring should be used throughout.

Congenital glaucoma

Glaucoma is a condition of raised intraocular pressure which causes impaired capillary blood flow to the optic nerve with resulting loss of tissue and function.

Eighty percent of cases of congenital glaucoma are inherited in an autosomal recessive pattern and 75% are bilateral. Infantile glaucoma occurs at any time from birth to 5 years and the juvenile type from 6 to 30 years. Childhood glaucomas may also be associated with various eye diseases or developmental anomalies. It is very important to make an early diagnosis and affected babies may present with epiphoria, photophobia, blepharospasm and irritability. Ocular enlargement (buphthalmos) and corneal oedema may be noted. Management requires frequent examinations to measure intraocular pressure, corneal diameter and to check for disc cupping. If any of these indicates a raised pressure, surgery is performed to provide drainage for the aqueous – either a goniotomy or a trabeculectomy, both of which will take at least 30 min.

Preoperative assessment is important as there may be associated congenital abnormalities that will affect anaesthesia; if the baby was premature, retinopathy of prematurity is associated with infantile glaucoma. Anti-glaucoma medication may be in use and have systemic side-effects. Premedication is atropine 0.02 mg/kg orally in infants, and EMLA should be used whenever possible, and temazepam 0.5 mg/kg orally with atropine in older children. Sedation is often required in young children preoperatively when they have to undergo frequent procedures. Intramuscular ketamine in a dose of 7 mg/kg will provide suitable conditions for intraocular pressure measurements in approximately 10 min and allow examination of the eyes for other features of raised pressure. Intravenous access should always be established and full monitoring is employed.

If it is necessary to proceed to surgery, the anaesthetic proceeds with a small dose of thiopentone or propofol and a muscle relaxant such as vecuronium 0.1 mg/kg, and the child is intubated with the appropriate-sized preformed endotracheal tube. Ventilation is controlled and anaesthesia maintained with a small dose of inhalational anaesthetic, such as isoflurane or enflurane, plus a small dose of opiate, such as alfentanil 0.01 mg/kg. Postoperative analgesia can be provided with a diclofenac suppository 1–2 mg/kg.

Strabismus surgery

Strabismus surgery is the most common ophthalmic operation performed on children. Full details of the associated problems and anaesthetic management will be found in Chapter 11.

Some concerns for the anaesthetist are that very young children may present for surgery and that squints may be associated with congenital anomalies, so a careful preoperative assessment is important. The high incidence of masseter spasm and susceptibility to malignant hyperthermia on subsequent testing associated with strabismus surgery means that most anaesthetists would wish to avoid the combination of halothane and suxamethonium even without a previous history of anaesthesia problems. Suxamethonium should be avoided if the surgeon wishes to perform forced duction tests under anaesthesia prior to surgery, as it produces sustained tonic contraction of the extraocular muscles. Intraoperative monitoring is vital during strabismus surgery, as the oculocardiac reflex and the oculorespiratory reflexes are strongly elicited by traction on the extraocular muscles. Prophylactic administration of an anticholinergic at induction of anaesthesia is recommended. The incidence of postoperative nausea and vomiting following strabismus surgery is very high, especially in children. It is important to select an anaesthesia technique that reduces this incidence and to use prophylactic anti-emetics if indicated. Strabismus surgery is considered suitable for day-case management and it is vital that hospital admission is not precipitated because of intractable vomiting postoperatively.

Lacrimal surgery

Nasolacrimal duct obstruction may present in a young child as a persistently watery eye, possibly with infection. The patency of the system will need to be investigated under anaesthesia with the passage of a lacrimal probe through the lacrimal puncta along the canaliculi and into the lacrimal sac. Sterile saline or fluorescein may then be injected and its passage into the nasopharynx looked for. A silicone tube (Lester-Jones tube) may be inserted if two to three probings fail to open the obstruction.

These are short procedures and can be managed on a day-case basis. The child should be premedicated with EMLA cream and atropine 0.02 mg/kg if inhalational induction is thought likely. Induction is preferentially intravenous with alfentanil 0.02 mg/kg and propofol 3 mg/kg to allow intubation with a preformed tube. If intravenous access is not possible prior to induction, intubation can be achieved under inhalational anaesthesia with halothane, or access may be obtained after induction and reduced intravenous induction doses given. A throat pack should be inserted to absorb the fluid injected via the lacrimal probe. Maintenance of anaesthesia is spontaneous with isoflurane or enflurane. Full monitoring is necessary throughout.

In some cases of acquired nasolacrimal duct obstruction, the child will need a dacryocystorrhinostomy, when the lacrimal sac is anastomosed to the nasal mucosa. This is a more major undertaking and requires measures to reduce intraoperative bleeding. Intubation with a throat pack to protect the larynx from blood is mandatory. A balanced technique with controlled ventilation and intraoperative opiates is usually used, as the removal of bone is surgically stimulating. Although formal hypotension is not usually employed, a head up tilt will reduce venous congestion and ooze at the operation site. Vasoconstrictors such as cocaine and adrenaline may be used topically to reduce bleeding, and the doses used must be checked to avoid possible arrhythmias.[67] (The maximal total dose of cocaine applied to the nasal mucosa is 1.5 mg/kg, and the total dose of adrenaline used topically is 0.5 mg.). Postoperative analgesia might be provided with diclofenac 1–2 mg by suppository with a small dose of an intramuscular opiate to provide some sedation. The throat pack must be removed and pharyngeal toilet performed prior to extubation, as blood clots may be concealed behind the soft palate. Extubation should be performed in the awake state to prevent inhalation of blood or laryngeal spasm.

Tumour surgery

Orbital tumours that may present in young children can be benign, such as capillary haemangiomas or lymphangiomas, or malignant, such as rhabdomyosarcomas or retinoblastomas. Although rare (1:20 000 live births), retinoblastoma is the most common malignant eye tumour in children and is usually diagnosed and treated in the first 3 years of life. Treatment may involve cryotherapy, photo-coagulation, enucleation, chemotherapy and radiation alone or in combination depending on the grade of tumour and treatment protocol. Altogether 30% of cases are bilateral; 30–40% are familial and children in at-risk families have to have an EUA every 3 months for the first 5 years of life.

The anaesthetist is faced with all the problems of repeated anaesthesia in a very young child. Ketamine may not provide adequate surgical conditions if the EUA proceeds to photocoagulation and a technique involving securing of the airway with a laryngeal mask or endotracheal tube is used with spontaneous or controlled ventilation via a T-piece with an inhalational anaesthetic such as isoflurane. If intravenous induction is not possible, repeated inhalational inductions with halothane may be necessary. Obviously, it would be preferable for the same anaesthetist to be available for each anaesthesia to reduce the anxiety of parent, child and anaesthetist.

Anaesthesia for radiotherapy involves short anaesthetics with the anaesthetist remote from the child, sometimes at daily intervals for weeks. Monitoring that is readily visible to the anaesthetist is vital and various anaesthesia techniques have been used. Ketamine in a dose of 4–8 mg/kg intramuscularly was popular but it may produce movements that make accurate delivery of radiation difficult. With the introduction of the laryngeal mask airway, a clear airway without the hazards of repeated intubation can be obtained and the child allowed to breath spontaneously on an inhalational anaesthetic.

Enucleation may be required and the traction on the extraorbital muscles and pressure on the orbit will be very strong stimuli of the oculocardiac reflex. Atropine 0.02 mg/kg or glycopyrrolate 0.01 mg/kg should be used prophylactically at induction of anaesthesia.

Congenital cataracts

The principles of anaesthesia for intraocular surgery are the same as for those in the adult. There must be complete akinesis of the eye and control of the intraocular pressure. If complete congenital cataracts are present, they must be removed as soon as possible or proper visual development will not take place; if a unilateral complete cataract is present, it must be removed in the first few months of life to prevent amblyopia. The child presenting for cataract extraction may therefore be very young and associated systemic disease must be looked for (Table 10.8). Premedication will be with atropine 0.02 mg/kg (usually intramuscularly) in a neonate to ensure absorption, with EMLA cream if possible, and sedation in older children.

Table 10.8   Some causes of cataracts in children

Idiopathic (50%)
Chromosomal disorders
Inborn errors of metabolism
Intrauterine infections
Trauma
Drugs (steroids)

Crying will raise intraocular pressure, and should be avoided if possible during induction of anaesthesia; this can be intravenous (if venous access is available), or inhalational. Intubation should be performed under muscle relaxation such as vecuronium 0.1 mg/kg and respiration controlled on a small dose of inhalational agent. Surgical stimulus is not very great but complete akinesia is necessary, as surgery will be performed under the microscope and consists of anterior chamber aspiration of the lens. The pupil will need to be maximally dilated with preoperative mydriatics and intraoperative intraocular infusions of adrenaline; the concentration of this irrigating infusion is 1:1 000 000 and usually has no systemic effects. Full monitoring is used throughout.

To avoid coughing and straining on the endotracheal tube following surgery, the child is extubated deep on his side following reversal of residual muscle blockade and the airway maintained carefully until reflexes return.

The penetrating eye injury

Penetrating eye injuries pose two conflicting problems: the first is the possibility of a full stomach and the need for a rapid sequence induction of anaesthesia, and the other is the need to protect the eye from the rise in intraocular pressure. Suxamethonium causes a transient but definite rise in intraocular pressure and in the author's opinion should be avoided. Crying, struggling or vomiting will also cause a rise in intraocular pressure and no attempt should be made to empty the stomach preoperatively. Laryngoscopy and intubation will also produce a significant rise in intraocular pressure which must be attenuated.

In a situation where early surgery is necessary in a penetrating eye injury to prevent further damage from crying and rubbing by the child, a rapid sequence induction with vecuronium may be used. Following EMLA cream, intravenous access is obtained. Alfentanil 0.02 mg/kg is given followed by vecuronium 0.15 mg/kg; as muscle weakness appears, propofol 3 mg/kg is given and cricoid pressure applied. Intubation can be performed without coughing at about 90 s following the vecuronium. A peripheral nerve stimulator will indicate when full paralysis has taken place. Preoxygenation should be performed if possible, but crying and struggling and pressure on the injured eye from the facemask must be avoided.

Maintenance of anaesthesia is by controlled ventilation with inhalational anaesthetic, and a nasogastric tube should be passed following surgery before reversal of anaesthesia. To avoid coughing on the endotracheal tube, extubation should be performed deep and on the side to prevent problems with regurgitation.

APPENDIX I

PAEDIATRIC RESUSCITATION

With the increasing popularity of day-case surgery for children, it is important that those involved in their care are trained in paediatric resuscitation. This is of particular importance in stand-alone day-case units where support from paediatric teams is not available. It also means there must be careful preoperative assessment to exclude children who might have potentially fatal postoperative complications, such as apnoea in premature infants. The parents of the children selected for day-case management must be able to provide adequate postoperative care and be able to recognize problems if they arise and obtain appropriate help. To enable parents to provide this care, they must be given comprehensive postoperative instructions both verbally and written in a language they can understand.

The causes of cardiac arrest in children are not usually primarily cardiac as they are in adults and the resuscitation protocols reflect this. Resuscitation is usually required following a problem with the airway or breathing in children. The resulting hypoxia if not corrected will result in bradycardia and ultimately asystole. The second most common cause of cardiac arrest in children is circulatory failure secondary to fluid or blood loss or to sepsis.

PAEDIATRIC BASIC LIFE SUPPORT

This refers to the maintenance of the airway and support of respiration and circulation without the use of equipment. The Working Party on Paediatric Resuscitation of the European Resuscitation Council have published its recommendations on basic and advanced life support.[63] The following guidelines are based on these recommendations (Fig. 10.6).

There is a difference in the recommended protocols for infant resuscitation and child resuscitation, the cut-off point being 1 year of age. In an infant, the brachial pulse is the easiest to feel. It is located on the inside of the middle of the upper arm and with the arm abducted and externally rotated can be felt with a finger hooked over the arm. Slow heart rates in infants do not support the circulation and, if the rate falls to 60 beats/min, chest compression should be started. As the child becomes older and larger, the resuscitation methods will progress to those used in adult basic life support, namely two-handed chest compression, a compression depth of 4–5 cm, a rate of 80 beats/min and a compression to ventilation ratio of 15:2.

PAEDIATRIC ADVANCED LIFE SUPPORT

In any day-case unit, the nursing and medical staff must be able to perform paediatric advanced life support and have the appropriate equipment to do so. The priorities in advanced life support are ECG monitoring and arrhythmia diagnosis, provision of a clear airway, effective ventilation with high concentrations of oxygen, establishment of venous access and administration of fluid and drugs (Fig. 10.7).

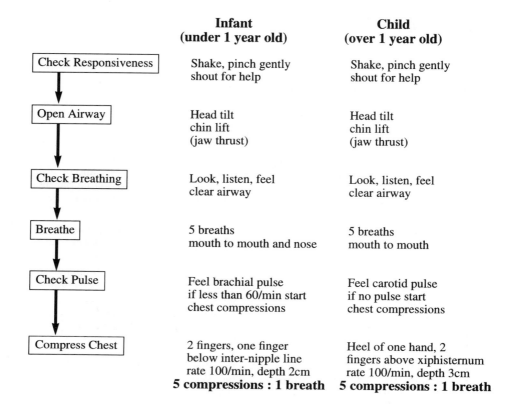

	Infant (under 1 year old)	Child (over 1 year old)
Check Responsiveness	Shake, pinch gently shout for help	Shake, pinch gently shout for help
Open Airway	Head tilt chin lift (jaw thrust)	Head tilt chin lift (jaw thrust)
Check Breathing	Look, listen, feel clear airway	Look, listen, feel clear airway
Breathe	5 breaths mouth to mouth and nose	5 breaths mouth to mouth
Check Pulse	Feel brachial pulse if less than 60/min start chest compressions	Feel carotid pulse if no pulse start chest compressions
Compress Chest	2 fingers, one finger below inter-nipple line rate 100/min, depth 2cm **5 compressions : 1 breath**	Heel of one hand, 2 fingers above xiphisternum rate 100/min, depth 3cm **5 compressions : 1 breath**

After one minute activate emergency medical services

Fig. 10.6.   Paediatric basic life support. (Based on European Resuscitation Guidelines.)

Airway and ventilation

The full range of endotracheal tube sizes and a selection of straight and paediatric curved laryngoscope blades must be readily available. Plain plastic uncuffed endotracheal tubes are the most useful for resuscitation and should have 15-mm international standard connectors to allow direct connection to a self-inflating resuscitation bag. Appropriate tube size is calculated by the following formula.

$$\text{Internal diameter (mm)} = 4 + \text{age (years)}/4$$

It may also be estimated from aids such as the Oakley chart and the Brasslow tape[64,65] or another useful guideline is to use a tube of about the same diameter as the child's little finger.

A self-inflating resuscitator bag of 500 ml (child) or 1600 ml (adult) should be available and fitted with a reservoir bag and attached to an oxygen supply of

Protocol 1.   ASYSTOLE

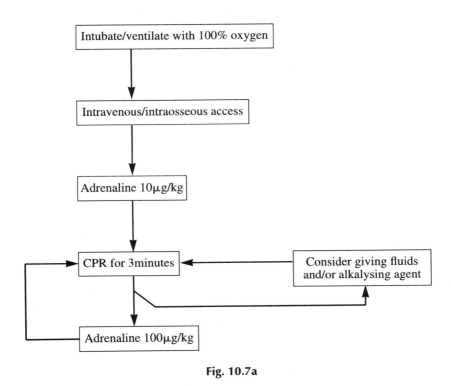

Fig. 10.7a

Fig. 10.7. Paediatric advanced life support protocols. (Based on European resuscitation guidelines.)

10–12 l/min to ensure delivery of oxygen concentrations of over 90%. A T-piece and open-ended bag is not recommended for the less experienced operator, but has advantages in that the operator can gain an impression of lung compliance.

Venous access

Peripheral venous access in small children with circulatory arrest is difficult to obtain. It is important therefore that venous access is secured at induction of anaesthesia in a child, even for a minor procedure. If an inhalation induction has been used, venous access should be secured as soon as possible following this. Central venous access in an emergency is for experts only and can be hazardous. The administration of drugs such as adrenaline and atropine via the endotracheal tube is a possibility using 10 times the intravenous dose, but large volumes of fluid or caustic drugs such as sodium bicarbonate cannot be given this way. An

Protocol 2.   VENTRICULAR FIBRILLATION

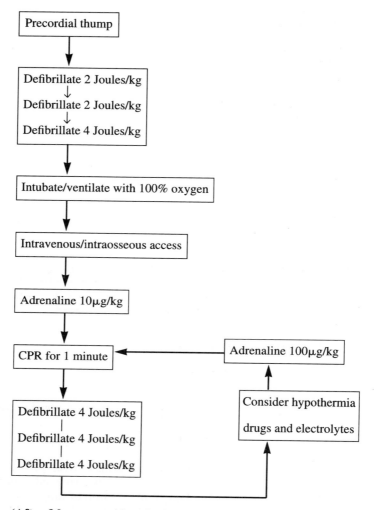

(After 3 loops consider alkalysing and/or antiarrhythmic agents)

Fig. 10.7b

alternative is the intraosseous route and this should be attempted if peripheral venous access is not gained within 90 s of circulatory collapse. The intraosseous needle (Fig. 10.8) is placed directly into the tibia, 1 cm below the tibial tuberosity. Resuscitation drugs, fluid and blood can safely be given by this route and reach the heart within 20–30 s.

Complications such as drug extravasation, skin infection and osteomyelitis are

Protocol 3.   ELECTROMECHANICAL DISSOCIATION

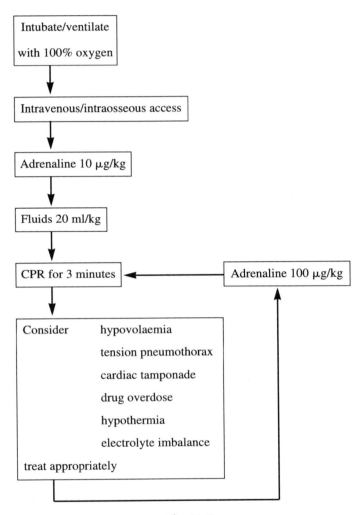

Fig. 10.7c

uncommon and are related to prolonged use or poor technique. The intraosseous route is for emergency access only and venous access should be obtained as soon as possible, which may necessitate a cutdown.

Drug and fluid administration

The correct drug doses and fluid volumes are calculated from the child's weight or if not available, from the child's length. All children that require anaesthesia –

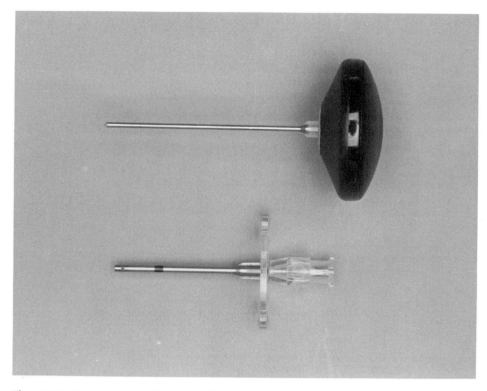

Fig. 10.8.   Intraosseous infusion needle for emergency paediatric vascular access via the intraosseous route.

even for minor procedures – must be weighed preoperatively, as drug doses for anaesthesia and resuscitation will be based on body weight (Table 10.9).

Adrenaline

Adrenaline is the first-line drug in paediatric resuscitation as it is in adult resuscitation. To restart the heart in cardiac arrest, the myocardial cells have to receive enough oxygen. The coronary arteries are perfused during diastole and the pressure required is at least 10–20 mmHg. Adrenaline has powerful alpha- and beta-adrenergic effects, but it is the alpha effects resulting in an increase in peripheral vascular resistance that are important in cardiac arrest. The resulting increase in aortic diastolic pressure will produce perfusion of the coronary arteries. The recommended dose is 10μg/kg initially, but there is some evidence to show that higher doses result in improved outcome in paediatric arrests.[68] Second and further doses of adrenaline are therefore 100μg/kg.

Atropine

Atropine is used for the treatment of bradycardias only. Hypoxia is the most common cause of bradycardia in children, so optimal oxygenation should be

Table 10.9   Weight-based paediatric resuscitation chart

	Weight of child (kg)					
	5	*10*	*20*	*30*	*40*	*50*
Endotracheal tube						
internal diameter (mm)	3.5	4	5.5	6.5	7	7.5–8
length (cm)	10	12.5	15	17	18	18–21
Adrenaline i.v./i.o.						
initial (ml of 1:10 000 solution)	0.5	1	2	3	4	5
subsequent (ml of 1:1000 solution)	0.5	1	2	3	4	5
Atropine i.v./i.o.						
(ml of 100 µg/ml solution)	1	2	4	6	8	10
Bicarbonate i.v./i.o.						
(ml of 8.4% solution)	5	10	20	30	40	50
Calcium chloride i.v./i.o.						
(ml of 10% solution)	1	2	4	6	8	10
Lignocaine i.v./i.o.						
(ml of 1% solution)	0.5	1	2	3	4	5
Salbutamol i.v./i.o.						
(ml of 50(µg/ml solution)	0.5	1	2	3	4	5
Glucose i.v./i.o.						
(ml of 10% solution)	25	50	100	150	200	250
(ml of 25% solution)	10	20	40	60	80	100
Diazepam i.v./i.o.						
(ml of 5 mg/ml solution)	0.25	0.5	1	1.5	2	2
Defibrillation (Js)						
initial	10	20	40	60	80	100
subsequent	20	40	80	120	160	200
Fluid infusion (ml)						
in hypovolaemia	100	200	400	600	800	1000

Abbreviations: i.o., intraosseus; i.v., intravenous.

achieved before using atropine. To block vagally mediated reflexes during airway manipulation or stimulation of the oculocardiac reflex during ophthalmic procedures a dose of 0.02 mg/kg, with a minimum of 0.1 mg and a maximum of 1 mg in children and 2 mg in adolescents, is administered.

Bicarbonate

Alkalizing agents are of unproven benefit and should only be used in the face of profound acidosis in cardiac or respiratory arrest if the first dose of adrenaline has been without effect. The dose is 1 mmol/kg by slow intravenous injection.

Calcium

Calcium is no longer recommended in cardiac arrest except in proven hypocalcaemia, hypermagnesaemia or hyperkalaemia. If indicated, calcium chloride is more effective than calcium gluconate and the dose is 10–30 mg/kg intravenously.

Fluid therapy

Any drugs used during resuscitation in children must be followed by a bolus of normal saline to ensure flushing into the circulation from a peripheral venous site or intraosseous site of injection. Depending on the size of the child, 5–20 ml should be used. If cardiac arrest has resulted from hypovolaemia and there is no response to adrenaline, a larger bolus of fluid should be given. This might be appropriate in the setting of prolonged fluid deprivation prior to anaesthesia and surgery. Crystalloid or colloid may be used in a volume of 20 ml/kg. Overloading must be avoided, as a raised right atrial pressure will reduce coronary perfusion pressure.

Glucose

Hypoglycaemia may be a problem in very small children who have been fasted for a prolonged period preoperatively. If this is suspected during a cardiac arrest, the blood glucose must be measured. Proven hypoglycaemia can be treated with 0.5 g/kg of glucose as a 10% or 25% infusion solution. Hyperglycaemia is thought to make ischaemic brain injury worse, so glucose solutions should not be given without good indication.

Post-resuscitation care

Any child who has required resuscitation must be cared for afterwards in a paediatric intensive care unit. This will involve transporting the child either within a hospital or to another hospital. It is important that the protocols to achieve this transfer as rapidly and as safely as possible are in place before an emergency occurs.

APPENDIX II

MANAGEMENT OF MALIGNANT HYPERTHERMIA

Malignant hyperthermia (MH) is an inherited condition that does not affect the general health of the patient and only becomes apparent on exposure to certain anaesthetic agents. On exposure to these trigger agents, signs of a greatly increased body metabolism, muscle rigidity and a rise in body temperature at the rate of 2–6°C per hour take place. Most cases develop during anaesthesia, but MH can arise up to 24 h postoperatively. Of those who develop fulminant MH, up to 10% may die. Death is due to cardiac arrest, brain damage, internal bleeding or intractable failure of other body systems.

The incidence of MH is probably in the order of 1:10 000 trigger general anaesthetics given in the UK. It occurs more commonly in the age range 10–30 years, it is very rare under 5 years and the incidence declines gradually after 30 years. In most cases it is inherited as an autosomal-dominant condition. Not everyone who is susceptible develops an MH episode during every trigger anaesthetic.

The aetiology of the metabolic crisis that takes place during an MH episode is thought to be an uncoupling of the excitation–contraction mechanism in skeletal muscle brought about by exposure to the trigger agents. This produces a massive rise in intracellular Ca^{2+} ions which causes sustained muscle contraction and rigidity.

Trigger agents include all volatile anaesthetic agents and suxamethonium.

TREATMENT OF AN MH CRISIS

The mortality from MH has dropped from 80% when the condition was first identified in 1960 to less than 20%. This has been due to the introduction of dantrolene and the greater awareness and earlier diagnosis by the anaesthetist with more aggressive treatment.

Be prepared

In all areas where general anaesthetics are given the following should be readily available:

1. A written treatment plan (such as the British Malignant Hyperthermia Association poster).
2. The UK telephone Hotline number (01345-333-111, pager no. 0525420, leave message with indication of urgency).
3. Monitors to allow continuous monitoring of end-tidal CO_2, oxygen saturation and core body temperature.
4. A hypothermia blanket, ice-making machine and refrigerator to store at least 3000 ml of cold intravenous fluids.
5. The following drugs should be immediately available on a trolley:
   Dantrolene sodium i.v. × 36 vials
   Sterile water for injection (without bacteriostatic agent) × 2000 ml
   Sodium bicarbonate 8.4% 50 ml × 10
   Mannitol 20% 500 ml × 2
   Hydrocortisone 100 mg × 10
   Frusemide 20 mg × 5
   Glucose 50% 50 ml × 2
   Soluble insulin 100 units/ml × 1 (refrigerated)
   Heparin 1000 units/ml × 3
6. Cooling equipment:
   50-ml syringe × 2
   Nasogastric tube × 2

Large clear plastic bags for ice
Bucket for ice
7. Other equipment:
Blood pump × 2
CVP line set × 2
Arterial line set × 2
Urinary catheters in several sizes
Anaesthetic breathing circuits
Fluid transfer sets or spikes for reconstituting dantrolene
Blood sample tubes for electrolyte, enzyme, myoglobin determinations and coagulation studies × 6
Blood gas sampling syringes × 6
Specimen containers for urine myoglobin measurements
Urine dip sticks for haemoglobin

Clinical signs

The clinical signs associated with an MH reaction are:

1. Masseter muscle spasm after suxamethonium
2. Generalized muscle rigidity
3. Unexplained tachycardia and dysrhythmias
4. Unexplained rise in end-tidal CO_2 or tachypnoea
5. Rapid rise in body temperature (2–6°C per hour)

Laboratory abnormalities

The laboratory abnormalities found are:

1. Metabolic acidosis
2. Hyperkalaemia
3. Very raised muscle creatine phosphokinase (CPK)
4. Myoglobinuria

Management of an MH crisis

1. Discontinue all volatile anaesthetics and hyperventilate with 100% O_2 at 2–3 times the estimated minute volume.
2. Stop surgery as soon as possible and obtain assistance.
3. Start reconstituting the dantrolene. Give initial dose of 1 mg/kg i.v. immediately. Response should occur within minutes. Judge response by heart rate, muscle rigidity and temperature. If no response give more dantrolene; the average successful dose is about 2.5 mg/kg but up to 10 mg/kg or more may be needed.
4. Cool patient by various routes, i.v. iced 0.9% saline, surface cooling, lavage of pleural and peritoneal cavities, iced fluids via nasogastric tube. Peritoneal dialysis with cold fluids and femoro-femoro cardiopulmonary bypass if necessary and available.
5. Take blood to estimate pH and potassium, but do not delay treatment waiting

for results. Give sodium bicarbonate 8.4% 1–2 ml/kg initially and dextrose 50% 50 ml with soluble insulin 10 units.

6. If dysrhythmias do not respond to treatment of acidosis and hyperkalaemia, beta-adrenergic blocking drugs may be needed. Avoid calcium channel blockers with dantrolene.

7. Change anaesthetic tubing and soda-lime. A separate anaesthetic machine is not needed, as high flows of oxygen will purge it of volatile anaesthetics in about 10 min.

8. Establish invasive monitoring and record all events.

9. Once stable the patient will need to be transferred to intensive care for further monitoring and treatment. Convert to oral dantrolene and give a total dose of 4 mg/kg/day in divided doses for 48 h following the crisis. Watch for disseminated intravascular coagulopathy (DIC) and myoglobinuria and renal failure.

10. Refer patient and family for MH testing.

ANAESTHESIA FOR THE MH SUSCEPTIBLE PATIENT

Remove or drain and disconnect all vaporizers on the anaesthetic machine. Put an oxygen flow of 10 l/min through the circuit for 20 min with the ventilator set to inflate a bag at the Y-piece of the circle system. Use a new or a disposable breathing circuit. Put a cooling blanket on the operating table.

Take a preoperative CPK level. Dantrolene prophylaxis is not recommended routinely but advice should be sought. If used, the dose is 2 mg/kg i.v. infusion starting 30 min prior to anaesthesia. Dantrolene can make muscle weakness worse in patients with muscle disease. The anaesthetic of choice is a regional or local block as all local anaesthetic agents are safe. If a general anaesthetic is necessary, suxamethonium and all inhalation anaesthetics must be avoided. All other agents are safe. Atropine is sometimes avoided because a tachycardia may make the early diagnosis of an MH crisis more difficult. A popular technique is to use a propofol infusion with or without a non-depolarizing muscle relaxant as indicated by the surgery. Full and invasive monitoring should be used and continued into the postoperative period for several hours if the anaesthetic has been uneventful. If any of the signs of MH appear, treat as for an MH crisis.

REFERENCES

1. Campling EA, Devlin HB, Lunn JN. *The Report of the National Confidential Enquiry into Perioperative Deaths* 1989. HMSO: London, 1990.
2. *Welfare of Children and Young People in Hospital*. HMSO: London, 1991.
3. Sumner E, Hatch DJ. *Textbook of Paediatric Anaesthetic Practice*. Baillière Tindall: London, 1989.
4. Morselli PL. Clinical pharmacokinetics in neonates. In *Handbook of Clinical Pharmacokinetics* (edited by Gibaldi M, Prescott L). Adis Health Science Press: New York, 1983: 79
5. Jessner L, Blom GE, Waldfogel S. Emotional implications of tonsillectomy and adenoidectomy on children. *Psychoanalytic Study of the Child*. 1952; **III**: 126.

6. American Society of Anesthesiologists. New classification of physical status. *Anesthesiology* 1963; **24:** 111.
7. *Recommendations for Standards of Monitoring during Anaesthesia and Recovery.* The Association of Anaesthetists of Great Britain and Ireland: London 1988.
8. Commission on the Provision of Surgical Services. *Guidelines for Day Case Surgery,* revised edn. Royal College of Surgeons of England: London 1992.
9. Sims C. Thickly and thinly applied lignocaine–prilocaine cream prior to venepuncture in children. *Anaesth Intens Care* 1991; **19:** 343.
10. Thornes R. *Just for the Day: Children Admitted to Hospital for Day Treatment.* Caring for Children in the Health Services: London 1991.
11. Steward DJ. Experiences with an outpatient anaesthesia service for children. *Anesth Analg* 1973; **52:** 877
12. Davenport HT, Valman B. Parents in the anaesthetic room. *Lancet* 1987; **i:** 45.
13. Schofield NMacC, White JB. Interrelations among children, parents, premedication, and anaesthetists in paediatric day stay surgery. *Br Med J* 1989; **299:** 1371.
14. Williams OA, Hills R, Goddard JM. Pulmonary collapse during anaesthesia in children with respiratory tract symptoms. Case report. *Anaesthesia* 1992; **47:** 411.
15. Levy L, Pandit UA, Randel IH, Lewis IH, Tait AR. Upper respiratory tract infections and general anaesthesia in children: Peri-operative complications and oxygen saturation. *Anaesthesia* 1992; **47:** 678.
16. Tolksdorf W, Eick C. Rectal, oral and nasal premedication using midazolam in children aged 1–6 years. A comparative clinical study. *Anaesthetist* 1991; **40:** 661.
17. Feld LH, Negus JB, White PF. Oral midazolam preanesthetic medication in pediatric outpatients. *Anesthesiology* 1990; **73:** 831.
18. McClusky A, Meakin GH. Oral administration of midazolam as a premedicant for paediatric day-case anaesthesia. *Anaesthesia* 1994; **49:** 782.
19. Manuksela E-L, Korpela R. Double-blind evaluation of a lignocaine–prilocaine cream (EMLA) in children. *Br J Anaesth* 1986; **58:** 1242.
20. Doyle E, Freeman J, Im NT, Morton NS. An evaluation of a new self-adhesive patch preparation of amethocaine for topical anaesthesia prior to venous cannulation in children. *Anaesthesia* 1993; **48:** 1050.
21. Aun CST, Panesar NS. Paediatric glucose homostasis during anaesthesia. *Br J Anaesth* 1990; **64:** 413.
22. Miller DC. Why are children starved? (Editorial). *Br J Anaesth* 1990; **64:** 409.
23. Splinter WM, Stewart JA, Muir JG. Large volumes of apple juice preoperatively do not affect gastric pH and volume in children. *Can J Anaesth* 1990; **37:** 36.
24. Phillips S, Daborn AK, Hatch DJ. Preoperative fasting for paediatric anaesthesia. *Br J Anaesth* 1994; **73:** 529.
25. Finholt DA, Henry DB, Raphaely RC. Factors affecting the leak around tracheal tubes in children. *Can Anaesth Soc J* 1985; **32:** 326.
26. Brain AIJ. The laryngeal mask – a new concept in airway management. *Br J Anaesth* 1983; **55:** 801
27. Wilson IG. The laryngeal mask airway in paediatric practice (Editorial II). *Br J Anaesth* 1993; **70:** 124.
28. Bhatt SB, Kendall AP, Lin ES, Oh TE. Resistance and additional inspiratory work imposed by the laryngeal mask airway. *Anaesthesia* 1992; **47:** 343.
29. Mizushima A, Wardall GJ, Simpson DL. The laryngeal mask airway in infants. *Anaesthesia* 1992; **47:** 849.
30. Dureuil M, Laffon M, Plaud B, Penon C, Ecoffey C. Complications and fiberoptic assessment of size 1 laryngeal mask airway. *Anesth Analg* 1993; **76:** 527.
31. Marjot R. Pressure exerted by the laryngeal mask airway cuff on the pharyngeal mucosa. *Br J Anaesth* 1993; **70:** 25.
32. O'Meara ME, Jones JG. The laryngeal mask: Useful for spontaneous breathing, controlled ventilation, and difficult intubations. *Br Med J* 1993; **306:** 224.

33. Hatch DJ, Miles R, Wagstaff M. An anaesthetic scavenging system for paediatric and adult use. *Anaesthesia* 1980; **35**: 496.
34. Bosomworth PP, Ziegler CH, Jacoby J. The oculocardiac reflex in eye muscle surgery. *Anesthesiology* 1958; **19**: 7.
35. Schwatz L, Rockoff MA, Koka BV. Masseter spasm with anaesthesia: Incidence and implications. *Anesthesiology* 1987; **61**: 772.
36. Carroll JB. Increased incidence of masseter spasm in children with strabismus anesthetized with halothane and succinylcholine. *Anesthesiology* 1987; **67**: 559.
37. Christian AS, Ellis FR, Halsall PJ. Is there a relationship between masseteric spasm and malignant hyperpyrexia? *Br J Anaesth* 1989; **62**: 540.
38. Hassall E, Israel DM, Gunasekaran T, Steward D. Halothane hepatitis in children: Case report. *J Pediat Gastroent Nutr* 1990; **11**: 553.
39. Wark HJ. Postoperative jaundice in children. *Anaesthesia* 1983; **38**: 237.
40. Battersby EF, Bingham R, Facer E *et al.* Halothane hepatitis in children. *Br Med J* 1987; **295**: 117.
41. Watcha MF, Simeon RM, White PF, Stevens JL. Effect of propofol on the incidence of postoperative vomiting after strabismus surgery in paediatric outpatients. *Anesthesiology* 1991; **75**: 204.
42. Parke TJ, Stevens JE, Rice ASC, Greenaway CL, Bray RJ, Smith PJ, Waldmann CS, Verghese C. Metabolic acidosis and fatal myocardial failure after propofol infusion in children: Five case reports. *Br Med J* 1992; **305**: 613.
43. Adams AK. Ketamine in paediatric ophthalmic practice. *Anaesthesia* 1973; **28**: 212.
44. Meyers EF, Charles P. Prolonged adverse reactions to ketamine. *Anesthesiology* 1978; **49**: 39.
45. Warran P, Radford P, Manford MLM. Glycopyrrolate in children. *Br J Anaesth* 1981; **53**: 1273
46. Meakin G, Walker RWM, Dearlove OR. Myotonic and neuromuscular blocking effects of increased doses of suxamethonium in infants and children. *Br J Anaesth* 1990; **65**: 816.
47. Craythorne NWB, Rottenstein HS, Dripps RD. The effect of succinylcholine on intraocular pressure in adults, infants and children. *Anesthesiology* 1960; **21**: 59.
48. Libonati MM, Leahy JJ, Ellison N. The use of succinylcholine in open eye injury. *Anesthesiology* 1985; **62**: 637.
49. Rodney GE, Reichert CC, O'Regan DN, Blackstock D. Propofol or propofol/alfentanil compared to thiopentone/succinylcholine for intubation of healthy children (Abstract). *Can J Anaesth* 1992; **39**: A129.
50. Steyn MP, Quinn AM, Gillespie DC, Miller DC, Best CJ, Morton NS. Tracheal intubation without neuromuscular block in children. *Br J Anaesth* 1994; **72**: 403.
51. Goudsouzian NG, Alifimoff JK, Everly C, Smeets R, Griswold J, Miler V, McNulty BF, Saverese JJ. Neuromuscular and cardiovascular effects of mivacurium in children. *Anesthesiology* 1989; **70**: 237.
52. Mirakhur RK. Newer neuromuscular blocking drugs. *Drugs* 1992; **44**: 182.
53. Youngberg JA, Subaiya C, Graybar GB. Alfentanil for day-stay surgery in children: An evaluation. *Anesth Analg* 1984; **63**: 213.
54. Hatch D, Fletcher M. Anaesthesia and the ventilatory system in infants and young children. *Br J Anaesth* 1992; **68**: 398.
55. Steward DJ. Outpatient paediatric anesthesia. *Anesthesiology* 1975; **43**: 268.
56. Baer GA, Roarius MFG, Kolehmainen S, Selin S. The effect of paracetamol or diclofenac administered before operation on postoperative pain and behaviour after adenoidectomy in small children. *Anaesthesia* 1992; **47**: 1078.
57. Dahl JB, Kehlet H. The value of pre-emptive analgesia in the treatment of postoperative pain. Review article. *British Journal of Anaesthesia* 1993; **70**: 434.
58. Watcha MF, Jones MB, Laguerula RG, Schweiger C, White PF. Comparison of ketorolac and morphine as adjuvants during paediatric surgery. *Anesthesiology* 1992; **76**: 368.

59. Lerman J, Eustis S, Smith DR. Effect of droperidol pretreatment on postanesthetic vomiting in children undergoing strabismus surgery. *Anesthesiology* 1986; **65**: 322.
60. Kraus GB, Giebner M, Palackal R. The prevention of postoperative vomiting following strabismus surgery in children. *Anaesthetist* 1991; **40**: 92.
61. Stevens RF. The role of ondansetron in paediatric patients: a review of three studies. *Eur J Cancer* 1991; **27**(suppl I): s 20.
62. Tomkins DP, Gaukroger PB, Bently MW. Hypoxia in children following general anaesthesia. *Anaesth Intens Care* 1988; **16**: 177.
63. Zideman D, Bingham R, Beattie T, Bland J, Blom C *et al.* Guidelines for Paediatric Life Support: A statement by the Paediatric Life Support Working Party of the European Resuscitation Council 1993. *Resuscitation* 1994; **27**: 91.
64. Oakley PA. Inaccuracy and delay in decision making in paediatric resuscitation and a proposed reference chart to reduce error. *Br Med J* 1988; **297**: 817.
65. Luten RC, Wears RL, Broselow J *et al.* Length-based endotracheal tube and emergency equipment selection in pediatrics. *Ann Emerg Med* 1992; **2**: 900.
66. Gronert GA. Malignant hyperthermia. *Anesthesiology* 1980; **53**: 395.
67. Nicholson KEA, Rogers JEG. Cocaine and adrenaline paste: a fatal combination? *Br Med J* 1995; **311**: 250.
68. Goetting MG, Paradis NA. High-dose epinephrine improves outcome from pediatric cardiac arrest. *Ann Emerg Med* 1991; **20**: 22.

CHAPTER 11

Strabismus

CAROLINE A CARR ————————————————————

INTRODUCTION

Strabismus surgery is the most common ophthalmic operation carried out in children. Malalignment of the visual axes occurs in about 5% of the population and may be accompanied by diplopia, amblyopia and loss of stereopsis.[1] Treatment may be non-surgical, involving glasses, prisms, patching and botulinum toxin injection, but many will need surgical correction and more than one operation may be required to achieve best correction. Adults, too, may require strabismus surgery, due to thyroid eye disease, trauma, sixth cranial nerve palsy, and following previous strabismus surgery as a child. Surgery usually involves weakening an extraocular muscle by moving its insertion on the globe (recession) and/or strengthening an extraocular muscle by removing a short piece of the tendon or muscle (resection).[2]

Infantile strabismus occurs in the first 6 months of life and may be noted in the first few weeks. The treatment is surgical and the timing of surgery is influenced by two opposing considerations: the avoidance of anaesthesia in an infant and the importance of developing binocular vision. The eyes should be aligned before the age of 2 years to give the child the optimal chance of developing some binocular vision.[3]

ANAESTHESIA CONSIDERATIONS (Table 11.1)

Day-case anaesthesia

Surgical correction of strabismus is considered an appropriate ophthalmic operation to be undertaken in both children and adults as a day-case procedure.[4] The patient, adult or child, must be medically fit (ASA I or II), and have suitable social circumstances for discharge to be treated on this basis.[5] Anaesthesia techniques and agents should be selected to ensure rapid recovery with as few sequelae as possible.[6]

Paediatric anaesthesia

This is dealt with in detail in Chapter 10. It is important to remember that the anaesthetist should not undertake occasional paediatric practice.[7]

Table 11.1   Special concerns with strabismus surgery

Day-case anaesthesia
Paediatric anaesthesia
Associated anomalies
Malignant hyperthermia
Use of suxamethonium
Topical adrenaline
Oculocardiac reflex
Oculorespiratory reflex
Postoperative nausea and vomiting

Associated anomalies

Although most children and adults with strabismus are healthy, the incidence of strabismus is increased in individuals with central nervous system dysfunction, such as cerebral palsy, and with various muscle disorders and myopathies.

Malignant hyperthermia

Malignant hyperthermia (MH) was first described in 1960 by Denborough and is a metabolic crisis triggered by anaesthetic agents.[8] It is a familial disorder probably inherited as an autosomal dominant. It is a disorder of skeletal muscle; the specific site of pathology is not known, but it is thought to concern calcium metabolism, as in a crisis there is a massive rise in intracellular calcium. Triggers include all inhalational anaesthetics and depolarizing muscle relaxants (suxamethonium). Controversial agents for use in MH patients are ketamine, phenothiazines and atropine, not because they trigger the syndrome but because they confuse the clinical diagnosis by causing hyperpyrexia and tachycardia. Lignocaine was originally thought to increase intracellular calcium but is now considered safe in MH. Stress is also thought to play a part in the triggering of MH.

The incidence has been reported as 1:260 000 general anaesthetic exposures, 1:60 000 if suxamethonium is used, 1:12 000 if masseter spasm is included in the diagnosis of MH, and 1:5000 if unexplained tachycardia and fever are also included (in anaesthetics using suxamethonium and an inhalational agent).[9] Duchenne's muscular dystrophy, Becker's muscular dystrophy, central core disease, neuroleptic malignant syndrome, myotonia congenita and arthrogryposis all have a strong association with MH. It is thought that even mild muscle problems could have a greater risk of MH, such as in inguinal hernia, ptosis or strabismus.

Masseter spasm

Associated with anaesthesia, masseter spasm is a phenomenon that is particularly triggered when suxamethonium is administered after halothane induction. It involves a transient masseter spasm lasting 3–5 min.[10] During this time the mouth cannot be opened but the lungs can be ventilated easily by mask. The incidence of masseter muscle spasm in children following this anaesthetic technique has been reported as 1:100.[11] This rises to 2.8:100 in the paediatric strabismus population.[12] What is interesting is that of the patients who have masseter spasm, 48% have a positive caffeine contracture test and are defined as belonging to the MH-susceptible group.[13] This would on the face of it make MH a much more common occurrence than it is. Systemic absorption will occur from conjunctiva and rapidly from the nasal mucosa via drainage through the nasolacrimal duct and it is important to be aware of the dose of adrenaline being used.

Management of masseter spasm is debatable.[14] Some authorities advocate that the surgery can proceed if there are no other signs of MH, full monitoring is available and the anaesthetist changes to a non-triggering technique. Others advise cancelling the operation and investigating the patient for MH susceptibility with halothane–caffeine contracture studies.[15]

The successful management of MH depends on being prepared, early detection and aggressive treatment.

Use of suxamethonium

The possibility of triggering MH is one good reason for avoiding the use of suxamethonium in anaesthesia for strabismus surgery. Another is the effect on the extraocular muscles, themselves. Suxamethonium causes a tonic contracture of the extraocular muscles which are physiologically similar to avian muscles, with many endplates scattered over the surface of each muscle fibre. Depolarization of these endplates with suxamethonium results in widespread depolarization in the extraocular muscles and sustained contracture. The clinical disadvantage of this phenomenon, apart from a rise in intraocular pressure, is interference with forced duction testing. This test is to differentiate between a paretic muscle and a restrictive force impeding ocular movement. It is performed by grasping the sclera of the eye with forceps near the limbus and moving the eye into each field of gaze, assessing tissue and elastic properties. This is abnormally altered for 15 min following suxamethonium.[16] If forced duction testing is to be performed, suxamethonium is contraindicated for 20 min prior to testing or a technique should be employed that avoids its use.

Topical adrenaline

Adrenaline solutions are frequently used topically in strabismus surgery to produce conjunctival vasoconstriction and reduce bleeding at the site of operation. The conjunctiva is a good site for systemic absorption and it is important to be aware of the dose of adrenaline being used and the maximum dose that should be used according to the weight of the patient under operation. Common adrenaline solutions available for use during ophthalmic surgery are 1:1000 (0.1%) and 1:10000 (0.01%). One drop of these solutions would contain approximately 50 μg and 5 μg of adrenaline, respectively. The maximum dose of adrenaline for topical application is 500 μg or about 10 drops of 1:1000 adrenaline solution. In a small child, it is better to use the 1:10000 adrenaline solution and to monitor carefully the amount instilled and the ECG at this period.

The oculocardiac reflex

The oculocardiac reflex was first described by Aschner and Dagini in two simultaneous but independent reports in 1908.[17,18] The reflex pathway is via the long and short ciliary nerves to the ciliary ganglion, terminating in the trigeminal sensory nucleus in the floor of the 4th ventricle. The efferent pathway is by the vagus nerve. The reflex is triggered by pressure on the globe, traction on the extraocular muscles, and traction or pressure on the conjunctiva or orbital structures. It is seen in vitreoretinal surgery, scleral banding, can be elicited by injection of retrobulbar and peribulbar local anaesthesia, and may occur in the empty socket if there is pressure on the remaining orbital tissues, such as a haematoma following enucleation.[19]

Although the most common manifestation of the reflex is sinus bradycardia, virtually any cardiac dysrhythmia may occur, from asystole to ventricular tachycardia.[20] Reported incidences are about 70% in adults and up to 90% in unpremedicated children.[21] It is also suggested that traction on the medial rectus is the most likely to provoke the reflex, although this may be just that this muscle is operated on more frequently.[20]

Management

Prophyaxis. Oral or intramuscular atropine or glycopyrrolate as premedication prior to strabismus surgery are not very effective in blocking the oculocardiac reflex compared to intravenous administration at induction of anaesthesia.[21] A dose of 0.02 mg/kg of atropine prior to surgery will reduce the incidence of the reflex to 5–15% in children, although intravenous glycopyrrolate 0.01 mg/kg may be preferred as it causes less tachycardia. Hypercarbia increases sensitivity to the reflex and an anaesthesia technique such as controlled ventilation rather than spontaneous ventilation might be preferred.[22]

Treatment. Stop the surgical stimulus and in the face of a severe bradycardia give intravenous atropine 0.01 mg/kg and wait for the rate to pick up before resuming surgery. If the dysrhythmia is fast or ventricular, stop surgery and wait for it to return to normal before giving atropine in case of provoking ventricular tachycardia or fibrillation. With repeated manipulation, bradycardia is less likely to recur due to fatigue of the reflex arc at the cardioinhibitory centre.[23]

The oculorespiratory reflex

First described in animals, the oculorespiratory reflex was reported in humans by Petzetakis in 1915.[24] It is frequently seen in strabismus surgery in the spontaneously breathing patient and traction on the extraocular muscles results in shallow breathing, slowing of the respiratory rate, or even respiratory arrest. The reflex afferent pathway is as for the oculocardiac and ends in the trigeminal sensory nucleus. The efferent pathway is thought to be via the pneumotaxic centre in the pons and respiratory centre in the medulla. Obviously, respiration should be monitored during strabismus surgery and it has been suggested that patients should have their ventilation controlled to avoid the problems of hypoventilation.[25]

Postoperative nausea and vomiting

Vomiting is the most frequent postoperative complication following strabismus surgery. In children over 2 years of age, the incidence of postoperative nausea and vomiting (PONV) is reported as ranging from 40 to 88%.[26] It appears that the incidence is much lower in younger children: 28% in the 4–30 months age group compared with 57% in the 3–18 year age group.[27] Postoperative nausea and vomiting may be missed following strabismus surgery, as it rarely occurs in the immediate postoperative period.[28] It usually occurs after return to the ward, during the journey home or at home between 2–8 h postoperatively, and may continue for up to 24 h.

Aetiology

There are several possible reasons put forward for the high incidence of PONV associated with strabismus surgery. These are: traction on the extraocular muscles, distorted visual images, early postoperative fluid intake and involvement of labyrinthine pathways. The oculoemetic reflex is stimulated by traction on the extraocular muscles, the afferent loop being via the trigeminal nerve to the vomiting centre.[29] The stresses maintained in the extraocular muscles of the squint-corrected eye appear to stimulate the oculoemetic reflex very strongly postoperatively. The acute realignment of the visual axes following strabismus surgery might result in distorted visual images and stimulate PONV. However, covering the operated eye makes no difference to the incidence of PONV following strabismus surgery.[29]

Mandatory administration of oral fluids to children recovering from strabismus surgery increases the incidence of PONV compared with children who drink only when they ask to.[28] The significance of this is that in day-case units with a policy of mandatory oral fluid intake prior to discharge of children, the incidence of PONV and delayed discharge will be greater. However, of the children discharged without drinking, many vomited after their first drink at home and the overall incidence of PONV was the same. Withholding oral fluids in the early postoperative recovery period following strabismus surgery merely shifts the PONV from the day-case unit to the home or the journey home.

It might be that with a vomiting centre already stimulated by traction on the extraocular muscles, stimulation of vestibular afferents to the centre by sudden head movements or motion such as on a hospital trolley will precipitate vomiting.[27]

Prevention and treatment

There is no doubt that the anaesthetic technique will affect the incidence of PONV following strabismus surgery.[30–33] The avoidance of opiates both intraoperatively and postoperatively, the avoidance of inhalational agents and nitrous oxide, and the use of propofol for induction and maintenance, will all reduce the incidence of PONV. Prophylactic use of various anti-emetics has been tried. Droperidol in a dose of 0.075 mg/kg reduces the incidence of PONV from 60% to 25%.[34] Smaller doses are less effective in reducing PONV, but the larger dose is associated with some sedation and extrapyramidal symptoms and dysphoria. Metoclopramide in a dose of 0.25 mg/kg is as effective as droperidol 0.075 mg/kg in reducing the emesis and discharge times following strabismus surgery.[35] Hyoscine as a transdermal patch has been shown to reduce the incidence of PONV in children following strabismus surgery.[36] Procedures such as acupressure or acupuncture appear to have a small effect on PONV.[37,38] Newer anti-emetics such as ondansetron have yet to be evaluated in PONV following strabismus surgery.

A careful overview has to be taken when considering the management of the nausea and vomiting associated with strabismus surgery. In most children, a single vomit usually after the first drink does not delay their departure from the day-case ward or result in an unexpected admission to hospital. A choice of anaesthesia technique and avoidance of opiate analgesia will avoid the possible side-effects of routine antiemetic use without unacceptable morbidity from PONV. In adults and children with a previous history of severe PONV after strabismus surgery, the prophylactic use of anti-emetics intraoperatively should be employed.

ADJUSTABLE SUTURES

The use of sutures that may be adjusted after surgery with the patient awake will allow the surgeon to prevent immediate undesirable over-corrections or under-corrections in the postoperative period. They may be used on one or more muscles, and if on testing postoperatively the alignment is unsatisfactory, the muscle or muscles may be moved to a new position. Adjustments are made within 24 h of surgery. This technique may be used in patients who have had previous strabismus surgery, in paralytic strabismus, when there are mechanical limitations to muscle movement as in thyroid eye disease, and when the muscles have aberrant innervation as for example in Duane's syndrome.

In preparation for adjustment, local anaesthetic is instilled in both eyes, usually 5 drops of 1% amethocaine over a 5-min period. The alignment of the eyes is checked with the patient seated and then a drop of 0.1% adrenaline solution, instilled in the eye to be adjusted, to reduce any bleeding that might occur with handling of the tissues. With the patient lying flat, a lid speculum is placed in the eye to allow access to the muscles. The muscles are moved as appropriate and the sutures tied off and covered by the conjunctiva. It may be necessary to recheck the alignment several times before finally tying off the sutures. This is carried out as a sterile procedure with a pack containing the necessary ophthalmic instruments and good overhead lighting. Although the local anaesthetic drops reduce the pain and can be augmented by local pressure with a cotton wool bud soaked in the local anaesthetic solution, this procedure can be fairly unpleasant for the patient.

The problems encountered due to patient factors are lack of cooperation, either because the patient is too upset or scared or is not sufficiently recovered from general anaesthesia. It is very important for the surgeon to have a thorough discussion with the patient prior to surgery about the adjustment procedure. A general anaesthetic technique should be employed that allows a rapid recovery. Most adults and children over 12–13 years will be suitable for adjustable sutures, although some younger children may well be sensible enough.

Very rarely suture slippage or breakage may result in retraction of an extraocular muscle so that it cannot be retrieved under local anaesthesia alone. This will mean a return to the operating theatre and a repeat general anaesthetic.

BOTULINUM TOXIN INJECTIONS

Botulinum toxin type A is a large protein molecule that is bound to the receptor sites on motor nerve terminals within 24 h of intramuscular injection. Here it will inhibit release of acetylcholine resulting in a functional denervation of the muscle. If therapeutic doses of botulinum toxin are injected into the extraocular muscles, weakness or paralysis will occur within 3–5 days. Extrajunctional acetylcholine receptors may develop in the denervated muscle, which can then become reinnervated and eventually recover. Although in most cases of extraocular muscle paralysis produced in this way the muscle recovers in 2–8 weeks, a permanently changed ocular alignment may result as the paralysed muscle lengthens and the antagonist shortens. This is a technique used in selected cases which can augment traditional surgery and sometimes eliminate the need for surgery.

In adults, the injection of botulinum toxin is an outpatient procedure performed under topical anaesthesia. Topical adrenaline is also used to prevent bleeding at the site of injection. An electromyogram (EMG) electrode needle is attached to a 1 ml syringe containing 0.1 ml of toxin. The needle is connected to an audible EMG amplifier. The needle is passed transconjunctivally and posteriorly along the surface of the globe into the belly of the extraocular muscle. The needle tip should be approximately 2.5 cm from the muscle insertion at the location of the motor endplate. The patient is then asked to move the eyes so the muscle contracts and a typical signal is heard from the amplifier; this confirms correct needle placement and the toxin injection is given.

Some older children will be able to cooperate and can have injection of botulinum toxin performed under topical anaesthesia in the same way as adults. Less cooperative children and the very young will need their treatment under a form of sedation. Intravenous ketamine in doses of 0.1–1.0 mg/kg is ideal for this and can produce a level of sedation where the injection is possible with topical anaesthesia but an EMG response is still obtained.[39] The child recovers fairly rapidly from this and can be treated on a day-case basis.

LOCAL ANAESTHESIA FOR STRABISMUS SURGERY

As with other forms of ophthalmic surgery, strabismus surgery may be performed under local anaesthesia. This may take the form of topical anaesthesia, retrobulbar block, peribulbar block or a sub-Tenon block.[40–43] In a cooperative adult in whom straightforward surgery is anticipated, topical anaesthesia would have the advantage of allowing adjustment of muscle sutures at the time of surgery to obtain optimal visual alignment. The oculocardiac reflex is not blocked by topical anaesthesia and ECG monitoring and intravenous access with the possible use of atropine or glycopyrrolate would have to be available. The other forms of local anaesthesia all provide protection from the oculocardiac reflex.

The choice between general anaesthesia and local anaesthesia will depend on a number of factors relating to the patient and to the surgery planned. Possible complications, local and systemic, of the anaesthesic itself, local or general, must be weighed against the degree of potential discomfort and the patient's ability to cooperate. As with all local anaesthetic techniques, strabismus surgery is limited to cooperative adult patients.

SUGGESTED ANAESTHESIA TECHNIQUES

Premedication

EMLA cream should be used in all children if a suitable vein is visible on the back of the hands. If an adult or child is particularly anxious, an oral dose of temazepam 0.5 mg/kg to a maximum of 20 mg is given 30 min preoperatively. If an inhalation induction is anticipated due to lack of venous access, oral atropine 0.02 mg/kg is given 30 min preoperatively. Atropine should also be used prior to ketamine solution for botulinum toxin injection to reduce salivation and possible airway obstruction.

Induction

An intravenous indication is used whenever possible. A preferred technique is: glycopyrrolate 0.01 mg/kg, alfentanil 0.01–0.02 mg/kg, propofol 2–3 mg/kg i.v. followed by insertion of the appropriate sized reinforced laryngeal mask airway. If the laryngeal mask is unsuitable for certain cases, or if it is anticipated that the surgery is to be prolonged (longer than 1 h), intubation with an appropriately sized preformed endotracheal tube is accomplished using vecuronium 0.1 mg/kg.

Maintenance

Spontaneous respiration with the laryngeal mask using a T-piece, coaxial Bain circuit or circle system appropriate to the size of the patient, with oxygen, nitrous oxide and isoflurane 1–3% may be used or controlled ventilation if the patient is intubated. Alternatively, a propofol infusion may be used following induction at a rate of 10 mg/kg/h for the first 10 min, reducing over the next 10 min to 5–6 mg/kg/h, combined with controlled ventilation with vecuronium and nitrous oxide and oxygen; this can be discontinued about 10 min before the end of surgery. Monitoring consists of non-invasive blood pressure measurement, oxygen saturation, ECG, end-tidal CO_2 concentration and peripheral nerve stimulator where appropriate. Intravenous ketorolac 0.75 mg/kg to a maximum of 10 mg unless contraindicated, or usually in children diclofenac 1–2 mg/kg by suppository can be given as pre-emptive analgesia. Droperidol 0.025–0.075 mg/kg given intravenously should be used in high-risk cases for PONV.

Postoperative

Paracetamol 15 mg/kg orally in children or 1 g in adults is usually sufficient for postoperative analgesia. Ketorolac or diclofenac can be used if stronger analgesia is required. Postoperative nausea and vomiting may be treated with intramuscular metoclopramide 10 mg in adults or in smaller doses of 1–5 mg in children if vomiting is severe.

REFERENCES

1. Reinecke RD. Current concepts in ophthalmology: Strabismus. *New Engl J Med* 1979; **300:** 1139.

2. Richards R. *A Text and Atlas of Strabismus Surgery.* Chapman and Hall: London, 1991.
3. Ing MR. Early surgical intervention for congenital esotropia. *Ophthalmology* 1983; **80:** 132.
4. Commission on the Provision of Surgical Services. *Guidelines for Day Case Surgery,* revised edn. The Royal College of Surgeons of England: London, 1992.
5. American Society of Anesthesiologists. New classification of physical status. *Anesthesiology* 1963; **24:** 111.
6. Dob DP, Whitwam JG. Pharmacology and day-case anaesthesia. In *Day-case Anaesthesia and Sedation* (edited by Whitwam JG). Blackwell Scientific: Oxford, 1994.
7. Campling EA, Devlin HB, Lunn JN. *The Report of the National Confidential Enquiry into Perioperative Deaths,* 1989. HMSO: London, 1990.
8. Denborough MH, Lovell RRH. Anasthetic deaths in a family. *Lancet* 1960; **34:** 395.
9. Ording H. Incidence of malignant hyperthermia in Denmark. *Anesth Analg* 1985; **64:** 700.
10. Ellis ER, Halsall PJ. Suxamethonium spasm: A differential diagnostic conundrum. *Br J Anaesth* 1984; **56:** 381.
11. Schwartz L, Rockoff MA, Koka BV. Masseter spasm with anesthesia: Incidence and implications. *Anesthesiology* 1984; **61:** 772.
12. Carroll JB. Increased incidence of masseter spasm in children with strabismus anaesthetised with halothane and suxamethonium. *Anesthesiology* 1987; **67:** 559.
13. Marsden CD, Rosenberg H, Fletcher JE. Masseter muscle rigidity and malignant hyperthermia susceptibility. *Anesth Analg* 1986; **65:** 161.
14. Grohert GA. Management of patients in whom trismus follows succinylcholine. *Anesthesiology* 1988; **68:** 653.
15. Rosenberg H. Trismus is not trivial. *Anesthesiology* 1987; **67:** 453.
16. France NK, France TD, Woodburn JD *et al.* Succinylcholine alteration of the forced duction test. *Ophthalmology* 1980; **87:** 1282.
17. Aschner B. Ueber einen bisher noch nicht beschriebenen Reflex von Auge auf Krieslauf und atmung: Verschwinden des Radialispulses bei Druck auf das Auge. *Wein Klin Wochenschr* 1908; **21:** 1529.
18. Dagnini G. Intorno ad un riflesso provacato in alcuni emiplegici cllo stimolo della cornea e colla pressione sul bulbo oculare. *Boll Sci Med* 1908; **8:** 380.
19. Ginsburg RN, Cartwright MJ, Murad SS, Nelson CC. Oculocardiac reflex in the anophthalmic socket. *Ophthalmic Surg* 1992; **23:** 135.
20. Alexander JP. Reflex disturbances of cardiac rhythm during ophthalmic surgery. *Br J Ophthalmol* 1975; **59:** 518.
21. Mirakhur RK, Jones CJ, Dundee JW, Archer DB. IM or IV atropine or glycopyrrolate for the prevention of the oculocardiac reflex in children undergoing squint surgery. *Br J Anaesth* 1982; **54:** 1059.
22. Blanc VF, Hardy JF, Milot J, Jacob JL. The oculocardiac reflex: A graphic and statistical analysis in children. *Can Anaesth Soc J* 1983; **30:** 360.
23. Moonie GT, Rees DI, Elton D. Oculocardiac reflex during strabismus surgery. *Can Anaesth Soc J* 1964; **11:** 621.
24. Petzetakis M. Effets reflexes de la compression oculaire a l'etet normal. Reflexes oculo-cardiaque, oculo-respiratoire, oculo-vasomoteur. *J Physiol Paris* 1915; **16:** 1027.
25. Blanc VF, Jacob JL, Milot J, Cyrenne L. The oculorespiratory reflex revisited. *Can Anaesth Soc J* 1988; **35:** 468.
26. Lerman J. Surgical and patient factors involved in postoperative nausea and vomiting. *Br J Anaesth* 1992; **69:** 245 (Suppl.).
27. Woods AM, Berry FA, Carter BJ. Strabismus surgery and postoperative vomiting: Clinical observations and review of the current literature. A medical opinion. *Paediatr Anesth* 1992; **2:** 223.
28. Schreiner MS, Nicolson SC, Martin T, Whitney L. Should children drink before discharge from day surgery? *Anesthesiology* 1992; **76:** 528.

29. van den Berg AA, Lambourne A, Clyburn PA. The oculo-emetic reflex: A rationalisation of postophthalmic anaesthesia vomiting. *Anaesthesia*. 1989; **44:** 110.
30. Weir PM, Munro HM, Reynolds PI, Lewis IH, Wilton NCT. Propofol infusion and the incidence of emesis in paediatric outpatient strabismus surgery. *Anesth Analg* 1993; **76:** 760.
31. Larsson S, Asgeirsson B, Magnusson J. Propofol–fentanyl anaesthesia compared to thiopental–halothane with special reference to recovery and vomiting after paediatric strabismus surgery. *Acta Anaesthesiol Scand* 1992; **36:** 182.
32. Munro HM, Riegger LQ, Reynolds PI, Wilton NCT, Lewis IH. Comparison of the analgesic and emetic properties of ketorolac and morphine for paediatric outpatient strabismus surgery. *Br J Anaesth* 1994; **72:** 624.
33. Watcha MF, Simeon RM, White PF, Stevens JL. Effect of propofol on the incidence of postoperative vomiting after strabismus surgery in paediatric outpatients. *Anesthesiology* 1991; **75:** 204.
34. Lerman J, Eustis S, Smith DR. Effect of droperidol pretreatment on postanesthetic vomiting in children undergoing strabismus surgery. *Anesthesiology* 1986; **65:** 322.
35. Lin DM, Furst SR, Rodarte A. A double-blinded comparison of metaclopramide and droperidol for prevention of emesis following strabismus surgery. *Anesthesiology* 1992; **76:** 357.
36. Horimoto Y, Tomie H, Hanzawa K, Nishida Y. Scopolamine patch reduces postoperative emesis in paediatric patients following strabismus surgery. *Can Anaesth Soc J* 1991; **38:** 441.
37. Lewis IH, Pryn SJ, Reynolds PI, Pandit UA, Wilton NCT. Effect of P6 acupressure on postoperative vomiting in children undergoing outpatient strabismus correction. *Br J Anaesth* 1991; **67:** 73.
38. Yentis SM, Bissonnette B. Ineffectiveness of acupuncture and droperidol in preventing vomiting following strabismus repair in children. *Can Anaesth Soc J* 1992; **39:** 151.
39. Magoon EH, Scott AB. Botulinum toxin chemodenervation in infants and children: An alternative to incisional strabismus surgery. *J Pediatr* 1987; **110:** 719.
40. Diamond GR. Topical anesthesia for strabismus surgery. *J Pediatr Ophthalmol Strabismus* 1989; **26:** 86.
41. Szmyd SM, Nelson LB, Calhoun JH *et al*. Retrobulbar anesthesia in strabismus surgery. *Arch Ophthalmol* 1984; **102:** 1325.
42. Sanders RJ, Nelson LB, Deutsch JA. Peribulbar anesthesia for strabismus surgery. *Am J Ophthalmol* 1990; **109:** 705.
43. Lavrich JB, Nelson LB. Local anesthesia for strabismus surgery. *Ophthalmol Clin North Am* 1992; **5:** 131.

CHAPTER 12

Adnexal surgery

G BARRY SMITH

INTRODUCTION

The term 'adnexal surgery' comprises all operations not on the globe or extraocular muscles. It is conveniently divided into orbital, lacrimal and oculoplastic surgery, but its borders overlap with those of neurosurgery, otolaryngology, maxillofacial and plastic surgery. Anaesthesia borrows many techniques from these related fields.

ORBITAL SURGERY

Numerically, this field of surgery is small and highly specialized. It not only deals with the investigation and treatment of space occupying lesions in the orbit, but also with surgery and repair of the orbital walls. In spite of the great advances in imaging[4,7] which have been of enormous advantage to the orbital surgeon, they have only allowed certain diagnoses to be confirmed without surgery.[7] Among these the radiolucent dermoid, the partially calcified phlebolith in the orbital varix and the vastly enlarged muscle in thyroid eye disease are outstanding. In many other situations, the surgeon will need tissue for histology or will attempt to excise a circumscribed mass.

The surgeon may incise over any part of the orbital rim to gain access from the anterior aspect. But this is difficult as the globe fills the orbit and in spite of retraction may only provide a very narrow field in which to operate. The anaesthetist may assist the surgeon by producing a soft eye. This may be done by reducing the production of aqueous humour with acetazolamide or by reducing the arterial pressure in a controlled way using vasodilators and beta-blockers. At systolic pressures of 70 mmHg, very little aqueous is secreted by the ciliary body and intermittent pressure by the surgical retractor forces aqueous out of the drainage angle. Continuous pressure over several minutes may cause retinal ischaemia and should be avoided.

Surgical access may also be obtained through the lateral wall by removing the orbital rim and exposing the orbit through the temporal fossa. Neurosurgeons favour a superior approach through the frontal region and the roof of the orbit. Exposure is limited by the levator muscle.

It is not important for the anaesthetist to be aware of the many different types of orbital mass, which include dermoid cysts, pleomorphic adenoma, lymphoma, secondary carcinoma, neural tumours and vascular hamartomas. However, some diagnoses present special interest to the anaesthetist.[5]

Vascular tumours

These may be venous, arterial or arteriovenous. Venous anomalies occur as large varices with little blood flow. The large blood lakes have episodes of thrombosis and inflammation and may contain phleboliths or altered blood. They become more prominent on lying or bending down. These varices present little risk of haemorrhage unless pulsation is visible.

Cavernous haemangiomata (lymphangiomata) are among the most common benign tumours of the orbit. They are usually well encapsulated and are of a characteristic dark plum colour. These have a moderate blood supply from a vascular pedicle which is easily controlled surgically.

Arteriovenous lesions are extremely dangerous, as they often have major communications with the internal carotid artery and the cavernous sinus. There are often secondary varices, which present as a pulsating exophthalmos. Fortunately, a proportion undergo spontaneous regression. Others may be treated radiologically by embolization. Surgery is sometimes associated with torrential haemorrhage which may be difficult to control. This may be a justification for profound, controlled arterial hypotension using vasodilators, posture and beta-blockers.

Thyroid eye disease

This may present to the surgeon for several reasons. First, as a differential diagnosis of proptosis, as it may be limited to one side or even one muscle. The muscles may so choke the apex of the orbit that they compress the optic nerve, with subsequent rapidly diminishing colour vision and eventually total blindness. Decompression constitutes an emergency sight-saving procedure.[6]

The anaesthetist is presented with a patient whose thyroid status may be higher, lower or normal. The eye disease at this stage is unrelated to the activity of the thyroid gland but seems to be entirely caused by an autoimmune process which may have some pituitary input. Some patients will have had treatment with iodine-131, others will be taking thyroid hormones and others still will be stabilized on neomercazole. It is important to establish and stabilize the thyroid status. Those who still have a degree of hyperthyroidism also have an excess of circulating catecholamines and the use of beta-blockade should be considered.

Many of these patients will have been treated for some months with steroids in massive doses and may well have osteoporosis, hypertension, fluid retention, obesity or diabetes as a result. These factors must be taken into consideration. There is a definite association between thyroid eye disease and cigarette smoking in some patients and combined with obesity may present problems. During surgery, the optic nerve is decompressed into the ethmoid air cells, the antrum and sometimes the temporal fossa. Blood will find its way to the pharynx. It is extremely important that the cornea of the eye on the other side is protected from exposure or damage.

LACRIMAL SURGERY

The purpose of lacrimal surgery is to improve the drainage of tears from the conjunctival sac into the nose. Obstruction may cause infection with reflux of infected matter into the conjunctival sac, tears may run down the cheek and vision is poor as an excessive tear film interferes with normal refraction.

Congenital obstruction

This occurs frequently in the neonate, reducing in incidence with age during childhood. The obstruction is commonly at the lower end of the nasolacrimal duct and the sac itself is dilated to form a mucocoele. This may have recurrent abscesses and loculi may form. Spontaneous cure tends to occur, but this may be hastened by gentle and accurate probing under general anaesthesia. Obstruction is proved by reflux and patency proved by syringing or the injection of contrast medium into a punctal catheter. The resultant X-ray is called a dacryocystogram (DCG). The surgical hazards of probing are an inability to locate the nasolacrimal duct at the bottom of a large mucocoele and damage to the canaliculi by creating a false passage.

This procedure should be treated seriously by the anaesthetist with all the precautions of a full general anaesthetic, with serious risks to the airway from the release of mucopus, injection of saline or contrast. The child should be protected with a snug-fitting endotracheal tube and by posture. A pad under the shoulders not only lets the trachea drain cephalad, but it also avoids the chin down position. The child's face should be horizontal if 'through orbit' X-ray pictures are required. Some anaesthetists would also use a pharyngeal pack. During the procedure, standard monitoring should be used, and if staff leave the patient to avoid radiation, then auditory warning systems should be used. At the end of the procedure, the pharynx and nose are full of mucus and the child should be extubated in the semi-prone position.

Other types of obstruction in children are punctal atresia, congenital absence of part of the system and fistula from the common canaliculus opening at the inner canthus. Obstruction is common in congenital craniofacial anomalies and in Down's syndrome.

Lacrimal obstruction in the adult

Most of these patients have obstruction from adhesions, strictures and stones resulting from chronic infection. The cause is reputed to be the herpes simplex virus, although acute episodes of infection are rarely seen. Specific causes are varicella, actinomycosis or the use of eye cosmetics such as Kohl. Blockage may occur at any point in the system and adhesions with debris block the canaliculi and the sac. The lacrimal apparatus is often torn due to lacerations of the lids, avulsion of the medial canthal tendon and fractures of the nose.

Surgery aims to produce an epithelial-lined track between the conjunctiva and nose. In a classical dacryocystorhinostomy (DCR), the sac is marsupialized into the nasal cavity using a large rhinostomy lined with flaps of nasal mucosa and sac. This track is stented with polythene or silicone rubber tubing inserted through the canaliculi and retained for several months. In selected cases, the lacrimal sac can be opened and a silicone stent introduced into the nasolacrimal sac. Recently, a diode laser has been used inside the nose to create a passage to the lacrimal sac but the results await evaluation.

Canalicular surgery – particularly trauma repair – has sometimes been treated as an urgent operation. In spite of improved techniques and accurate apposition of the torn ends, the incidence of stricture remains high and many patients end up with a DCR or bypass tube. Bypass tubes (Jones' tubes) are glass tubes which drain the conjunctival sac through a rhinostomy into the nose. They need expert siting and supervision as they block, move or become dislodged. They are sometimes difficult to reinsert as the track closes down rapidly.

Anaesthesia for DCR, CDCR and Jones' tubes

The problem for the surgeon is one of access and vision. The operative site is small, deep and soon fills with blood. It is difficult to illuminate except with a headlight or coaxial illumination on a microscope.

Most of the bleeding during the first part of the operation is venous and arises from tributaries of the angular vein lying on the outside of the nose just under the skin. Surgical control by pressure, traction suture and diathermy are vital. If the angular vein itself is damaged, then ligature may be needed. The anaesthetist can help this part of the procedure by elevating the head and allowing venous pooling in the feet. Many agents and artificial ventilation tend to raise central venous pressure a little, but this can be overcome with posture.

Bleeding from the bone during the rhinostomy can be persistent but is dealt with by the use of bone wax. The nasal mucosa does not bleed much from its periosteal surface but once incised it pours blood from dilated arterioles. Most surgeons or their anaesthetists insert adrenaline or cocaine packs into the nose, although the toxic effects of these are well documented as considerable amounts are absorbed.[1,3] These packs also shrink the size of the mucosal flaps. In the UK, controlled hypotension has been used during the later part of the procedure to reduce blood loss which may be severe.

In America, many DCRs are performed with local anaesthesia with an added vasoconstrictor. This seems very satisfactory provided that the patient's airway is satisfactory and heavy sedation does not block the cough reflex and allow the inhalation of blood clot.

In small infants DCRs present the serious problem of major blood loss. Surgeons become accustomed to operating with a continuous sucker and seldom realize that the size of operative field and blood loss are similar in an adult to that in a neonate. Anaesthetists must be more prepared to measure loss, more eager to prevent it by the use of vasoconstriction, and more enthusiastic to replace blood loss by an equal volume of blood or volume expander.

OCULOPLASTIC SURGERY

This is a wide area of adnexal surgery concerned with the lids, the orbital walls and the socket. It overlaps with the specialities of neurosurgery, maxillofacial, paediatric, ENT (ear, nose and throat) and general plastic surgery, as well as the other ophthalmic subspecialities. The field is so wide that justice cannot be done to the surgery and points will be raised with special relevance to anaesthesia. Although it might be felt that as in all facial surgery the most important aspects are the maintenance of a clear airway and the reduction of blood loss, it is perhaps equally important to remember that these patients experience feelings of disfigurement, anger, fear and inadequacy. The building of the patient's confidence resides not merely in the surgeon but in the caring, optimistic and sympathetic approach of the whole team.

Surgery of the eyelids

This may be functional or cosmetic. Ptosis of the upper lid may be congenital or acquired. It may result from a third nerve lesion, muscle weakness or swelling. If there is some levator function, the surgeon will resect the muscle to achieve maximum function. When there is no muscular action, then he will be forced into using a brow suspension relying on the facial musculature. Although synthetic materials have been tried, the most satisfactory and long-lasting material is a sling made from fascia lata taken from the lateral aspect of the patient's thigh. The anaesthetist must be prepared to extend the anaesthetic tubing, place a sandbag under the buttock and remember that the patient may need additional analgesia.

Numerous lid operations are performed by surgeons using infiltration with local anaesthetic on an outpatient basis. These patients have minimal preoperative assessment, preparation, monitoring and the record-keeping may be very limited.[2] This may be a very satisfactory and economical method of treatment provided the surgeon limits his ambitions and the patients are graded ASA I or II. It is still essential to have full resuscitation facilities available including defibrillator, oxygen and drugs. Operations for the removal of benign lesions, curettage of chalazia, ectropion, entropion and blepharoplasty can all be dealt with in this way. Correct patient selection is the key to a successful outcome.

Blowout fractures

These result from blunt trauma and are often associated with other fractures of the facial skeleton, ocular trauma and intracranial injury. Enophthalmos results from implosion of the ethmoid air cells and depression of the globe from the herniation of orbital contents into the maxillary antrum through the orbital floor. There is frequently double vision and restriction of upper gaze caused by tethering or herniation of the inferior rectus.

Early surgery does not seem to improve the prognosis and most cases are now treated conservatively with a late repair of the orbital floor through an extraperiosteal approach and later correction of motility if this is possible. It is important to use sufficient bulk to correct the enophthalmos. A proportion of these patients require wire replacement of the medial canthal tendon to correct the telecanthus, pulling the lids medially.

Enucleation

In this operation a blind, painful or diseased eye is removed. The extraocular muscles are divided and the optic nerve is cut or snared. The globe is removed intact with any malignancy, infection and the uveal tract contained within it. In most cases, the extraocular muscles are stitched to a prosthesis which will move. To assist retention of this prosthesis, it is often covered in Teflon mesh or donor sclera before Tenon's fascia and conjunctiva are carefully closed over it.

Evisceration

When the eye has been destroyed by infection, the sclera may be left as a barrier. The contents of the globe are cleaned out through a circumcorneal incision. Great care is taken to remove all traces of uveal tissue and to arrest bleeding. Traditionally, the collapsed sclera is then left to granulate, but some surgeons introduce a small acrylic ball and close the eye with ample antibiotic cover.

Exenteration

This is removal of the orbital contents contained in the periorbita and the conjunctiva. Frequently, the lids are removed and the bare bone of the socket is left to granulate for several months, being repacked as necessary. If the lids are not involved in the disease process, then they may be split and joined in a tarsorrhaphy. Although skin grafts and flaps have been used to speed healing, the end result is not satisfactory, as the skin becomes macerated and evil smelling.

Secondary procedures

Orbital prostheses may be too small or they may extrude. The conjunctival sac may shrink and the fornices become obliterated. This leads to poor lid movement and an inability to retain the glass eye. The anaesthetist should be aware that the surgeon having freed up the structures may need to use mucus membrane grafts from the mouth to improve the lining of the socket. It is as well to be prepared for this by having a pharyngeal pack already placed.

Any operation which requires the removal of an eye requires the identity and side of operation to be checked and double-checked before and after the patient is rendered unconscious. Particular danger exists when the eye is apparently normal but has a malignant melanoma of the choroid or a retinoblastoma. In these patients, it is usual to dilate the pupil and examine the fundus before proceeding.

All orbital procedures are likely to be associated with vagal reflexes, which may continue into the postoperative period.

REFERENCES

1. El-Din Asmak, Mostafa SM. Severe hypertension during anaesthesia for dacryocystorhinostomy. *Anaesthesia* 1985; **40:** 787.
2. Elkington JR, Khaw PT. Eyelid and lacrimal disorders. *Br Med J* 1988; **297:** 473.
3. Meyers EF. Cocaine toxicity during dacryocystorhinostomy. *Arch Ophthalmol* 1980; **98:** 842.
4. Moseley I, Sanders M. *Computerized Tomography in Neuro-ophthalmology.* WB Saunders: London, 1982.

5. Stewart WB, Krohel GB. Evaluation of orbital diseases. In *Ophthalmic, Plastic and Orbital Surgery*. American Academy of Ophthalmology Manual: New Orleans, 1988.
6. Trokel SL, Jakobiec FA. Correlation of CT scanning and pathologic features in ophthalmic Graves' disease. *Ophthalmology* 1981; **88:** 553.
7. Zimmerman RA *et al*. Orbital magnetic resonance imaging. *Am J Ophthalmol* 1985; **100:** 312.

CHAPTER 13

Ocular trauma

G BARRY SMITH ———————————————————————

INTRODUCTION

Damage to the eye is frequently associated with other injury, particularly head injury, sometimes with damage to the cervical spine and with multiple injuries elsewhere. It is important to bear other injuries in mind and to ensure neurological and cardiovascular stability before attempting any form of general anaesthesia. If possible, the eye should be gently examined with the aid of a few drops of local anaesthetic at an early stage before gross swelling of the eyelids renders this impossible. Trauma is conveniently divided into blunt trauma and perforating injuries.

BLUNT TRAUMA

The numerous causes of blunt trauma include sports injuries, assault and motor accidents. The orbital walls may be fractured and classically 'blow out' fractures occur in the thinnest bones, which are the ethmoid sinuses and the roof of the maxilla. Enophthalmos is obvious; the eye may be depressed and, if the inferior rectus is trapped in the fracture, there may be restriction of upward rotation of the globe. Unless there is gross disruption of the facial bones, fractured nose or a depressed malar fracture, these injuries are usually treated symptomatically with late secondary repair with implants to the orbital floor and correction of diplopia with muscle surgery.

The globe may rupture at any point, particularly at the site of previous surgery. When the rupture is posterior, it is often necessary to explore the exterior of the sclera, as the eye usually has blood in the anterior chamber or the vitreous which prevents ophthalmoscopic examination. The indication for this is a very low tension in the globe. Blunt trauma may lead to dislocation of the lens, retinal detachment and a contracoup injury to the macular region called commotio retinae. Diagnosis is assisted by ultrasound.

PENETRATING INJURY

The use of seatbelts has reduced the incidence of injuries from vehicle accidents involving the face and eye. A number of injuries of the lids, lacrimal drainage system and anterior part of the eye result from assaults with broken bottles and glasses. However, the most common injury is from construction and activities involving hammering or grinding, when high-speed fragments pass into the unprotected eye and imbed themselves in the lens or retina. These may be either metallic or non-metallic. Metals are highly toxic inside the eye and minute fragments of copper, brass or iron will poison the retina in a few weeks. The entry site may be minute and only visible to microscopy on a slit lamp. The particles themselves may be visible or a track may be seen in the lens with an impending cataract. Once again, haemorrhage may conceal the diagnosis which may be confirmed by computed tomography scan. Magnetic resonance imaging may be used for non-metallic particles but may cause metallic particles to move. Similar injuries are found in patients who have been exposed to explosions.

Gunshot wounds involving small shot or airgun pellets are common injuries. Sticks, branches, thorns and bamboo canes may well injure the globe, though many enter the soft tissues of the orbit and are frequently associated with severe cellulitis or purulent infection.

ANAESTHETIC PROBLEMS

General problems of multiple injury, neurological deficit, a full stomach and recent intake of alcohol are potentially life-threatening and can be approached by the usual methods. It is desirable in the presence of a suspected ruptured globe to avoid elevating the venous pressure by causing the patient to cough, strain or vomit. It is not appropriate to pass a gastric tube or to attempt an awake endotracheal intubation.

Although there is some increased risk of infection, delay is often a safer option than operating out-of-hours when proper assistance, full investigation and recovery facilities are unavailable. Unfortunately in many hospitals, theatre space is at a premium and there is some pressure to treat emergencies rapidly.

The precise induction technique is controversial and several techniques can be recommended. The aim of all of them is to avoid external pressure on the eye and to prevent rises in intraocular, venous and blood pressure, and at the same time to maintain full oxygenation and avoid aspiration.

After a full clinical examination and investigation, the patient may be prepared with metoclopramide and a hydrogen ion antagonist.

INDUCTION OF ANAESTHESIA

All anaesthetic agents with the exception of ether and ketamine tend to lower intraocular pressure. For emergencies and sick patients, there is often safety in using familiar agents with well-documented actions and reactions. Sleep doses of thiopentone, etomidate or propofol are all safe to use.

Thiopentone 2–7 mg/kg is cheap, well-tolerated and seldom provokes anaphylaxis. Slow injection avoids the cardiac or respiratory depression caused by a bolus. The possible disadvantages are that it may provoke bronchospasm in patients with asthma, leading to temporary reduction in pulmonary compliance. The strongly alkaline solution may cause tissue damage or arterial thrombosis if it is extravasated or accidently injected into an artery, and it may be unsuitable for restless patients.

Etomidate 0.3 mg/kg is an excellent agent which can be used in patients who are reputed to be allergic to thiopentone. It produces a smooth induction of unconsciousness with low intraocular pressure and good cardiovascular stability. Uncontrolled muscle movements may occur, but these can be controlled by narcotic analgesics. Occasionally, convulsions occur and this drug should be avoided in known epileptics. Etomidate depresses adrenal cortical function for some hours and adrenal failure has been reported. Its use should be avoided in patients with poor adrenal function or who have had recent steroid therapy. Only one dose should be used and it should not be used for maintenance of anaesthesia, sedation or repeated anaesthesia within a short time scale.

Propofol 2.0–2.5 mg/kg produces smooth induction and a sensation of well-being during recovery with little nausea. Injection into small veins may be associated with local pain or discomfort which may be avoided by the addition of 1 ml of lignocaine 1–2% immediately before injection. Some patients have a transient period of apnoea or respiratory depression and preoxygenation will avoid any reduction in oxygen saturation. This may be associated with moderate hypotension, which seems to be entirely benign and recovers within 10 min. The vital signs should be carefully observed at the onset of positive pressure respiration or during the introduction of anaesthetic vapours. It seems to be a particularly safe agent, but a smaller dose may be appropriate for the elderly or other sick patients with a reduced minimum anaesthetic concentration (MAC).

INTUBATION

If the patient has taken food or fluid in the 4 h before induction, or if stomach emptying has been delayed by shock or narcotics, or if the patient is pregnant, morbidly obese or has a history of hiatus hernia, then precautions must be taken to avoid reflux of gastric contents. The patient should be prepared with a hydrogen ion antagonist, possibly a soluble antacid and an intravenous injection of metoclopramide to aid gastric emptying.

At induction, suction must be immediately available to perform toilet of the pharynx. Firm pressure on the cricoid cartilage as consciousness slips away will occlude the oesophagus. There is a small risk of oesophageal rupture if active vomiting should occur, which has to be weighed against the much greater risk of inhalational pneumonitis. Cricoid pressure should continue until the endotracheal tube is positioned and the airway is secure.

Relaxants for intubation

Unnecessary heat is generated in the controversy over the choice between suxamethonium and nondepolarizing relaxants. Suxamethonium is the ideal agent for endotracheal intubation when the anaesthetist is inexperienced or in the patient in whom difficulties with intubation may be anticipated even in experienced hands. It causes a transient rise in intraocular pressure, produced by a contraction of the slow fibres in the extraocular muscles and other mechanisms, which might in a few patients lead to further loss of ocular contents. As the rise in pressure is only 8–10 mmHg and lasts for about 12 min, it is hardly significant compared with the pressure caused by squeezing with the eyelids or the changes on intubation. It may last longer in patients who have abnormal or deficient plasma cholinesterase. The rise in pressure is not blocked by lignocaine, narcotics or small doses of nondepolarizing drugs.

Suxamethonium commonly causes severe delayed muscular pains in the back or chest, which are a diagnostic hazard postoperatively. Neuromuscular blockade may last for 4–8 h which necessitates artificial ventilation. The most serious danger is malignant hyperthermia which, fortunately, is rare. The principal safeguards are a high index of suspicion, good monitoring including temperature, and dantrolene should be available within a few minutes. For further details, the reader is referred to Chapter 10.

Many experienced anaesthetists have abandoned the use of suxamethonium and rely on one of the new nondepolarizing muscle relaxants such as atracurium, mevacurium or vecuronium, whose time of onset is about 2.5 min to 80% neuromuscular blockade. These agents cannot be hurried as it is important to avoid any gagging or straining during intubation. The disadvantage of these agents is that it becomes essential to pass a tube with absolute certainty and that artificial ventilation will be required during surgery.

Intubation reflexes

Laryngoscopy and endotracheal intubation raise the blood pressure and intraocular pressure more than any drug. Good topical anaesthesia might be expected to block this reflex, but it may stimulate coughing and in any case is only partly successful. Parenteral lignocaine has its advocates and there are many papers advocating its use. Other anaesthetists prefer to administer a small dose of narcotic such as alfentanyl.

MAINTENANCE

This consists of the usual techniques of balanced anaesthesia. If air or gas is introduced into the eye to produce internal tamponade, then nitrous oxide may have to be discontinued and replaced with air, narcotics and anaesthetic vapours. Some vitreoretinal centres have abandoned the use of the DC magnet for extracting ferrous foreign bodies from the eye, as these travel at speed in a magnet field and inflict more uncontrolled damage on the eye. When a magnet is used, it is important to remove all electronic equipment to a safe distance with all steel instruments. Internal cardiac pacemakers are an absolute contraindication to the use of this instrument without consulting the manufacturers of the device.

CHAPTER 14

Day-case surgery

CAROLINE A CARR

INTRODUCTION

Day-case surgery in the USA is a well-established practice in either hospital-based or free-standing units. Up to 60% of all elective operations are performed on a day-case basis. Virtually all cataract extractions are performed under local anaesthesia and the hospital stay rarely exceeds 2 h.[1] In the UK, the growth of day-case surgery has been much slower; only 16.4% of surgical admissions were day-case in 1983.[2] Following the publication of documents by the Royal College of Surgeons of England, the Audit Commission for local authorities, and the National Health Service Management Executive, this percentage has increased to about 32%.[3-5] Day-case surgery is now considered the best option for 50% of all patients undergoing elective surgical procedures, although this proportion will vary between specialities.[6]

Advances in techniques of surgery and anaesthesia have both made this increase in day-case surgery possible, and been brought about, because of the pressure to increase day-case surgery.[7,8]

ADVANTAGES OF DAY-CASE SURGERY

This trend towards day-case surgery was primarily in response to economic pressures, but has also been shown to offer advantages for the patient and the health care system. Patients like day-case surgery because it disrupts their home life to a much lesser extent and decreases their chance of postoperative infection or complications.[9] Waiting lists can be reduced because an increased volume of surgery can be undertaken and routine operations do not have to compete with urgent operations for operating time. A date for surgery, which is most unlikely to be cancelled can be given at the time of outpatient consultation; this makes it much easier for the patient to organize working or domestic life to fit in with the intended surgery.[6]

Although cost savings from day surgery are well documented, costs may in fact rise as more patients are being treated in a given time period and, unless wards are closed, inpatient numbers will also rise.[10] The workload and work patterns of hospital and community staff will change with a move from inpatient to day-case surgery and these require planning.[11]

FACILITIES FOR DAY-CASE SURGERY

Day surgery is not a subspecialty of surgery, but is appropriate surgery performed on a day basis and it is essential that the quality of hospital service and facilities provided should be at least equivalent to that for inpatient surgery.[6] The most efficient service is provided by a self-contained unit designed to integrate day patient accommodation and operating facilities. It will need to provide changing facilities for the patients, a waiting room for escorts, facilities for medical and ophthalmic examination of the patients, and a mixture of beds and reclining chairs depending on the form of anaesthesia employed. Full facilities for resuscitation must be readily available. Parking spaces nearby for the patients' escorts should be provided. It is recommended that the unit should be linked to a general hospital that can provide back-up facilities such as blood tests or inpatient beds should a day-case unexpectedly require admission. To minimize postoperative complications, a high level of expertise is required in both the operating surgeon and the anaesthetist. Day-case surgery and anaesthesia must be performed or closely supervised by experienced staff. Nursing staff, too, will need to be experienced in day-case care of patients and are of importance in the initial selection of patients.

A less satisfactory but workable alternative is a day-case ward within a hospital from which the patients go to the main operating theatres for their surgery on day-case lists. These operating lists in practice become mixtures of inpatient and day-case surgery making them less efficient, as patients have to come from different wards.

A third possibility where day beds are on inpatient surgical wards is unsatisfactory for patients and staff. The two main advantages of a day-case ward – booked beds that are not blocked by emergency admissions and closure of the ward at night – are no longer possible. The administration and clerical back-up for day-case surgery has to be organized and efficient as the usual procedures of reception, admission, preparation, surgery, recovery and discharge are compressed into a single day.

DAY-CASE SURGERY IN OPHTHALMOLOGY

In ophthalmology, a distinction should be made between outpatient surgery and day-case surgery.[12]

Outpatient surgery

The term 'outpatient surgery' covers simple operations which do not carry the risk of serious postoperative complications. Minor plastic surgery of the eyelids, excision of eyelid cysts, removal of corneal graft sutures, cryotherapy and laser therapy are examples of suitable procedures that might be managed on this basis. These patients are not formally admitted to hospital and remain ambulant in their own clothes.

Day-case surgery

Day-case surgery covers the more complex procedures that may be performed on a day-case basis, as well as any procedure in children that requires general anaesthesia to obtain the necessary conditions. Procedures recommended for ophthalmic day-case surgery are included in the Guidelines for Day Case Surgery of the Royal College of Surgeons of England (Table 14.1).[6] These patients are formally admitted to hospital for the day and given a hospital bed or reclining chair. Local or general anaesthesia may be used for these procedures.

Age-related cataract constitutes the main surgical workload of ophthalmic services and the bulk of ophthalmic waiting lists in the UK.[13] Day-case surgery is proving to be the most efficient and cost-effective way of managing cataract surgery. Although there were initial reservations about the suitability of intraocular surgery for day-case treatment the successful management of routine intraocular surgery in this way is widely reported.[14–17] It has even been suggested that selected cases of vitreoretinal surgery could be performed as day-cases.[18,19]

Table 14.1   Ophthalmic operations and procedures suitable for day-case treatment

Adults	*Children*
Cataract surgery	Correction of strabismus
Corneal transplant surgery	Examination under anaesthetic for
Procedures on the eyelid or tarsal plate	conditions such as buphthalmos and
Operations on the lacrimal apparatus	retinoblastoma
Correction of strabismus	Electrodiagnostic tests
Refractive surgery	

SELECTION OF PATIENTS FOR OPHTHALMIC DAY-CASE SURGERY

The selection of patients for day-case surgery depends on three sets of criteria: surgical, medical and social (Table 14.2). These criteria will differ in detail from unit to unit but must be agreed on and adhered to at a local level to prevent unnecessary cancellations and unexpected inpatient admissions. Assessment and selection of patients involves the teamwork of the professionals involved in the day-case unit. Many of the patients who present for cataract extraction are elderly and have poor vision, so communication may be slow and difficult. It is very important for successful day-case management to take the time to ensure that the patient and his escort understand what is going to happen and what is expected of them. Information booklets explaining procedures are useful and should be available in the patient's native language. The use of video- and audio-tapes can also be very useful in informing the patient about the intended surgery.[20]

Assessment of the patient will usually take place at three separate stages, at which times the relevant selection criteria for day-case surgery should be

Table 14.2   Selection criteria for ophthalmic day-case surgery

Surgical criteria

Routine surgery anticipated
Minor postoperative complications
Mild or no postoperative pain
Mild or no postoperative nausea and vomiting
Surgery of short duration (30–60 min)

Medical criteria

American Society of Anesthesiologists (ASA) class I
ASA class II
ASA class III acceptable if the underlying medical condition is well controlled
No history of anaesthesia problems (difficult intubation, malignant hyperthermia)
Not morbidly obese
Age limit – premature infants should not be treated as day-cases until at least 60 weeks
    postconceptual age, otherwise no upper age limit as long as other selection criteria
    fulfilled
Must not be pregnant

Social criteria

Distance and ease of travel to hospital
Responsible adult escort available
Responsible adult supervision on postoperative night
Telephone readily available
Registered with a general medical practitioner

applied: at the initial surgical clinic visit, at a preoperative assessment clinic shortly before surgery, and on the day of surgery itself.

Initial clinic visit

The initial selection of the patient and of the surgical treatment is made by the surgeon who has the responsibility to determine whether the patient is suitable and willing to be treated as a day-case. There are various protocols and questionnaires available as examples of patient assessment.[6,21] Many patients for routine cataract extraction will have medical problems that require consultation with their medical practitioner to ensure optimal treatment prior to surgery. On occasion, consultation with the anaesthesia staff may be necessary to determine the optimal management of a problem patient. The form of anaesthesia should also be considered and discussed with the patient. The choice between local and general anaesthesia will depend on many factors, but contraindications to local anaesthesia must be considered to avoid cancellations on the day (Table 14.3). Most children will require general anaesthesia for ophthalmic procedures.

Patients for intraocular surgery or for any operation requiring general anaesthesia should be booked into an assessment clinic 2–4 weeks prior to surgery.

Table 14.3   Contraindications to ophthalmic local anaesthesia

Patient refusal
Unable to cooperate due to dementia, deafness or language barrier
Unable to lie still due to uncontrolled cough or tremor
Unable to lie flat as breathless at rest due to respiratory or cardiac disease
Unstable medical condition (cardiac ischaemia or arrythmias)
Coagulation defect
Allergy to local anaesthetic agents

Assessment clinic

The aim of a preoperative assessment clinic is to obtain the relevant medical and social information about the patient, to educate the patient and reduce anxiety. This is best carried out in the day-case unit itself. Ideally, an experienced anaesthetist would perform the medical assessment but this is not possible in many busy units. Experienced nursing staff using a standard questionnaire and consultation with the anaesthesia staff can perform this role. A full medical history, including current medication and allergies, should be taken. Routine measurements should be made and results outside a predetermined range initiate referral back, either to the booking surgeon, to the patient's medical practitioner or to the anaesthesia department (Table 14.4). A height–weight nomogram has been constructed to show a reasonable threshold of height–weight combinations acceptable for day-case general anaesthesia (Fig. 14.1). The nomogram should be considered as a guide only and should not substitute for good clinical judgement.

Morbidly obese patients, or those who are just outside the acceptable height–weight criteria but with other complications such as chronic obstructive airway disease (COAD), are not suitable for day-case management under general anaesthesia. Routine urine testing can be performed simply and cheaply by dipstick to detect unsuspected diabetes or renal disease in asymptomatic patients. Patients with glycosuria or proteinuria need further investigation. Unacceptably high blood pressure readings will require referral to the patient's medical practitioner for treatment prior to booking for day-case surgery.

Table 14.4   Routine preoperative measurements for ophthalmic day-case surgery

Height
Weight
Blood pressure
Urinalysis
Peak flow rate
Biometry in cataract patients

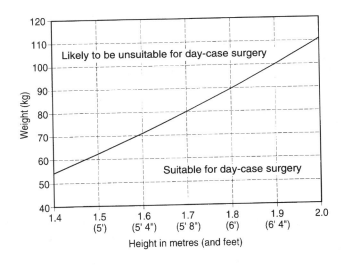

Fig. 14.1.   Height/weight nomogram for day-case surgery suitability.

Investigations

Further investigations should not be performed routinely but only as indicated by guidelines drawn up locally and based on abnormalities discovered in the medical history and on examination of the patient (Table 14.5). If there is any doubt, an anaesthesia opinion should be sought. When routine screening of active elderly patients was performed, only 0.1% of all tests led to a change in management.[22] In a study of the results of screening tests in ambulatory surgical patients, the abnormalities discovered could have been predicted on the basis of history and examination and the abnormal results did not affect patient outcome.[23]

Full blood count

A full blood count (FBC) is usually requested to detect anaemia, which may place a patient at risk from a general anaesthetic. However, routine screening of FBC contributes little to the patient's management.[24] Most cases of anaemia which may alter patient management can be detected by a full history and examination, and routine FBCs for day-case patients for minor surgery are unnecessary.

Sickle cell testing

Sickle cell anaemia affects those of African, Afro-Caribbean, Middle Eastern, Indian and Mediterranean descent. In the UK, about 5000 people have sickle cell disease and a much larger number have sickle cell trait. The carrier trait rarely gives rise to problems, especially for day-case ophthalmic surgery, and the racial background and clinical history should indicate those individuals at risk. Patients with sickle cell disease are unsuitable for day-case general anaesthesia.

Table 14.5   Indications for preoperative investigations for ophthalmic day-case surgery

Full blood count

Only in patients with signs or symptoms of anaemia

Sickle cell testing

If sickle disease indicated from racial origin or history

Coagulation screen

Patients on anticoagulants or with signs or symptoms of a coagulopathy

Urea and electrolytes

In patients taking diuretics, those with signs or symptoms of renal disease or with diabetes

ECG

Signs and symptoms of cardiac disease or ischaemia
Systemic disease known to be associated with cardiac problems (hypertension, diabetes etc.)
Age – many day-case units take 60 years as an indication for routine preoperative ECG

Chest X-ray

In patients with a history suggestive of active lung disease or physical signs such as a low oxygen saturation. These patients will not be suitable for day-case surgery

Coagulation screening

Routine preoperative coagulation screening is unreliable and produces a large number of false-positive results. It should only be requested when a coagulopathy is clinically suspected or the patient is on anticoagulants.

Blood chemistry

In healthy patients under 50 years of age, routine urine testing is all that is necessary to pick up unsuspected disease that might alter management. The pick-up rate of biochemical abnormalities in surgical patients has been shown to vary according to the designated ASA class.[25] The incidence of abnormalities was 1.5% in ASA I patients, 17% in ASA II patients and 50% in ASA III patients or those taking diuretics. Urea and electrolyte estimates need only be made in patients taking diuretics or with diabetes or renal disease.

Electrocardiography

Routine preoperative electrocardiograms (ECGs) commonly show abnormalities which correlate with increasing age, male gender and ASA class. However, of the patients with abnormal ECGs, very few experience adverse cardiovascular events and in even less is the preoperative ECG of help.[26] A resting ECG has low sensitivity as a detector of ischaemic heart disease and if it shows signs of a previously unrecognized myocardial infarction, it gives no indication of the timing of the infarction. Many day-case units have a policy of doing routine ECG on those over 60 years as the pick-up rate of abnormalities is high, although management is rarely altered unless the patient has clinical signs of heart disease.

Chest radiography

Reasons for taking a preoperative chest X ray are to make a diagnosis suspected from the history and examination, to detect asymptomatic pathology and to establish a baseline for comparison with postoperative films. In the first instance, a patient with symptomatic heart or lung disease is probably inappropriate for day-case surgery. In the second instance, a national study found that the radiologist's report was not available until after the operation in over 27% of patients who had a preoperative chest X-ray.[27] The baseline value of the preoperative chest X-ray could not be proved or correlated with postoperative pulmonary complications.

Social assessment

A full social assessment should be made at this time. It is advised that patients should not use public transport following intraocular surgery and should be taken home by car or by taxi. If there are problems with travel home or with support at home on the postoperative night, hostel accommodation should be available. Patients selected for hostel stay must be independently mobile and have sufficient vision in the unoperated eye to allow them to look after themselves. The form of anaesthesia should be carefully discussed, as patients may not understand what is involved with a local or a general anaesthetic. Tuition on the instillation of eyedrops is given. Instructions as to preoperative food and fluid restriction and the taking of usual medication should be given verbally and in written form. If the assessment is satisfactory, the patient is given the date of surgery and time of arrival on the day-case unit. Patients for general anaesthesia are usually given morning or early afternoon times of surgery and are asked to attend at least an hour before that.

Day of surgery

On the day of surgery, the patient is formally admitted to the hospital in the day-case unit and a number of preoperative checks made. The day ward staff take routine observations of pulse, blood pressure and temperature, check that the patient is appropriately fasting and has an escort available and someone to supervise on the first postoperative night.

The surgeon checks the operation to be performed, that all preoperative measurements relevant to the eye surgery have been made, that the correct eye is marked if appropriate, and that the consent form is signed.

The anaesthetist checks the patient's current health and medication and that the patient is appropriately listed for general or local anaesthesia. Premedication may be prescribed if necessary.

ANAESTHESIA FOR OPHTHALMIC DAY-CASE SURGERY

The form of the anaesthesia will depend on the surgeon, the patient, the anaesthetist and the operation. In most cases, children will require general anaesthesia. In the UK, most adult strabismus surgery is carried out under general anaesthesia. For uncomplicated cataract extraction performed on a day-case basis, either local or general anaesthesia will provide good operating conditions in appropriately selected patients.

Anaesthesia techniques for day-case surgery must be ones that provide rapid recovery, give good postoperative analgesia, and result in the minimum of adverse sequelae, of which postoperative nausea and vomiting are the most serious.

Optimal anaesthesia techniques for all the ophthalmic operations that are suitable for day-case treatment are described in detail in other chapters. However, the introduction of new agents (propofol, alfentanil, mivacurium and desflurane), the laryngeal mask, improvements in monitoring and procedural safety have all contributed to the development of day-case anaesthesia.

Premedication

Premedication in day-case patients is uncommon, as sedation is avoided to ensure a rapid recovery, and patients are often only admitted to the day ward just prior to surgery. In children, the application of a eutectic mixture of local anaesthetics (EMLA) prior to anaesthesia makes a painless intravenous induction possible in most cases.[28] If anxiolysis is thought necessary midazolam is as effective as temazepam in adults although some depression in psychomotor function was found at 4 h.[29] For children, the presence of a parent at induction of anaesthesia is effective in reducing anxiety.[30] Oral midazolam in a dose of 0.5 mg/kg is effective in about 20 min and does not prolong the child's stay in the day ward.[31]

Patients considered to be at risk of aspiration of gastric contents despite adequate preoperative starvation, such as those with hiatus hernia or oesophageal reflux, may present for day-case general anaesthesia. Histamine receptor (H_2) antagonists such as ranitidine with or without metoclopramide can be prescribed to increase gastric pH and reduce gastric fluid volume.[32] In patients having their surgery under local anaesthesia this might also be of help in preventing the discomfort of reflux while lying flat for the operation.

Other premedicants of interest are the alpha-2 agonists. Clonidine produces sedation, reduces anxiety and improves cardiovascular stability in elderly patients undergoing general anaesthesia for intraocular surgery.[33] The shorter-acting dexmedetomidine may be of value in day-case surgery and initial studies have shown a reduction in the minimal alveolar concentration of volatile anaesthetics required, attenuation of the haemodynamic response to intubation, a reduction in postoperative nausea and fatigue and in the need for opioids.[34,35]

Propofol

Propofol is established as the anaesthetic agent of choice for day-case anaesthesia. It produces a high-quality induction of anaesthesia and a rapid high-quality recovery from anaesthesia.[8] A comparison of thiopentone with propofol for induction of anaesthesia followed by maintenance with isoflurane and nitrous oxide showed a much faster recovery time with propofol.[36] Propofol can be used as an infusion to provide total intravenous anaesthesia (TIVA), which will give rapid high-quality recovery.[37] Propofol also has antiemetic properties which are of value in ophthalmic day-case surgery, especially strabismus surgery.[38]

Opioids

Opioid analgesics are often used as part of day-case anaesthesia to reduce the incidence of complications at induction and provide smoother anaesthesia, especially in unpremedicated patients. Alfentanil has a rapid onset time of 90 s and an elimination half-life of 1–2 h, and as a single dose with propofol–enflurane anaesthesia does not delay recovery or increase the incidence of postoperative nausea and vomiting.[39] It is also suitable for administration as an infusion, the recommended rate being 1 µg/kg/min. Alfentanil causes less postoperative nausea and vomiting than fentanyl, another widely used opioid in day-case anaesthesia, due to its shorter elimination half-life.[40]

Sufentanil is widely used in the USA for day-case anaesthesia and has a slightly shorter elimination half-life than fentanyl (2–4 h compared with 3–4 h).

Inhalational agents

The inhalational agents commonly in use for day-case anaesthesia are halothane, enflurane and isoflurane. Desflurane and sevoflurane are newer agents that are still being evaluated.

Desflurane

Desflurane is a new methyl ether derivative with potential for day-case anaesthesia. It has a low lipid solubility (oil:gas partition coefficient of 19), and a high minimal alveolar concentration (MAC) value (6–7.2% in oxygen), which means it provides a rapid onset of anaesthesia and a rapid recovery. It is minimally metabolized (0.02%). The main disadvantages of desflurane are that it causes coughing, laryngospasm and excitement on inhalation induction, it has a boiling point of 23.5°C, requires pressurized vaporizers and it is expensive. However, used with propofol it offers very rapid recovery from anaesthesia.[41]

Sevoflurane

Sevoflurane is a methyl propyl ether in clinical use in Japan. It has a low blood:gas solubility (coefficient of 0.6) and a MAC of 1.7–2% in oxygen, and although onset and recovery are not as quick as with desflurane, they are much faster than with halothane or isoflurane. It can be used in a conventional vaporizer. Sevoflurane has a big advantage in that it is pleasant to inhale and could replace halothane for inhalation inductions. Unfortunately, it may not be stable in soda-lime and it produces high concentrations of fluoride ions, although no renal problems have been reported yet.[42,43]

Isoflurane and enflurane

Isoflurane and enflurane are both widely used for day-case anaesthesia. Recovery times are similar and both are faster than halothane. Isoflurane is an irritant and difficult to use for inhalation induction but is only metabolized to a small extent (0.2%). Enflurane is metabolized to free fluoride ions but has not caused problems clinically. It is a cheap, safe alternative agent for day-case anaesthesia. Halothane remains the anaesthetic agent of choice for inhalation induction in children, but its potential for hepatic necrosis means that safer alternatives should be used in day-case anaesthesia.

Muscle relaxants

Suxamethonium

Suxamethonium was widely used in day-case anaesthesia because of its rapid onset and short duration of action. Its main serious drawback was the high incidence of postoperative suxamethonium myalgia, especially in ambulatory patients. However, it has now become largely redundant, due to the use of the laryngeal mask and techniques with alfentanil and propofol for intubation.

Atracurium and vecuronium

Atracurium and vecuronium are very extensively used in day-case anaesthesia where muscle relaxation is required and can be easily reversed after 20–30 min.

Mivacurium

Mivacurium is a new short-acting muscle relaxant that is partially metabolized by plasma cholinesterase. It has a duration of action of about 10–20 min that is not affected by prolonged infusion, so antagonism of blockade is rarely necessary. The recommended dose is 0.07–0.15 mg/kg in adults.[44] Its main drawbacks are that it has prolonged action in patients with pseudocholinesterase deficiency, and it is associated with histamine release and falls in blood pressure.

Rocuronium

Rocuronium is an analogue of vecuronium with an onset time similar to suxamethonium for providing good intubating conditions. Its duration of action in a dose of 0.6 mg/kg is similar to that of vecuronium. It is without autonomic side-effects.

Laryngeal mask airway

The laryngeal mask airway (LMA) has become well established in anaesthesia as a more secure airway than a conventional airway with many of the advantages of endotracheal intubation without many of the disadvantages.[45] Its use should be avoided in patients at risk of aspiration, i.e. those with hiatus hernia or oesophageal reflux in the day-case population of patients. Studies on its use in intraocular surgery have shown it to be particularly beneficial in reducing the frequency of postoperative coughing, straining, breath-holding and sore throat.[46] The LMA is also increasingly used in paediatric practice and has the advantage of avoiding intubation in day-case paediatric ophthalmic anaesthesia, when the airway has to be secured to allow surgical access.[47]

LOCAL ANAESTHESIA

Local anaesthesia for cataract extraction is indicated in routine uncomplicated cases. It should be seen as an alternative method of anaesthesia for the more fit and healthy and not as a means of operating on those unfit for general anaesthesia.[1] It is a prerequisite for local anaesthesia for cataract surgery that the patient can lie still and flat comfortably. If they are unable to do this or have other contraindications to local anaesthesia, such as an inability to cooperate or a language difficulty, then general anaesthesia may provide the best operating conditions (Table 14.3).

Management of patients for local anaesthesia

Traditionally, the operating surgeon has inserted the local anaesthetic block and proceeded to operate on the patient without the assistance of an anaesthetist. Potentially life-threatening complications have arisen on occasion and it is now recommended that an anaesthetist should be available for resuscitation should this be necessary and be responsible for the monitoring of the patient's general condition throughout the operation.[48]

Patients should be selected and prepared in the same way as they are for general anaesthesia, and preoperative investigations performed if clinically indicated. Their medical condition should always be optimal as for general anaesthesia. Practice with regard to preoperative fasting varies, ranging from full fasting as for general anaesthesia to normal food intake. A middle way is probably appropriate with patients advised to take a light meal a few hours prior to surgery. This could be varied in individual cases, such as insulin-dependent diabetics or patients with oesophageal reflux following food. A responsible escort should be available to take the patient home following surgery. All patients undergoing ophthalmic local anaesthesia should have intravenous access secured prior to administration of the block. This is then ready for resuscitation or if necessary for sedation.

The patient is made comfortable on the operating table and a means of communication provided in case of distress. This is ideally the hand of a member of the nursing staff that can be squeezed if the patient wishes to speak. Monitoring consists of arterial oxygen saturation (SaO_2), ECG and noninvasive blood pressure measurement.

Techniques of local anaesthesia

Techniques and their complications are described in detail in other chapters but the principles will be outlined below.

Retrobulbar anaesthesia

Retrobulbar anaesthesia is still widely practised.[49] It was first performed in 1884 using cocaine.[50] The technique involves the introduction of a needle percutaneously from an inferotemporal entry point aiming for the apex of the orbit. A small volume (2 ml) of local anaesthetic is deposited within the extraocular muscle cone. To prevent contraction of the orbicularis oculi muscle, a facial nerve block must also be performed. The onset of this block is usually rapid. Rare but serious complications have occurred. Local complications such as retrobulbar haemorrhage, globe perforation and optic nerve damage are well documented.[51] Systemic complications are due to the spread of local anaesthetic along the dural sheath of the optic nerve to the brainstem, or to direct intravascular injection. This will result in a variety of symptoms from drowsiness, blindness of the contralateral eye, convulsions, loss of consciousness to cardiopulmonary arrest.[52,53]

Peribulbar anaesthesia

Peribulbar anaesthesia was first described in 1986,[54] and is a technique designed to give good operating conditions while avoiding the serious complications of retrobulbar block.[55] It is well accepted by the patient, as there is little discomfort during insertion of the block when the transconjunctival approach is used and a facial nerve block is unnecessary. From inferolateral and medial sites of injection, up to 10 ml of local anaesthetic are placed around the globe outside the muscle cone with the needle tip no further back than the equator of the eye. The local anaesthetic spreads back to the apex and all compartments of the orbit through the network of orbital connective tissue. Onset of the block is relatively delayed and a pressure device of some sort is required to ensure spread of local anaesthetic and to reduce intraocular pressure.

Sub-Tenon's infiltration

The sub-Tenon's block seeks to avoid all the complications of a sharp needle being passed into the orbit. After making a small entrance wound in the conjunctiva, a curved blunt cannula is passed under Tenon's capsule to the back of the eye and a small volume of local anaesthetic deposited directly behind the globe.[56]

Topical anaesthesia

The topical application of local anaesthetic such as amethocaine completely dispenses with akinesia as part of the operating conditions for cataract extraction. It is a recognized technique that avoids all the complications of needles in the orbit, sharp or blunt. It works well with selected patients for small-incision cataract surgery performed by an experienced ophthalmic surgeon.

RECOVERY FROM DAY-CASE ANAESTHESIA

Recovery from general anaesthesia in the context of day-case surgery may be considered in three separate phases. The first phase is the recovery of the vital reflexes and should take place in a fully equipped and staffed recovery area as for inpatient surgery. In day-case anaesthesia, the use of rapidly metabolized agents should make this a rapid phase. The second phase of recovery takes place on the day-case ward in bed or on a trolley and consists of mobilization of the patient, control of postoperative pain, nausea and vomiting and checking for immediate postoperative complications of surgery. The third phase is recovery to 'street fitness' and is discussed in the final section of this chapter.

Postoperative pain control

Good postoperative pain control is vital in day-case surgery. Intraocular surgery is not very painful postoperatively and simple analgesics such as paracetamol are sufficient to control patients' symptoms. Very severe pain associated with nausea and vomiting following cataract surgery is probably an indication of a raised intraocular pressure which will require treating with oral acetazolamide. If long-acting local anaesthetics such as bupivacaine are used for local anaesthesia, pain relief will last for some hours postoperatively. The main problem with this is that the patient will also be unable to close the eye for this period and it will have to be kept closed with a pad to prevent corneal exposure. For surgery that is anticipated to be more painful postoperatively, such as strabismus surgery, it is now considered good practice to provide pre-emptive analgesia.[57] Non-steroidal anti-inflammatory drugs (NSAIDs) are popular for postoperative pain relief and may be used for their opiate sparing effect or as an adjunct to simple oral analgesics. These drugs inhibit prostaglandin synthesis and the formation of the mediators involved in pain perception. If they are given preoperatively or perioperatively prior to the start of surgery they are more effective.[58] Well-known side-effects which may limit their use are bronchoconstriction in asthmatics, stomach ulceration and haemorrhage, renal failure in those with compromised renal function and an anticoagulant effect due to inhibition of platelet function. The NSAIDs commonly in use for postoperative analgesia are diclofenac, ibuprofen, indomethacin and ketorolac.

Ketorolac

Ketorolac is a new potent NSAID, 30 mg of which is equivalent to 10 mg morphine if given by intramuscular injection. It has a relatively slow onset of action, taking over 30 min to take effect, but has a long duration of action with a half-life of over 7 h. Ketorolac can provide analgesia equivalent to morphine without the side-effects of respiratory depression and nausea and vomiting. It may be given orally, by intramuscular injection and by intravenous injection. Recently, the recommended starting dose for parenteral administration in adults has been reduced from 30 to 10 mg.[59] Its use in children under 16 years of age is not recommended but has been used successfully via the intravenous route during paediatric surgery.[60]

Diclofenac

Diclofenac is another commonly used NSAID in day-case surgery, and can be administered orally, intramuscularly and by suppository. This last route is particularly useful in providing postoperative analgesia in children following strabismus surgery when a dose of 1–2 mg/kg is given as a suppository after induction of anaesthesia.[61] It is important to discuss this with the parents beforehand and obtain their permission. As with other NSAIDs, diclofenac should not be used if there is a history of asthma, peptic ulceration, bleeding diathesis, hypersensitivity to NSAIDs or aspirin, renal impairment or in hypovolaemia, dehydration or operations with a high risk of haemorrhage.

Postoperative nausea and vomiting

Vomiting is common after eye surgery and is the most frequent postoperative complication of strabismus surgery. In children over 2 years of age, the incidence of postoperative nausea and vomiting (PONV) following strabismus surgery has been reported as ranging from 40 to 88%.[62] Obviously, this has implications for the rapid discharge of children from the day-case ward after surgery. Various causes have been put forward for this high incidence of PONV, including traction on the extraocular muscles stimulating the oculoemetic reflex, early postoperative fluid intake and involvement of the labyrinthine pathways. There is no doubt that anaesthetic technique affects the incidence of PONV and the use of propofol for induction of anaesthesia or as an infusion for maintenance greatly reduces it.[63] Routine use of an anti-emetic such as droperidol in a dose of 0.075 mg/kg will reduce PONV, but is associated with sedation, extrapyramidal symptoms and dysphoria.[64] Ondansetron is a 5-hydroxytryptamine ($5HT_3$) antagonist that has been used in adults for the prevention and treatment of severe PONV either orally (8 mg) 1 h preoperatively or intravenously (4 mg) at induction and is of use in day-case surgery in patients with a history of severe PONV.[65]

DISCHARGE

The third phase of recovery is recovery to 'street fitness' and discharge from the day-case unit. Patients will have to fulfil certain predetermined criteria that should be documented prior to discharge (Table 14.6). Discharge policies will vary between units and will involve the nursing staff, the surgeon and the anaesthetist. On discharge, patients must be given verbal and written advice about restriction of activities following the anaesthetic, specific instructions relating to surgical care (e.g. instillation of eye drops) and instructions regarding postopera-

Table 14.6   Discharge criteria following general anaesthesia or sedation

---

Can walk unaided
Adequate control of pain and nausea
No early complications of surgery
Tolerating oral fluids
Stable observations of pulse, BP, respiration, temperature
Responsible adult escort available
Suitable transport available
Given written postoperative instructions with emergency contact number

---

tive medication, including painkillers. They should be discharged into the care of a responsible adult who will stay with them the first postoperative night. A means of contact in emergency should be clearly explained and details of postoperative appointments given. Following general anaesthesia or sedation, patients are advised not to drink alcohol, drive a car, ride a bicycle, operate machinery or make any important decisions for 24–48 h.

The move to day-case ophthalmic surgery is proceeding at a rapid rate. To ensure patient safety and a good opthalmic outcome, it is vital that corners are not cut. Time and money must be spent on patient assessment and education. Ward and theatre facilities need to be up to inpatient standard with the added facilities for escorts. Clerical staff and facilities to deal with the administrative load involved must be provided. Both surgical and anaesthesia techniques must be of a high standard and provide a rapid return to normality for the patient with a minimum of complications. This will mean the involvement of experienced senior staff along with available up-to-date equipment and anaesthetic agents. Audit of day-case activity is important to ensure patient satisfaction and to ensure that appropriate patients are being selected for appropriate operations. Postoperative surgical and anaesthesia complications resulting in admission of patients to hospital should be kept to a minimum. If a high standard of care is provided at all stages, day-case ophthalmic surgery is a very efficient way of dealing with routine cases and results in increased patient and staff satisfaction.

REFERENCES

1. Rubin AP. Anaesthesia for cataract surgery – time for a change? *Anaesthesia* 1990; **45:** 717.
2. Department of Health. *Statistical Bulletin*. Government Statistical Service: London, 1994.
3. Commission on the Provision of Surgical Services. *Guidelines for Day Case Surgery*. Royal College of Surgeons of England: London, 1985.
4. Audit Commission. *A Short Cut to Better Services – Day Surgery in England and Wales*. HMSO: London,1990.
5. NHS Management Executive Value For Money Unit. *Day Surgery – Making it Happen*. HMSO: London, 1991.
6. Commision on the Provision of Surgical Services. *Guidelines for Day Case Surgery*, revised edn. Royal College of Surgeons of England: London, 1992.
7. Acheson JF, McHugh JD, Falcon MG. Changing patterns of early complications in cataract surgery with new techniques: A surgical audit. *Br J Ophthalmol* 1988; **72:** 481.
8. Heath PJ, Kennedy DJ, Ogg TW, Dunling C, Gilks WR. Which intravenous induction agent for day surgery? A comparison of propofol, thiopentone, methohexitone and etomidate. *Anaesthesia* 1988; **43:** 365.
9. Audit Commission. *Measuring Quality: The Patient's View of Day Surgery*. HMSO: London, 1991.
10. Haworth EA, Balarajan R. Day surgery: Does it add to or replace inpatient surgery? *Br Med J* 1987; **294:** 133.
11. Stott NCH. Day case surgery generates no increased workload for community based staff. True or false? *Br Med J* 1992; **304:** 825.
12. College of Ophthalmologists. Advice on day case surgery in ophthalmology. *J One-Day Surg* 1993; **2:** 14.
13. Courtney P. The national cataract surgery survey: 1. Method and descriptive features. *Eye* 1992; **6:** 487.

14. Watts MT, Pearce JL. Day-case cataract surgery. *Br J Ophthalmol* 1988; **72:** 897.
15. Strong NP, Wigmore W *et al.* Daycase cataract surgery. *Br J Ophthalmol* 1991; **75:** 731.
16. Strong NP, Wigmore W *et al.* Ophthalmic day case surgery: The role of the dedicated day-case unit. *Health Trends* 1992; **24:** 148.
17. Eason J, Seward H, Mount A. Daycare cataract surgery – Croydon experience. *J One Day Surg* 1993; **2:** 9.
18. Leaver P. Prospects for day-case vireoretinal surgery (Editorial). *Br J Ophthalmol* 1992; **76:** 65.
19. Cannon CS, Gross JG, Abramson I *et al.* Evaluation of outpatient experience with vit-reoretinal surgery. *Br J Ophthalmol* 1992; **76:** 68.
20. Baskerville PA, Heddle RM, Jarrett PEM. Preparation for surgery: Information tapes for the patient. *Practitioner* 1985; **229:** 677.
21. Pollard BJ. Assessment of fitness for day-case surgery under general anaesthesia. In *Anaesthesia for Day Case Surgery: Clinical Anaesthesiology, International Practice and Research* (edited by Healy TEJ). Ballière Tindall: London, 1990: 615.
22. Domoto K, Ben R, Wei JY, Pass TM, Komanoff AL. Yield of routine annual laboratory screening in the institutionalized elderly. *Am J Public Health* 1985; **75:** 243.
23. Johnson H Jr, Knee-Ioli S, Butler TA, Muoz E, Wise L. Are routine preoperative labo-ratory screening tests necessary to evaluate ambulatory surgical patients? *Surgery* 1988; **104:** 639.
24. Narr BJ, Hansen TR, Warner MA. Preoperative laboratory screening in healthy Mayo patients: Cost-effective elimination of tests and unchanged outcomes. *Mayo Clinic Proc* 1991; **66:** 155.
25. McCleane GJ. Urea and electrolyte measurement in preoperative surgical patients. *Anaesthesia* 1988; **43:** 413.
26. Rabkin SW, Horne JM. Preoperative electrocardiography: Effect of new abnormalities on clinical decisions. *Can Medl Assoc J* 1983; **128:** 146.
27. Royal College Working Party on the Effective Use of Diagnostic Radiology. Preoperative chest radiology: National study by the Royal College of Radiologists. *Lancet* 1979; **ii:** 83.
28. Manuksela E-L, Korpela R. Double-blind evaluation of a lignocaine–prilocaine cream (EMLA) in children. *Br J Anaesth* 1986; **58:** 1242
29. Nightingale JJ, Norman J. A comparison of midazolam and temazepam for premedica-tion of day-case patients. *Anaesthesia* 1988; **43:** 111.
30. Schofield NMacC, White JB. Interrelations among children, parents, premedication and anaesthetists in paediatric day stay surgery. *Br Med J* 1989; **299:** 1371.
31. McClusky A, Meakin GH. Oral administration of midazolam as a premedicant for pae-diatric day-case anaesthesia. *Anaesthesia* 1994: **49:** 782.
32. Escolano F, Castano J, Lopez R, Bisbe E, Alcon A. Effects of omeprazole, ranitidine, famotidine and placebo on gastric secretion in patients undergoing elective surgery. *Br J Anaesth* 1992; **69:** 404.
33. Kumar A, Bose S, Bhattacharya A, Tandon OP, Kundra P. Oral clonidine premedica-tion in elderly patients undergoing intraocular surgery. *Acta Anaesthesiol Scand* 1992; **36:** 159.
34. Peden CJ, Prys-Roberts C. Dexmedetomidine – a powerful new adjunct to anaesthesia (editorial II). *Br J Anaesth* 1992; **68:** 123.
35. Virkkila M, Ali-Melkkila T, Kanto J, Turunen J, Scheinin H. Dexmedetomidine as intramuscular premedication in outpatient cataract surgery: A placebo-controlled dose-ranging study. *Anaesthesia* 1993; **48:** 482.
36. Gupta A, Larsen LE, Sjoberg F. Thiopentone or propofol for induction of isofllurane-based anaesthesia for ambulatory surgery? *Acta Anaesthesiol Scand* 1992; **36:** 670.
37. Nightingale JJ, Lewis IM. Recovery from day-case anaesthesia: Comparison of total IV anaesthesia using propofol with an inhalational technique. *Br J Anaesth* 1992; **68:** 356.

38. Watcha MF, White PF. Postoperative nausea and vomiting. *Anesthesiology* 1992; **77:** 162.

39. White PF, Coe V, Shafer A, Snug ML. Comparison of fentanyl and alfentanil for out-patient anaesthesia. *Anesthesiology* 1986; **64:** 99.

40. Bagshaw ONT, Singh P, Aitkenhead AR. Alfentanil in daycase anaesthesia: Assessment of a single dose on the quality of anaesthesia and recovery. *Anaesthesia* 1993; **48:** 476.

41. Ghouri AF, Bodmen M, White PF. Recovery profile after desflurane nitrous oxide versus isoflurane nitrous oxide in outpatients. *Anesthesiology* 1992; **74:** 419.

42. Wrigley SR, Jones RM. Inhalational agents – an update. *Eur J Anaesth* 1992; **9:** 185.

43. Holaday DA, Smith FR. Clinical characteristics and biotransformation of sevoflurane in healthy human volunteers. *Anesthesiology* 1981; **54:** 100.

44. Wrigley SR, Jones RM, Harrop-Griffiths AW, Platt MU. Mivacurium chloride: A study to evaluate its use during propofol nitrous oxide anaesthesia. *Anesthesiology* 1992; **74:** 646.

45. Brain AIJ. The laryngeal mask – a new concept in airway management. *Br J Anaesth* 1983; **55:** 801.

46. Akhtar TM, McMurray P, Kerr WJ, Kenny GNC. A comparison of laryngeal mask airway with tracheal tube for intra-ocular ophthalmic surgery. *Anaesthesia* 1992; **47:** 668.

47. Wilson IG. The laryngeal mask airway in paediatric practice (Editorial II). *Br J Anaesth* 1993; **70:** 124.

48. Report of the Joint Working Party on Anaesthesia in Ophthalmic Surgery. Royal College of Anaesthetists and College of Ophthalmologists: London, 1993.

49. Hodgkins PR, Luff AJ *et al*. Current practice of cataract extraction and anaesthesia. *Br J Ophthalomol* 1992; **76:** 323.

50. Knapp H. On cocaine and its uses in ophthalmic surgery. *Arch Ophthalmol* 1884; **13:** 402.

51. Morgan CM, Schatz H *et al*. Ocular complications associated with retrobulbar injections. *Ophthalmology* 1988; **95:** 660.

52. Meyers EF, Ramirez RC, Boniuk I. Grand mal seizures after retrobulbar block. *Arch Ophthalmol* 1978; **96:** 847.

53. Javitt JC, Addiego R *et al*. Brain stem anaesthesia after retrobulbar block. *Ophthalmology* 1987; **94:** 718.

54. Davis DB II, Mandel MR. Posterior peribulbar anaesthesia – an alternative to retrobulbar anaesthesia. *J Cataract Refract Surg* 1986; **12:** 182.

55. Wang HS. Peribulbar anaesthesia for ophthalmic procedures. *J Cataract Refract Surg* 1988; **14:** 441.

56. Stevens JD. A new local anaesthesia technique for cataract extraction by one quadrant sub-Tenon's infiltration. *Br J Ophthalmol* 1992; **76:** 670.

57. Bush D. Pre-emptive analgesia (Editorial). *Br Med J* 1993; **306:** 285.

58. Baer GA, Rorarius MGF, Kolehmainen S, Seun S. The effect of paracetamol or diclofenac administered before operation on postoperative pain and behaviour after adenoidectomy in small children. *Anaesthesia* 1992; **47:** 1078.

59. *Current problems in pharmacovigilence. Ketorolac: New restrictions on dose and duration of treatment.* Committee on Safety of Medicines (UK), 19 June 1993: 5–6.

60. Watcha MF, Jones MB, Laguerula RG, Schweiger C, White PF. Comparison of ketorolac and morphine as adjuvants during paediatric surgery. *Anesthesiology* 1992; **76:** 368.

61. Bone ME, Fell DA. A comparison of rectal diclofenac with intramuscular papaveretum or placebo for pain relief following tonsillectomy. *Anaesthesia* 1988; **43:** 277.

62. Lerman J. Surgical and patient factors involved in postoperative nausea and vomiting. *Br J Anaesth* 1992; **69:** 245 (Suppl. 1).

63. Weir PM, Munro HM, Reynolds PI, Lewis IH, Wilton NCT. Propofol infusion and the incidence of emisis in paediatric outpatient strabismus surgery. *Anesth Analg* 1993; **76:** 760.

64. Lerman J, Eustis S, Smith DR. Effect of droperidol pretreatment on postanaesthetic vomiting in children undergoing strabismus surgery. *Anesthesiology* 1986; **65:** 322.
65. Leeser J, Lip H. Prevention of postoperative nausea and vomiting using ondansetron, a new, selective, 5-HT3 receptor antagonist. *Anesth Analg* 1991; **72:** 751.

CHAPTER 15

General anaesthesia for vitreoretinal surgery

G BARRY SMITH —————————————————————————

SURGICAL PROCEDURES

These operations are lengthy and complex. It is necessary for the anaesthetist to know something of the surgical approach so that he can provide a rational service for patient and surgeon.

RETINAL DETACHMENT

Retinal detachments (Fig. 15.1) are associated with trauma, high myopia, hypertension, Marfan's syndrome, age and vitreous disease. They are particularly likely to occur in big eyes with thin sclera and degenerate retina, which accounts for their association with myopia and with some types of glaucoma, especially congenital glaucoma with buphthalmos.

The retina splits between the pigmentary layer and the neuroepithelium and fluid collects between the layers. The word rhegmatogenous refers to those detachments which are associated with a break, tear or hole which allows fluid to pass through and strip up the retina. The detached retina loses its function and becomes fibrotic and shrunken, so that it is more difficult to reattach. If the retina can be reattached within a period of days or a few weeks, then some visual function returns. However, if the macula is detached, then fine vision and colour perception are lost permanently. Detachments in which only part of the retina is detached and the macula is threatened are considered to be urgent cases to be operated on at the first opportunity.

Conventional surgery for detachments consists of apposing the area near the break by the pressure of oversewn explants and sealing the hole by creating a sterile inflammation with cryotherapy. Sometimes the whole eye is made smaller by using a silicone rubber band to make a 2 mm circumferential indent. If the detached retina is so bullous that the areas cannot be brought into apposition, then subretinal fluid can be drained through an external sclerotomy. This carries some risk of choroidal haemorrhage or incarcerating retina in the drainage hole. Air, gas or saline may be injected to restore tone to the eye. The surgeon will

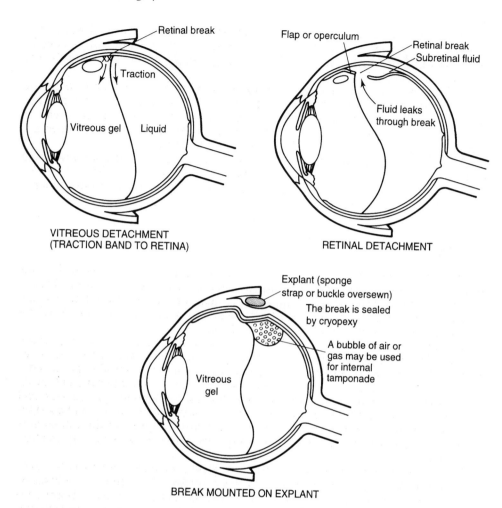

Fig. 15.1. A retinal detachment is started by a number of factors:
(a) Weakness or thinness of the retina such as lattice or holes. (b) Degeneration and liquifaction of the vitreous gel with remaining points of traction. (c) Contraction of remaining gel causing traction, particularly anteriorly. This may cause 'flashes'. 'Floaters' are red cells and pigment. (d) The break may be 'V'-shaped with an operculum or circumferential, when it may be called a 'Giant tear'. (e) Fluid enters the break and strips off the retina within hours or days, including the macula. The detached retina loses function (the patient sees curtain or darkness). (f) The retina forms a funnel attached anteriorly and at the optic disc. (g) Over the next few days, weeks or months, it fibroses, the eye becomes soft and new vessels may appear on the iris. If these produce excessive fluid, pressure may again rise to produce a painful, blind eye. Treatment is to localize, block and seal the break, sometimes draining off the fluid. The layers are held in apposition and a sterile inflammatory response created with a cryo-probe.

confirm that the retinal circulation has not been occluded before closure. It is important for the anaesthetist to maintain a normal blood pressure during detachment procedures, so that rises in intraocular pressure due to explants do not occlude the retinal circulation.

At the conclusion of the procedure, the surgeon may often wish to examine and provide prophylactic treatment to the retina of the other eye. This prophylaxis will be in the form of cryotherapy or laser to any breaks or thin areas of retina. Laser is highly effective in sealing breaks in attached retina, but does not seal holes when there is a layer of fluid between the layers.

There are a number of other types of retinal detachment which are much less common. Among these are traction detachments caused by vitreous bands, serous detachments resulting from low intraocular pressure and detachments caused by neoplastic deposits.

VITREOUS SURGERY

Surgery to the vitreous is a fast growing area of ophthalmic surgery which has developed from retinal detachment surgery with the aid of microsurgical techniques. When the vitreous is opaque, the surgeon cannot see the retina and the patient cannot see. Diagnosis will be dependent on the history, supported by ultrasound which will identify retinal detachment.

Vitreous opacity of sudden onset is usually caused by blood. In young people this usually results from severe trauma or intraocular foreign body and in older patients from retinal branch vein occlusion associated with arterial hypertension. At least a third of all vitrectomies are associated with retinal microvascular disease caused by diabetes. Repeated small bleeds from abnormal vessels and microaneurysms lead to the build up of multiple layers of fibrinous and collagenous membranes with a preretinal membrane closely applied to the retinal surface. The membranes contract and drag off the retina, creating traction detachments.

Even when the vitreous appears clear, it may be associated with retinal detachment. It shrinks away from the retina in middle life and the vitreous base loses its attachment to the anterior retina and in the process may cause breaks. Many retinal detachments can be treated more surely by vitrectomy than by conventional methods. Vitrectomy enables drainage of subretinal fluid by internal drainage through the break under direct vision and reduces the need for explants by providing internal tamponade with saline, gas, air or silicone oil.

The vitrectomy itself is performed under microscopic vision through a series of pars plana vitrectomies 4 mm behind the corneoscleral junction. Through these are introduced an infusion of balanced salt solution at a known pressure, a hydraulic suction cutter and a variety of fibre-optic cables, lasers, electrodes, scissors and picks. Debris, blood, gas and fluid are removed and exchanged by a blunt cannula with a side hole called a Charles flute needle, which is also used for draining subretinal fluid.

Vitreous replacement is with saline, silicone oil, air and a number of insoluble gases, such as sulphur hexafluoride (SF6), which provide a gentle tamponade on the retina from inside the eye. This is assisted by postoperative posture regimes for the patient so that the bubbles of foreign material press the detachment in the

correct direction. Recently, a heavy liquid, perflouro-*m*-octane has been introduced for intractable detachments.

THE ANAESTHETIC

So far, little has been said directly about the anaesthetist's role in these operations. It should be clear that these operations are extremely long (lasting several
hours) and very delicate. It follows that only a few patients can tolerate these
procedures under local anaesthesia. If local anaesthesia is used, a long-acting
agent such as bupivicaine must be used or some technique which allows 'top-
ping up' during the operation. The head must be rigidly immobilized on a hard
surface in a rigid frame. This means that access to the airway will be extremely
limited and only obtained by major surgical inconvenience. In general, access
to any part of the patient is minimal. It is essential that there is a perfect and
sure airway and that all monitoring probes and infusions are set up before
surgery.[2]

The intraocular part of the operation is done without external light and the
anaesthetists must ensure that they have sufficient light under their own control
to check apparatus, gas flows and monitors. They must be able to read the labels
on drug ampoules and ideally should have enough light to be able to observe nail
bed cyanosis in the hands of their patients. Adequate lighting screened from the
surgeon will provide a safer anaesthetic procedure and reduce the dangers of
needle stick injuries and other hazards.

Under these trying conditions, complete noninvasive monitoring of the patient
and the equipment is not merely desirable but essential. These include:

- ECG and heart rate with alarms
- pulse oximetry with alarms
- noninvasive blood pressure
- end-tidal capnography with alarms
- peripheral nerve stimulator
- inspired oxygen concentration with alarm
- high- and low-pressure (disconnect) alarms

In some countries, volatile agent analysers are legally demanded. I would not
myself wish to give an anaesthetic with a machine that did not have an oxygen
failure device or where I was solely dependent on machine-mounted cylinders
(gas bottles).

INTERNAL TAMPONADE

To occlude breaks or tears in the retina, the traditional repair of a retinal detachment used the patient's own vitreous to block the break and allow the subretinal
fluid to be reabsorbed. It is more efficient to use other substances to achieve this
objective and is essential when the vitreous has been removed. The gases or liquids used must be biologically inert, have a high surface tension and, if intended
for long-term use, be capable of transmitting light.

GAS/VITREOUS EXCHANGE

Filtered air is the easiest to use, but it is absorbed within 3 days. When mixed with an inert gas such as sulphur hexafluoride (SF_6), perfluoroethane (C_2F_6) or perfluoropropane (C_3F_8), the bubble persists for 3–4 weeks. These gases are very insoluble and were first used for inducing artificial pneumothorax. Pure gas gives an expanding bubble because nitrogen and oxygen diffuse into it until the partial pressures in the bubble are equal to those in the tissues. When a total vitreous replacement with 3–4 ml of gas is used, then a concentration of approximately 20% of gas in air produces a stable volume.

Gas provides an excellent internal tamponade and is particularly valuable for recent breaks in the upper part of the retina. Postoperatively, the patient needs careful posturing to keep the bubble pressing on the break.

The problems associated with the use of gas are related to Boyle's Law and Graham's Law of Diffusion. The volume of the bubble changes with atmospheric pressure. This may not be discernible with normal atmospheric fluctuations associated with depressions and anticyclones in the range 950–1040 torr, but becomes obvious on change in altitude. Flying in aircraft pressurized to a height of 3000 m is a major risk, as the bubble will tend to double in size and will render the retina ischaemic even if the globe does not rupture. This is a major disadvantage for patients who wish to fly home within a month of surgery.

Nitrous oxide being a very soluble gas has a similar effect by rapidly diffusing into the bubble to reach a partial pressure equal to that in the inspired gas. The bubble may increase in size by 250% within 30 min.[1,3] During vitreoretinal surgery, it is sound practice to avoid nitrous oxide or to turn it off a few minutes before the introduction of gas, substituting intravenous analgesia, anaesthetic vapour or other intravenous agents to replace the hypnotic and analgesic effects of the nitrous oxide. At this stage in the operation, the pressure in the eye is usually regulated by the surgeon using an infusion or an airline, but it is also at about this stage when gas is introduced that these are sealed off. If the bubble which is injected is allowed to contain a proportion of nitrous oxide from diffusion, then the size of the bubble will shrink rapidly in the postoperative recovery period as nitrous oxide washout from the body proceeds.[4]

A particular danger arises in the patient who has gas in the eye but who requires a general anaesthetic for some accident or unrelated condition. This second intervention may be managed by an anaesthetist who is unfamiliar with ophthalmic anaesthesia and the use of nitrous oxide in these circumstances may raise the intraocular pressure to such levels as to cause blindness or to rupture the globe. If anaesthesia is required for a second procedure (or even for the other eye), then it is worth considering the advantages of regional block. If general anaesthesia is required, then a total intravenous technique might be preferred or one which does not use nitrous oxide.

INTERNAL TAMPONADE WITH SILICONE OIL OR HEAVY LIQUID

When the retina is stiffened by fibrosis very large breaks are present or, if the patient is flying home, then silicone oil is used to support the retina permanently.

A total replacement of the vitreous is usually the aim. There are no particular anaesthetic problems, except that the retinal circulation should be maintained at or near the normal blood pressure for the patient.

Silicone oil interferes with the nourishment of the lens which develops a cataract within a year or two and the subsequent extraction is complicated by the loss of some oil and the possibility of posterior dislocation of the lens into the oil. In spite of the high surface tension of silicone oil, some emulsification may occur. This not only reduces visual function but small droplets pass through the zonule and tend to block the drainage angle leading to a rise in intraocular pressure. The oil may need to be removed or replaced in these circumstances.

Heavy organic liquids are sometimes used to treat breaks in the inferior retina. These are not soluble in silicone oil or water.

THROMBOEMBOLISM AND PROPHYLAXIS

The lengthy period on the operating table followed by several days relative immobility during postural closure of the breaks by internal tamponade, particularly in patients with diabetes, might be thought to promote venous thrombosis and the risk of pulmonary embolism. In practice, the risk seems to be small – so small that no up-to-date figures are available in the literature.

At Moorfields Hospital, all patients have ankle supports to prevent weight on the muscular parts of the calf. Those patients who have a history of previous deep vein thrombosis are provided with elastic stockings. The use of heparin is considered and discussed with the surgeon. Although some argue for its use, in some patients it may cause intraocular haemorrhage. For the moment, these questions remain unanswered, but any risk is small and largely theoretical.

REFERENCES

1. Merhige K, Lincoff H, van Poznak A. Effect of nitrous oxide on gas bubble volume. *Arch Ophthalmol* 1985; **103:** 1272.
2. Mirakhur RK. Anaesthetic management of vitrectomy. *Ann Roy Coll Surg* 1987; **67:** 34.
3. Smith RB, Carl B, Linn JG, Nemoto E. Effect of nitrous oxide on air in vitreous. *Am J Ophthalmol* 1974; **78:** 314.
4. Timpson TW, Donlan JV. The interaction of air and sulphur hexafluoride with nitrous oxide: A computer simulation. *Anesthesiology* 1982; **56:** 385.

CHAPTER 16

Audit

G BARRY SMITH

INTRODUCTION

The encouragement of good practice in ophthalmic anaesthesia is as important as it is elsewhere in medicine. It is necessary for practitioners engaged in this speciality to meet their colleagues in a formal and informal way at local, regional, national and international meetings, so that progress is made on a wide front. Until recently, the only formal arrangements were the delivery of papers at congresses and at a more local level the discussion of interesting individual problems at 'mortality and morbidity' meetings. Morbidity meetings in ophthalmic work not only concern the general well-being of the patient, but also encompass the operating conditions provided for the surgeon and those hazards, such as loss of vitreous or prolapse of the iris, for which the anaesthetist might bear some part of the responsibility.

Rapid change has occurred in the last few years, partly as the result of major surveys (such as the two confidential enquiries into perioperative deaths), but also from the backing given by the British Government to the work of the Audit Commission and the provision of central funds from the Health Services Board to provide formal opportunities during normal working hours for audit with the back-up of non-medical staff and computers.

The essence of all audit is the collection and analysis of relevant information. This may lead to the collection of rather less relevant information on large numbers of controls.[2,3] It is customary to divide the audit period into the subheadings of 'access', 'process' and 'outcome' (Fig. 16.1).

ACCESS

This refers to the ability of the system to select and triage patients into patterns appropriate to the facilities available for treatment. In ophthalmology, it is important to select only those patients who will benefit from a surgical intervention. For example, in a retirement home, there may be a number of patients with cataracts. Some will be unsuitable for surgery because of mental or physical handicap and may not be referred by the attending physician. It is reported by ophthalmologists that some patients who have been blind for a long period find the sudden restoration of vision stressful, having previously adapted to their

Patient's
Name
(Surname first)

ANAESTHETIC AUDIT

MOORFIELDS
EYE HOSPITAL

NOTE: Mark thus ⬜ NOT ☑️☒◯ Cancel thus: ⬛ **PLEASE REFER TO DEFINITIONS ON THE REVERSE** ─

DATE	START TIME	Th No	PRE-MED	ANAES 1	ANAES 2	DATE OF BIRTH	WEIGHT Kg	PATIENT NUMBER

(numeric grid columns with values: Day Month Year; Hrs Mins; etc.)

1 EYE			6 CEPOD CLASS'N	9 HYPNOTICS SEDATIVES	14 RELAXANTS	20 ADVERSE EVENTS
L [ ] R [ ] B/L [ ]			Emergency [ ]	Nil [ ]	Nil [ ] Vec [ ]	Nil [ ]
2 SURGEON			Urgent [ ]	Benzodiazepine [ ]	Sux [ ] DTC [ ]	Failed intubation [ ]
Consultant [ ]			Scheduled [ ]	Etomidate [ ]	Atracurium [ ] Panc [ ]	Patient injury [ ]
Senior Registrar [ ]			Elective [ ]	Ketamine [ ]	Other [ ]	Aspiration vomit [ ]
Registrar [ ]			Day case [ ]	Methohexitone [ ]	**15 REVERSAL**	Cardiovascular [ ]
S.H.O. [ ]			**7 CURRENT MED'N**	Neuroleptic [ ]	Nil [ ] Atrop [ ]	Respiratory [ ]
Fellow [ ]			Nil [ ]	Propofol [ ]	Glycopy [ ] Neostig [ ]	Drug reaction [ ]
Anaesthetist only [ ]			Analgesic (non opiate) [ ]	Thiopentone [ ]	Naloxone [ ] Other [ ]	Equipment failure [ ]
Other [ ]			Analgesic (opiate) [ ]	Other [ ]	**16 I V FLUIDS**	Recovery problem [ ]
3 PROCEDURE			Anti-anginal [ ]	**10 G A TECHNIQUE**	Nil [ ]	Other [ ]
Cataract [ ]			Anti-arrhythmic [ ]	Nil [ ]	Blood [ ]	**21 DISCHARGED TO**
Corneal [ ]			Antibiotic [ ]	Facemask [ ] LMA [ ]	Crystalloids [ ]	Ward [ ]
Glaucoma [ ]			Anti-coagulant [ ]	O/T tube [ ] N/T [ ]	Colloids [ ]	ICU/HDU [ ]
Lacrimal [ ]			Anti-convulsant [ ]	Larynx grade [1][2][3][4]	Drug Infusion [ ]	Died [ ]
Oncology [ ]			Anti-depressant [ ]	Spont res [ ] IPPV [ ]	Mannitol [ ]	
Orbit [ ]			Anti-diabetic (oral) [ ]	Circle [ ] Low flow [ ]	**17 MONITORING**	DEPT PERSONAL
Plastic [ ]			Anti-diabetic (insulin) [ ]	Hypotensive [ ]	Nil [ ]	
Squint [ ]			Anti-hypertensive [ ]	Other [ ]	ECG [ ] Vt [ ]	
Vitreo-Retinal [ ]			Anti-malignancy [ ]	**11 GASES**	NIBP [ ] Art L [ ]	
[ ]			Bronchodilator [ ]	Air [ ]	Sa O₂ [ ] % Vol AGT [ ]	
Other [ ]			Contraceptive (oral) [ ]	Oxygen [ ]	ETCO₂ [ ] CVP [ ]	
4 PRE-OP FACTORS			Digoxin [ ]	Nitrous Oxide [ ]	FiO₂ [ ] Vent alarm [ ]	
ASA [1][2][3][4][5]			Diuretic [ ]	CO₂ [ ]	PN stim [ ] Pa/w [ ]	
Sex: M [ ] F [ ]			Hypnotic/Anxiol'tic [ ]	Other [ ]	Stethosc [ ]	
Allergy [ ]			Steroid [ ]	**12 VOLATILES**	Temp [ ] Other [ ]	
Cardiac Ischaemia [ ]			Endocrine (other) [ ]	Nil [ ]	**18 ASSISTANT**	
Cardiac (Other) [ ]			Other [ ]	Enflurane [ ]	Nil [ ] Nurse [ ]	**END TIME**
Diabetes [ ]			**8 WARD PRE-MED**	Halothane [ ]	ODA [ ] Other [ ]	Hrs Mins
Endocrine (Other) [ ]			Nil [ ]	Isoflurane [ ]	**19 LOCAL TECHNIQUE**	
Haemoglobinopathy [ ]			Antiemetic [ ]	Other [ ]	Nil [ ]	
Hiatus hernia [ ]			Anticholinergic [ ]	**13 ANALGESICS**	Topical [ ]	
Hypertension [ ]			Benzodiazepine [ ]	Nil [ ]	Infiltration [ ]	
Obesity [ ]			Opiate [ ]	Alfentanil [ ]	Retrobulbar [ ]	
Renal [ ]			Trimeprazine [ ]	Fentanyl [ ]	Peribulbar [ ]	
Respiratory [ ]			EMLA [ ] Other [ ]	Morphine [ ]	Facial [ ]	
Other [ ]			Insuff [ ] Excess [ ]	NSAID [ ]	Other [ ]	
5 PROCEDURE CANCELLED because:				Papaveretum [ ]	Failed [ ]	
Poor clinical condition [ ]			Deteriorated surgical status [ ]	Pethidine [ ]	Reaction/Complication [ ]	
Improved surgical status (operation unnecessary) [ ]			Admin problem [ ]	Other [ ]	Local by Surgeon [ ]	Narrative comment Yes [ ]

blind state. It is a fact that 70% of patients presenting for cataract extraction in the inner London area live alone, while the majority of the remainder live with spouses or children. Very few patients are referred for operation who have suffered a stroke or who live in institutions.

Access in such situations is restricted not by the anaesthetist but by the interaction between the referring physician and the ophthalmologist, who together decide that surgical intervention is not required or might be 'risky' for the patient. There is a strongly conservative element that is opposed to altering the situation or accepting risk, and the arguments that patients might lead richer and more fulfilled lives are expressed only weakly. It is doubtful whether vision alone delays the onset of senile confusion, but it does allow access to that powerful panacea of the modern age, the television.

The anaesthetist seldom meets the patient before arrival in the hospital. A number of decisions will have already been made by the ophthalmologist, who will have strong views on the timing of operation and the type of anaesthesia. The decisions are partly guided by the patient's social circumstances, general health, the urgency of operation and partly by the resources available in terms of beds, operating time and anaesthetic services.

At Moorfields Hospital there are two internal departments which guide the ophthalmologist's decision. All patients due for elective surgery are reviewed by experienced members of the nursing staff designated as patient care coordinators. They investigate in depth the degree of social support required, the difficulties of travelling to the hospital and the general health of the patient, in particular noting the blood pressure and the blood sugar level. These care coordinators provide a counselling service for the patients and are able to utilize other specialist services in the hospital. They frequently call on a consultant anaesthetist to advise on the management of patients with severe respiratory or cardiac problems, so that more active steps can be taken to stabilize these before admission and so that after admission appropriate procedures can be adopted, such as preoperative physiotherapy, intraoperative monitoring or even the designation of the type of anaesthesia and the grade of anaesthetist.

The anaesthesia assessment clinic deals only with patients referred by ophthalmologists and sees a small number of patients, most of whom have severe disabilities. These are patients who have a poor anaesthesia history, neurological and metabolic diseases. The investigation of suspected malignant hyperpyrexia, sickle cell disease, myasthenia gravis and similar conditions is coordinated through this clinic, which liaises with appropriate centres in other hospitals.

From the point of view of audit, it is essential that the preoperative state is linked closely with the techniques used during the *process* and most importantly with the *outcome*. At present, these extensions of audit are still to be developed

---

Fig. 16.1. Anaesthetic audit form from an ophthalmology unit. The data collected can be fed into an optical mark reader, recorded on a computer database and networked with surgical and clinic data. It is unfocused on a specific objective and most of the data will remain valueless. Little emphasis is placed on recovery or outcome, which needs a separate form. Definitions of ASA status, CEPOD classification and grading of the larynx are printed for reference on the obverse of the form where there is space for manual recording of detail. There are some questions about the disposal of the forms once they have been read and there must be some monitoring of the completeness of the sample. A similar form could analyse local anaesthesia in greater detail.[11]

and refined. It should eventually be possible to make statements of probability of which the following is an unsubstantiated example. Ten male patients with a preoperative peak flow of 90/l min were given enflurane anaesthesia, four of whom required postoperative ventilation in an intensive care unit for more than 6 h. The same number and class of patients were given local anaesthesia. Five of these could not lie flat, one had uncontrollable cough and one lost vision through an expulsive haemorrhage. Such a spurious example, based on small numbers, might not be considered valid and a number of interpretations could be placed on such results. One conclusion might be not to operate on such patients, another might be to book intensive care beds in advance when general anaesthesia was chosen. It might also be valuable to look at the management of intractable cough under local anaesthesia or consider the monitoring and control of blood pressure during local anaesthesia to avoid the rare instances of expulsive haemorrhage. It is only by the collection and analysis of large numbers of such patients from many centres that truly valid conclusions can be reached and progress can be made. It is time for anecdotal medicine to be replaced entirely by scientific methods in this area.

PROCESS

Graphic records for general anaesthesia have improved considerably over the last 20 years. A number of vital signs are recorded for every patient, and the type and doses of drugs, the equipment used and the monitors, alarms and techniques are written up manually or provided in printout form. Computerized records are still mostly at the individual level, but will soon be routine in most departments. The missing element until now has been the coordination and analysis of this information, so that some useful conclusions can be drawn. There is a need for coordination between anaesthesia technique and surgical outcome. One outstanding example lies in expulsive haemorrhage, which is a surgical catastrophe whose relationship with pre-existing systemic hypertension, anaesthesia technique, ocular pathology or surgical manipulation remains entirely speculative.

Records of the administration of local anaesthesia, the doses used, routes of administration, results, monitoring and adverse reactions remain unsatisfactory, so that valid conclusions can seldom be drawn. There is a difference between anaesthetists and surgeons in the recording of these techniques and there is considerable need for convergence and standardization.

The immediate postoperative period is sometimes compared with Bunyan's Valley of the Shadow of Death. The improvement in training and expertise of recovery staff, improved record-keeping, pulse oximetry, the routine administration of oxygen and the recording of vital signs have done much to reduce the level of critical incidents in this area.

The term 'critical incident' is an important concept, as it not only includes points at which a disaster occurred, but also the times at which a disaster could have occurred if corrective action had not immediately been taken. Unfortunately, there is a grey area in which a critical incident undoubtedly happened but was instantly put right and hence was not recorded. Examples of this are a temporary accidental disconnection with immediate reconnection, or the passage of a tube into the oesophagus which was instantly withdrawn and reinserted into the larynx. Minor failures of monitoring equipment come into a similar category. No harm results and hence no overall corrective action is taken. It is very difficult to know at what level lines are to be drawn; the investigation of all critical incidents is a fruitful field for audit because, by the elimination of risk, more serious outcomes can be avoided.

OUTCOME

The anaesthetist may feel satisfied that the patient has recovered from the anaesthesia and has gone home. Outcome, however, is a much larger subject over a longer postoperative period and deals not only with the petty discomforts of general anaesthesia such as bruising, vomiting and sore throat, and the more serious but rare complications of thrombosis and chest infection, but it also examines the patients' degree of satisfaction with the procedures and how they re-adapt to life outside hospital – and, in younger patients, their return to work.

There is no doubt that for many patients hospital is frightening, that many elderly patients feel rushed and that there is a more or less suppressed fear of needles, pain and an unsatisfactory conclusion. Some patients find discomfort in starvation, claustrophobia under the drapes and expect more sympathy than they receive.

The problem of postoperative pain has received much attention recently and has historically been dealt with on a demand basis. The patient feels pain and is then given an analgesic drug which works some time later. Many eye operations produce severe discomfort which may be eased by reducing eye movement with a pad and bandage. Some patients require regular opiates, but these are few and the majority of patients are quite happy with simple analgesics. There seems to be no major requirement for patient-controlled analgesia in this type of surgery. Some anaesthetists have started to use analgesics, particularly non-steroidal anti-inflammatory agents (NSAIDS), routinely before, during and after surgery as a pain prophylaxis. I am not aware of any eye hospital which has arranged for postoperative pain scoring, but when this has been instituted it will become a proper subject for audit.

Audit is a powerful management tool for the intensive use of staff and other resources. When combined with costing, it can be used to produce more effective and cheaper techniques. Unfortunately, there are dangers in this approach if quality assurance is not given the priority it deserves. It is only by quality assurance in audit that patients will ultimately get the best treatment and the most satisfaction.[8,9,10,12]

AUDIT MEETINGS

Regular meetings of a department provide opportunities for colleagues to discuss the various topics outlined in this chapter. Training grades may be able to play a valuable part in the interpretation of the results of audit, and it is a stimulus to their seniors to produce guidance and recommendations as a result of the meeting.[1] Peer review may be misdirected and lead to the perpetuation of old-fashioned ideas without scientific foundation.[5-7] There are considerable problems about the confidentiality of audit, both for the staff concerned and also for the patient. It is important to implement a system without medico-legal implications, as some of the most valuable lessons arise out of apparent disasters. Ultimately, some benefit should accrue due to improvements in staffing, techniques or equipment.[13]

There are a number of different types of meetings. Medical audit is restricted to doctors and gives an opportunity for conversation between anaesthetists, ophthalmologists, radiologists and pathologists on matters of mutual interest. It should not necessarily be divided into anaesthetic and surgical audit. There must be many meetings in which nursing staff from the recovery ward or operating suite will have valuable contributions to make. These are usually designated 'clinical audit'. When special topics are discussed, then family doctors, community nurses, care coordinators and other staff may be invited to attend.

Financial or economic audit involving management to discuss productivity, financial savings and expenditure has a very real role to play, provided that quality assurance is not sacrificed and that managers can be persuaded that local anaesthesia is not without its dangers and anaesthetists will always be required in the monitoring and resuscitation team.

Audit depends a great deal on leadership, organization and tolerance to obtain the sometimes reluctant cooperation of all participants.[4, 14]

REFERENCES

1. Batstone GF. Educational aspects of medical audit. *Br Med J* 1990; **301:** 326.
2. Crombie IK, HTO Davies. Towards good audit. *Br J Hosp Med* 1992; **48:** 182.
3. Donabedian A. The quality of care: How can it be assessed? *JAMA* 1988; **260:** 1743.
4. Ellis BW, Sensky T. A clinician's guide to setting up audit. *Br Med J* 1991; **302:** 704.
5. Lomas J, Anderson GM, Domnick-Pierre K. Do practice guidelines guide practice? The effect of a consensus statement on the practice of physicians. *New Engl J Med* 1989; **321:** 1036.
6. McKee CM, Langlo M, Lessof L. Medical audit: A review. *J Roy Soc Med* 1989; **82:** 474.
7. Mitchell MW, Fowkes FGR. Audit reviewed: Does feedback on performance change clinical behaviour? *J Roy Coll Phys Lond* 1985; **19:** 251.
8. Moss F, Smith R. From audit to quality and beyond. *Br Med J* 1991; **303:** 199.
9. Royal College of Physicians. *Medical Audit: A First Report.* Royal College of Physicians: London, 1989.
10. Royal College of Surgeons. *Guidelines to Clinical Audit in Surgical Practice.* Royal College of Surgeons: London, 1989.
11. Samuel J. Personal communication.
12. Shaw CD. *Medical Audit: A Hospital Handbook.* King's Fund Centre: London, 1990.
13. Shaw CD, Costain DW. Guidelines for medical audit: Seven principles. *Br Med J* 1989; **300:** 65.
14. Smith T. Medical audit: Closing the feedback loop is essential. *Br Med J* 1990; **300:** 65.

Index